Pathology Made Ridiculously Simple

Aiman Zaher, MD, FCAP, FASCP
Clinical Professor
Dept. Pathology, School of Medicine
Case Western Reserve University
Cleveland, Ohio USA

MedMaster Inc.
Miami, Florida

Published by MedMaster, Inc.
P.O. Box 640028
Miami FL 33164

Cover by Richard March

Contributing Authors

Keith Bohman, M.D.
Summer Bohman, M.D.
Robert Conley, M.D.
Huma Fatima, M.D.
Lynda Gentchev, M.D.
George Koberlein
Anuradha Paturi, M.D.
Stacie Roshong-Denk, M.D.
Heather Sciambra
Todd Sheridan, M.D.
Sarah Steirman
Jean Thomas, M.D.
Jennifer Tserng, M.D.
Douglas Washing, M.D.
Jill Zyrek-Betts, M.D.

Special thanks to Edwin R. Phillips, M.D., for the illustrations.

Dedication

To my father Nizam and my son Nizam

Contents

Preface

This book aims to provide medical students and residents with a simple, updated, organized, and clear understanding of clinical pathology, correlating pathologic and molecular processes with their relevant clinical presentations. The information should be useful to students for Pathology courses, USMLE preparation, and patient care.

Humor and mnemonics are used throughout the book to facilitate learning and retention and should not be misconstrued as any disrespect for this important field. The book is supplemented by a CD with hundreds of normal and pathologic slides. These slides correlate closely with references to them in the text.

I thank the editor, Stephen Goldberg, for his helpful input and for programming the CD, as well as Phyllis Goldenberg for proofreading the manuscript.

Aiman Zaher, MD

1

Cellular Response to Injury

OVERVIEW

The basic concept is that the cell has adaptive responses to most forms of stress. When it cannot adequately adapt to the stress or it has no form of adaptation at all, then cell injury occurs. This injury can be reversible, leading to some level of remaining function, or it can be irreversible, resulting in cell death.

Causes of Injury

Cellular injury occurs when adaptation to stress is not sufficient. The potential etiologies (causes) of stress can be remembered by the following mnemonic: **Please Give Our Cells No Irreversible Injury!**

Physical: Examples include injury from exposure to electricity, radiation, barotrauma, mechanical stress, burns, and excessive cold.

Genetic: Cellular defects can result from DNA alteration that is either inherited or acquired (de novo).

Oxygenation: Too little O_2 (hypoxia), depletion of O_2 (anoxia), or too much O_2 can all be detrimental.

Chemical: Drugs and toxins can disrupt biochemical cell function or physical cell structure.

Nutritional: Deficiency or excess in vitamins, minerals, or proteins can result in cell injury.

Infectious: Cells can be affected by an organism, the molecular components of the organism (e.g. toxins), or the immune response to the organism.

Immunologic: A deficient or exuberant immune response may lead to cell damage. Also, an inability to distinguish self from non-self (autoimmune response) can lead to the injury of functional cells.

REVERSIBLE CELLULAR INJURY

Prolonged stress and repeated injury, in the form of the aforementioned mechanisms, can cause a cell to take action. The cell adopts mechanisms to more effectively handle the insult. Therefore, instead of constantly repairing itself, the cell would rather devote its time preventing the recurrent attacks (a true believer in the old saying "an ounce of prevention is worth a pound of cure"). These adaptations are either physical (morphological) or functional.

The most common types of change a cell can undergo to prevent future injury are **hypertrophy, hyperplasia, metaplasia, dysplasia,** and **atrophy**.

Fig. 1-1. Kinds of cellular adaptations:
1. **Hypertrophy**: Enlargement due to an increase in the size of cells (trophy for the biggest cell)
2. **Hyperplasia**: Enlargement due to an increased number of cells
3. **Metaplasia**: Reversible change from one type of fully mature cell to a different type of mature cell that is normally not found in the tissue involved
4. **Dysplasia**: Partially reversible change from a mature cell to a cell with abnormalities in both differentiation and maturation.
5. **Atrophy**: Decrease in size or number of cells.

How a cell responds may depend on many factors involving both the type of injury and the cell.

Physiology of Reversible Cell Injury

Fig. 1-2. The physiology of reversible cellular injury. The cell is stressed by one of the causes of injury mentioned above and adaptation is insufficient. Therefore, cell injury begins. There is dysfunction of normal activities and decreased energy supply. The plasma membrane loses its ability to be selectively permeable, and substances can rush in and out freely, causing a loss in volume control. This is quite pleasing to sodium (Na+) and potassium (K+), which are usually held back by the Na+/K+ ATPase pump. Sodium and water rush into the cell, and potassium runs out. This disrupts the osmotic balance, and the cell begins to swell. Calcium (Ca++) also enters the cell, and the endoplasmic reticulum (ER)

CELLULAR ADAPTATIONS

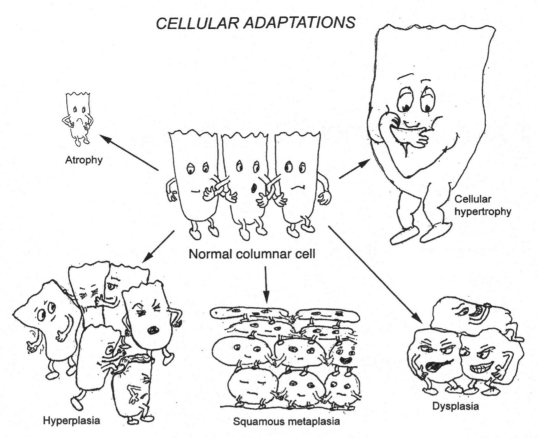

Atrophy

Cellular hypertrophy

Normal columnar cell

Hyperplasia

Squamous metaplasia

Dysplasia

Figure 1-1

releases its stockpile of calcium (Ca++). This results in changes involving the mitochondria, ER, lysosomes, and cytoskeleton.

Microscopic Appearance of Reversible Cell Injury

Since most of these changes are subtle, they are easier to appreciate by electron microscopy rather than light microscopy.

1. **Hydropic ER, and mitochondrial swelling**: The cell, ER, and mitochondria all increase in size.
2. **Mitochondrial densities**: Small densities form within the mitochondria.
3. **Lysosomal autophagy**: Lysosomes begin to ingest cell contents.
4. **Nuclear chromatin clumping**: Dark blue clumps of DNA are seen within the nucleus.
5. **Membrane blebbing**: The cell membrane develops outpouchings.
6. **Ribosomal detachment**: Rough ER membranes lose their ribosomal attachments, resulting in a pink cytoplasm (it is usually blue).

There is a point at which the injury is no longer reversible, **the point of no return**, after which the cell dies.

IRREVERSIBLE CELLULAR INJURY

Fig. 1-3. Two forms of cellular death. Cell death occurs by one of two mechanisms: **apoptosis** (programmed and/or premeditated) or **necrosis** (manslaughter, or more specifically, cell-slaughter). Cells that are preprogrammed to die, such as those destroyed during embryogenesis, undergo apoptosis. Other circumstances leading to programmed cell death include:

- hormone-dependent cells following loss of stimulation (lack of stimulation causes death)
- liver cells infected by viral hepatitis (a form of immune-mediated cell death)
- proliferative cells with a quick turnover rate (a proliferative need drives cell death).

Cells that acquire an irreversible injury may undergo apoptosis or necrosis, but necrosis is only seen after injury, i.e., it is **never physiologic**.

REVERSIBLE CELLULAR INJURY

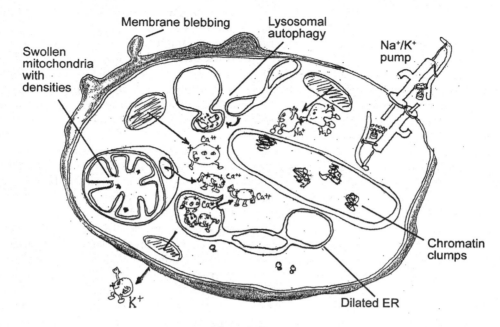

Figure 1-2.

TWO WAYS A CELL CAN DIE

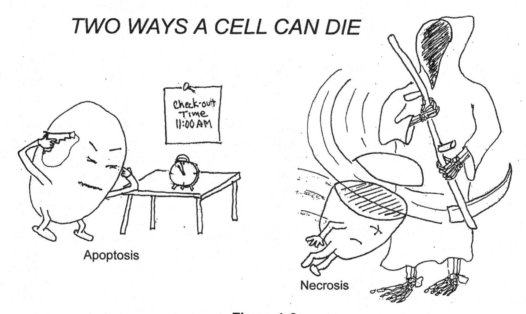

Figure 1-3

Physiology of Cell Death

The biochemical pathways that initially lead a cell to the point of no return (irreversible injury leading to cell death) vary among the etiologies of cell injury. The final physiological appearance of a dead cell is similar for apoptosis and necrosis; however, the mechanisms to which a cell reaches the final pathway differs between apoptosis and necrosis.

In necrosis, the influx of calcium activates enzymes to hydrolyze DNA, disrupt membranes, and digest the cytoskeleton. In apoptosis, enzymes are activated to hydrolyze proteins (via **caspases**), crosslink proteins (via **transglutaminases**), and cleave DNA (via **endonucleases**). The trigger that activates these enzymes is currently unknown. This signal takes its cue from the apoptotic environment in the form of a feedback mechanism.

Microscopic Appearance of Irreversible Cell Injury and Cell Death

Several specific details differentiate the microscopic appearance of apoptosis and necrosis (but don't worry; they're discussed below).

Morphologic changes associated with cell death develop over time. There is a 1–3 hour time delay between cell death and visible changes via electron microscopy. It takes 6-8 hours before a light microscope demonstrates alterations. Therefore, if heart cell (myocyte) necrosis results in patient demise within minutes, don't expect to immediately see necrotic heart cells, since the microscopic changes did not have a chance to develop.

Reversible cell injury can be microscopically distinguished from irreversible cell injury by the more dramatic alterations in the cellular cytoplasm and the nuclear changes specific to the latter. The following list can be easily compared to the preceding list for the microscopic appearance of reversible cell injury.

1. **Myelin figures**: Large masses of phospholipids that are phagocytosed or further degraded into fatty acids.
2. **Membrane defects**: The cell membrane become discontinuous and eventually ruptures.
3. **ER lysis**: Swelling progresses to the point of rupture.
4. **Mitochondrial swelling**: Severe swelling that increases mitochondrial size.
5. **Mitochondrial densities**: Large densities form within the mitochondria.
6. **Lysosomal rupture**: Lysosomal enzymes are released into the cytoplasm and digest cellular components, leading to a pink (eosinophilic) cytoplasm.
7. **Nuclear chromatin changes**: 3 patterns of DNA breakdown are possible: **pyknosis** (nuclear shrinkage with a darker blue appearance), **karyorrhexis** (nuclear fragmentation into multiple blue fragments), and **karyolysis** (fading of the nucleus with a lighter blue appearance).

Microscopic Appearance of Necrosis

Cell membrane rupture results in the release of cellular components into the extracellular space. The surrounding cells recruit trained professionals to clean up this type of debris (i.e., neutrophils and macrophages) and an acute inflammatory reaction begins (described below).

The morphology of necrosis varies with the type of cell, type of injury, and the speed of cell breakdown. The four most common types of necrosis can be remembered by the mnemonic: **Coagulation** of **Liquid Fat** results in lawsuit **Cases**.

Fig. 1-4. The four types of necrosis:

Coagulation necrosis: The cell maintains its outline for days, resulting in a well-defined, anuclear mass of pink cytoplasm. Therefore, the tissue **maintains its architecture**. This is seen in all cells that have undergone hypoxia, except for the brain. Grossly, gangrene can be seen (described below).

Liquefactive necrosis: The cell is transformed into a thick liquid without a defined shape (the cellular **outline is destroyed**). This is seen in bacterial infections, some fungal infections, and brain hypoxia. Grossly, thick yellowish fluid is seen (pus formation).

Fat (Enzymatic) necrosis: The fat cell is broken down, but it maintains its outline. Also, a bluish calcium layer deposits around the cells, and the fat cell becomes surrounded by neutrophils, lymphocytes and macrophages. This is seen in the pancreas and fatty tissues (breast, abdomen, and subcutaneous tissue). Grossly, white chalky areas are seen, known as fat saponification (described below).

Caseous necrosis: The cell becomes amorphous and loses its outline. Therefore, the tissue loses its architecture. Surrounding the necrotic area, a **granulomatous** inflammatory border is formed primarily by macrophages and lymphocytes. This is seen in **tuberculous** lung infections. Grossly, yellowish cheesy areas are seen.

A less common type of necrosis known as **fibrinoid necrosis** also occurs. The cell loses its outline and becomes homogenous and pink – like fibrin. However, there is **no fibrin** involved (depositions of fibrin are described as fibrinous – composed of fibrin). This is seen in the blood vessels of people with autoimmune diseases (e.g., systemic lupus erythematosus, polyarteritis nodosa, and rheumatic fever).

Microscopic Appearance of Apoptosis

Since the cell death is preprogrammed in apoptosis, the neighboring cells are aware of the changes occurring. Therefore, the apoptotic cells are quickly removed (via phagocytes and macrophages) without interrupting the surrounding tissue (i.e., there is minimal inflammation). This makes it difficult to microscopically visualize apoptosis unless a large area of tissue is involved.

The main differences when compared to necrosis include the following: the nuclear chromatin changes are pyknotic (dark and condensed); the cell shrinks and the organelles become more compact; and the cell membrane remains intact for a longer duration with cell fragmentation (**apoptotic bodies**).

Signs and Symptoms of Cell Death

So how do you know which cells are dead in your patient simply by looking at him or her? Like all of medicine, it depends on many factors. The type and quantity of cells affected are important factors. Also, the type of cell death (apoptosis or specific type of necrosis) plays an important role in clinical identification of pathology. The most evident gross changes are described below.

THE 4 FORMS OF NECROSIS

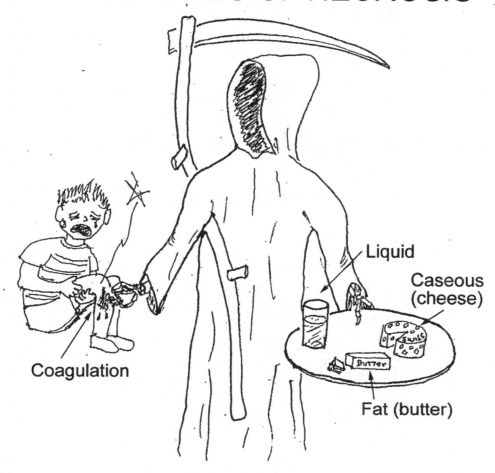

Liquid

Caseous (cheese)

Coagulation

Fat (butter)

Figure 1-4

Gangrene: Gangrene occurs in a necrotic tissue (usually a limb), which has undergone coagulation necrosis. It appears black, dry, and shriveled (known as **dry gangrene**) with a sharp demarcation from viable tissue. When a bacterial infection involves the necrotic area, the tissue appears swollen, dark red, and liquified. When a foul odor is present, and the border between dead and viable tissue is obscured, this is known as **wet gangrene**.

Fat saponification: White chalky areas are seen within fat, indicating fat necrosis.

Loss of function: Individual cell death can affect tissue function. The severity of clinically evident cell death depends on the quantity of cells involved, the type of tissue, and the ability of the surviving cells to continue functioning. For example, a few brain cells can die, resulting in seizure activity, muscle paralysis, or sensory loss. On the other hand, all of the cells of the kidney can die without consequence because the other kidney can compensate for the loss.

Blood: Bleeding into dead tissue can cause symptoms, such as coughing up blood (**hemoptysis**), with cellular demise in the lungs, or local hemorrhage secondary to a bleeding ulcer.

Fever: Necrotic cells can release pyrogens, resulting in an increased core body temperature.

Laboratory Diagnosis of Cell Death

Cellular death can have an associated acute inflammatory reaction, which may result in an increased number of neutrophils in the peripheral blood (**neutrophil leukocytosis**).

In addition, the bacteria seen in wet gangrene grow readily in necrotic tissue and may be cultured. These bacteria may also enter the blood stream (**bacteremia**) or lymphatic channels and may be cultured directly from a blood sample.

Irreversible cell injury results in cell membrane defects, from which the cytoplasmic enzymes can escape into the bloodstream. Once again, the type and

CELLS INVOLVED IN THE IMMUNE RESPONSE

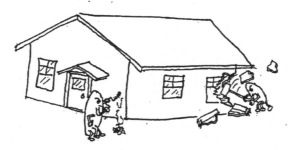

Inflammatory stimulus

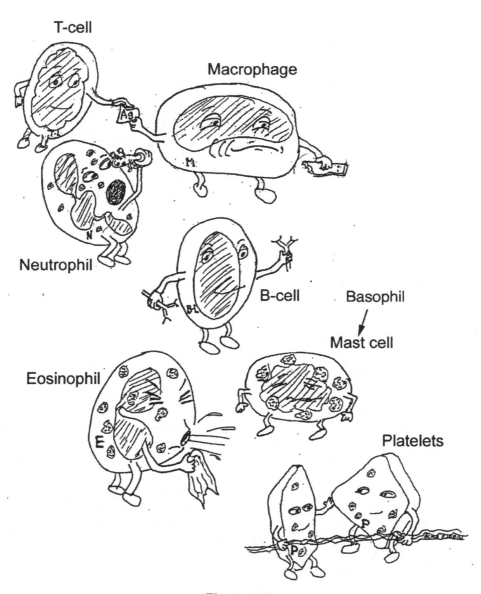

T-cell

Macrophage

Neutrophil

B-cell

Basophil

Mast cell

Eosinophil

Platelets

Figure 1-5

quantity of enzymes seen depends on the type and quantity of cells that have died. Some of the more common examples are included below.

1. **Alanine aminotransferase** (aka ALT or SGPT): Found in liver and skeletal muscle.
2. **Amylase:** Found in pancreas and salivary glands.
3. **Aspartate aminotransferase** (aka AST or SGOT): Found in liver, heart, and skeletal muscle.
4. **Creatine kinase** (aka CK): Different isoenzymes are found in different tissues. For example, CKMB: heart, CKBB: brain, and CKMM: heart and skeletal muscle.
5. **Lactate dehydrogenase** (aka LDH): Different isoenzymes are found in different tissues. For example, LDH1 - heart, RBCs, and skeletal muscle. LDH5 – liver and skeletal muscle.

INFLAMMATION
Purpose of Inflammation

Inflammation is an attempt to prevent further cell/tissue damage by attacking the cause of the insult. Inflammation is a wonderful way to kill, inactivate, detoxify, and clean up. However, like most things in life, it is possible to have too much of a good thing. In other words, sometimes an inflammatory response will lead to adverse effects, such as fistula formation (formed by tissue breakdown), contractures or keloids (secondary to increased scar formation), and adhesions (due to abnormal scar formation).

Important Cells Involved in Inflammation

Fig. 1-5. The most important cells in acute and chronic inflammation:

The **neutrophil** (polymononuclear cell, PMN): The paramedics of the body. They are the initial respondents to an acute injury. They contain numerous digestive enzymes, such as oxidase and protease. Also, they are the main phagocytic cells in bacterial infections.

Lymphocyte: These cells are usually associated with chronic inflammation. They can be subdivided into **T-cells** (70-80% of the circulating lymphs) and **B-cells**.

The **T-cells** can be further subdivided into **helper/inducer (T4) cells, suppressor/cytotoxic (T8) cells,** and **natural killer (NK) cells.** The T-cells are involved in the acute immune response.

The **B cells** differentiate into plasma cells that produce one specific type of immunoglobulin (IgG, IgM, IgA, IgE, or IgD). B-cells are the cells involved in the humoral immune response.

Macrophage: See *Slide 1.4*. These cells engulf foreign material and cellular debris, and process antigens for lymphocytes. They are also involved in granuloma

formation during chronic inflammatory states. Finally, they release many substances. Some of the most important ones include: colony-stimulating factor (CSF); tumor necrosis factor (TNF); interleukin-1 (IL-1); IL-8; IL-10; IL-12. Important subpopulations of macrophages include their blood derivative (monocyte) and fixed tissue derivative (histiocyte).

Eosinophil: These cells jump into action when you have an allergic reaction or parasitic infection, either acute or chronic. They function in phagocytosis and contain cytoplasmic granules filled with enzymes. These enzymes include antihistamines (necessary in allergic reactions) and **major basic protein**, which kills bacteria and parasites (helpful in certain infections). Major basic protein also induces mast cell degranulation, which continues the inflammatory process.

Basophil: These cells, as well as their tissue derivatives (mast cells), are involved in vasodilation and alteration of vascular permeability via the production of histamine and serotonin. Mast cells also play an important role in anaphylactic reactions and specific parasitic infections.

Platelet: These cells are known for their role in hemostasis. However, they are also important producers of chemical mediators for inflammation and coagulation, including serotonin, histamine, platelet activating factor (PAF) and thromboxane A_2 (T_xA_2), as discussed below.

Pathogenesis of Inflammation

Acute Inflammation

You've been injured and you want to get help there as soon as possible. Makes sense right? Your cells and tissues have the same reaction. They want to get supplies from the blood to the tissue, so they initiate vascular changes to accommodate these wishes. In order to increase blood flow, vascular dilation occurs (causing erythema and warmth). An increased vascular permeability allows protein-rich fluid and leukocytes to escape into the extravascular space (causing edema). Once out of the bloodstream, the leukocytes migrate to the site of injury via chemotaxis.

Leukocytes need to get from the blood vessel lumen to the site of tissue injury, and they do this via a four-step process. This process can easily be remembered by the mnemonic **M**arge **R**olls **A**long the **T**rack.

Fig. 1-6. Marge Rolls Along the Track:

Margination, to the wall of the blood vessel, is the process by which a cell moves from the center of flowing blood to the periphery of flowing blood.

Rolling along the endothelial surface, in which the inflammatory cells begin to interact with the blood vessel endothelium.

THE WBC RESPONSE TO INFLAMMATION

MARGE **R**OLLS
ALONG THE **T**RACK

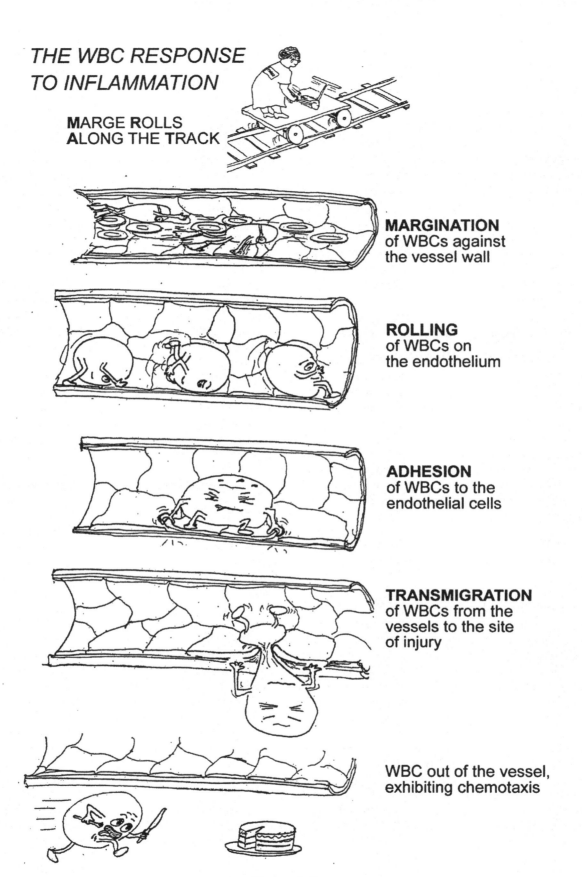

MARGINATION
of WBCs against
the vessel wall

ROLLING
of WBCs on
the endothelium

ADHESION
of WBCs to the
endothelial cells

TRANSMIGRATION
of WBCs from the
vessels to the site
of injury

WBC out of the vessel,
exhibiting chemotaxis

Figure 1-6

EFFECTS OF CHEMICAL MEDIATORS OF INFLAMMATION

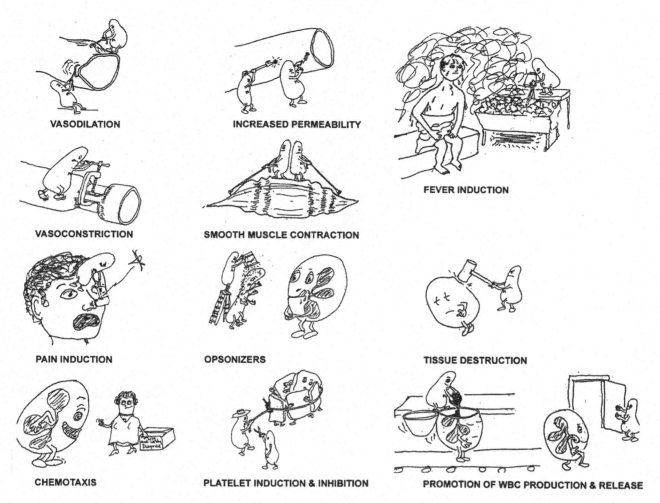

VASODILATION

INCREASED PERMEABILITY

FEVER INDUCTION

VASOCONSTRICTION

SMOOTH MUSCLE CONTRACTION

PAIN INDUCTION

OPSONIZERS

TISSUE DESTRUCTION

CHEMOTAXIS

PLATELET INDUCTION & INHIBITION

PROMOTION OF WBC PRODUCTION & RELEASE

Figure 1-7

Adhering to the endothelial lining via adhesion molecules (i.e., selectins, immunoglobulins, integrins, mucin-like glycoproteins).

Transmigration (also known as **diapedesis**) is the event of a cell moving through the endothelial cells of the blood vessels into the tissue.

Once at the site of injury, the leukocytes assess the environment, and a response is generated, based upon the damage. The goal is to return the tissue to a functional and productive state via removal of foreign material and cellular debris. Acute inflammation can lead to complete resolution, abscess formation, regenerative healing, scarring (connective tissue healing), or chronic inflammation.

Chronic Inflammation

Chronic inflammation (*Slides 1.5–1.6*) can be described as prolonged active inflammation with evidence of tissue destruction and repair. While chronic inflammation is usually preceded by acute inflammation, there are exceptions to every rule. The most common examples of chronic inflammation include granulomatous inflammation (TB, sarcoidosis), chronic lung disease, and autoimmune diseases (RA).

Chemical Mediators of Inflammation

The inflammatory response is mediated by numerous chemicals. These mediators can be preformed in the plasma (in an inactive state) or produced by various cells throughout the inflammatory process. Researchers have discovered how many of these chemical mediators function and where they are produced.

Fig. 1-7. Effects of the various chemical mediators of inflammation. The chemical mediators include:

GRANULOMA

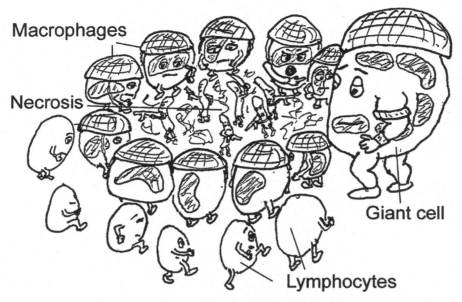

Figure 1-8

1. **Vasoactive amines**: Preformed and released quickly from mast cells (mostly histamine) and platelets (mostly serotonin).
   a. **Histamine**: Vasodilation, increases vascular permeability
   b. **Serotonin**: Vasodilation, increases vascular permeability
2. **Bradykinin**: Preformed in the plasma. It is involved in increasing vascular permeability, vasodilation, smooth muscle contraction, and it elicits pain.
3. **Components of the complement system**: Preformed in the plasma.
   c. **C3a**: Promotes histamine release, mediates chemotaxis, promotes opsonization
   d. **C5a**: Mediates chemotaxis, promotes histamine release
4. **Arachidonic acid metabolites**: Located on the lipid membrane and formed via the cyclooxygenase and lipoxygenase pathways.
   e. **Prostaglandins**: Vasodilation, increases vascular permeability, mediates chemotaxis
   f. **Prostaglandin E2 (PGE2)**: Elicits pain
   g. **Prostaglandins D2 (PGD2) and F2 alpha (PGF2 alpha)**: Vasodilation
   h. **Thromboxane A2 (TxA2)**: Promotes platelet aggregation
   i. **Prostacyclin (PGI2)**: Inhibits platelet aggregation
   j. **Leukotriene B4**: Mediates chemotaxis
   k. **Leukotrienes C, D, and E**: Increase vascular permeability

5. **Cytokines**: General term for a family of proteins produced by many cell types to mediate the function of other cell types.
   l. **IL-1**: Mediates chemotaxis, induces fever, induces WBC release from bone marrow, promotes histamine release
   m. **IL-6**: Induces fever
   n. **IL-8**: Promotes histamine release
   o. **TNF**: Induces fever, induces WBC release from bone marrow
   p. **Colony stimulating factors (CSFs)**: Increases WBC production in bone marrow
6. **Platelet activating factor (PAF)**: Released from mast cells, PMNs, macrophages, endothelial cells, and platelets and is involved in platelet aggregation, increasing vascular permeability, vasoconstriction, vasodilation (at very low concentrations), and chemotaxis.
7. **Nitric oxide (NO)**: Released from macrophages and endothelial cells. It is involved in tissue destruction (cytotoxin) and vasodilation.

Now let's review what we just read in another form (a good method of learning!):

Increases vascular permeability: bradykinin, C3a, C5, histamine, serotonin, PAF, prostaglandins, leukotrienes C, D, and E
Vascular dilators: bradykinin, histamine, serotonin, prostaglandins, NO, low dose PAF
Vascular constrictors: PAF

Smooth muscle contractors: bradykinin

Pain elicitors: bradykinin and PGE2

Histamine release promoters: C3a, C5a, IL-1, IL-8

Opsonization promoters: C3a

Chemotaxis mediators: C5a, C3a, IL-1, leukotriene B4, prostaglandins, PAF

Platelet aggregation promoters: thromboxane A2

Platelet aggregation inhibitors: prostacyclin

Fever inducers: IL-1, IL-6, TNF

Tissue destroyers: NO

Increase white blood cell release from bone marrow: IL-1, TNF

Increase white blood cell production in bone marrow: CSFs

Microscopic Appearance of Inflammation

Ouch! So you hurt yourself and want to see your injury under the microscope. The histologic appearance of your inflamed tissue depends on the cause of the inflammation, the time period since the injury, and your immune status. The etiologies of injury mentioned earlier (physical, genetics, chemical, nutritional, infectious, or immunologic) play a major role in which defenses your body initiates. Also, the microscopic appearance of inflammation evolves as time progresses. Acute (minutes to hours to days), subacute (days to weeks), and chronic (weeks to months) inflammation have different appearances. Finally, it is important to remember that immunocompromised individuals do not have enough cells to initiate the usual response to injury.

Microscopic Appearance of Acute Inflammation

The vascular changes previously described lead to the main morphological findings of acute inflammation: neutrophils and excessive interstitial fluid (**edema**). Since the reparative process starts soon after inflammation begins, early granulation tissue (inflammatory cells, mostly chronic, as well as fibroblasts and myofibroblasts) can also be seen. This includes proliferation of small blood vessels and increased connective tissue formation.

Microscopic Appearance of Chronic Inflammation

Mononuclear cells (lymphocytes, macrophages, and plasma cells) dominate the picture in chronic inflammation, similar to the neutrophil predominance seen in acute inflammation. Tissue destruction, in the form of necrosis, is seen secondary to the inflammatory cell reactions. **Angiogenesis** (proliferation of small blood vessels) and **fibrosis** (connective tissue), which are important components of wound healing and repair, are present as well. Multiple granulomas are evident in a specific form of chronic inflammation, known as **granulomatous inflammation**.

Fig. 1-8. Granuloma. This is composed of macrophages surrounding a central core of necrosis with a rim of lymphocytes. These macrophages may fuse to have multiple nuclei, at which point they are called **giant cells**. Granulomatous inflammation is seen in both infectious and noninfectious conditions where the irritant is poorly digestible or a T cell-mediated reaction occurs.

Signs and Symptoms of Inflammation

The classic signs of inflammation include loss of function, swelling, redness, warmth, and pain. They can be remembered as the 4 functionless (functio laesa) ten*ors*: tum*or*, rub*or*, cal*or*, and dol*or*.

Fig. 1-9. The four ten*ors* of inflammation: Tum*or*, Rub*or*, Cal*or*, and Dol*or*.

Proteins that are increased during injury and inflammation cause various reactions including the four mentioned above. These proteins also cause acute phase reactions, which include fever, anorexia, hypertension, tachycardia, and increased slow wave sleep. Also, the accumulation of leukocytes (mostly neutrophils) and cellular debris forms an inflammatory exudate commonly referred to as pus.

Laboratory Diagnosis of Inflammation

An immature neutrophil has a single-lobed, long nucleus and is called a **band** form.

Fig. 1-10. Band and mature neutrophils.

An increased number of "bands" in a blood sample indicates an infectious process. Since an increased number of neutrophils is needed to combat the infection, immature cells are released to help. An increase in the production and release of white blood cells from the bone marrow secondary to the chemical mediators of inflammation results in a leukocytosis.

Acute phase reactants, which cause the acute phase reactions described above, are a group of proteins that increase in response to inflammation and tissue injury. Interleukins are a key mediator of this process. **C-reactive protein** is the most important acute phase reactant.

Erythrocyte sedimentation rate (ESR), a non-specific marker for infection, is increased during inflammation due to acute phase reaction proteins. Therefore, a higher than normal ESR corresponds to an increase in acute phase reactants.

Treatment of Inflammation (Anti-inflammatories)

1. **Non-steroidal anti-inflammatory drugs (NSAIDs)**: Inhibits cyclooxygenase (COX) function. The lack of COX inhibits the arachidonic acid pathway and thus prevents prostaglandin production.

The 4 TenORs of Inflammation

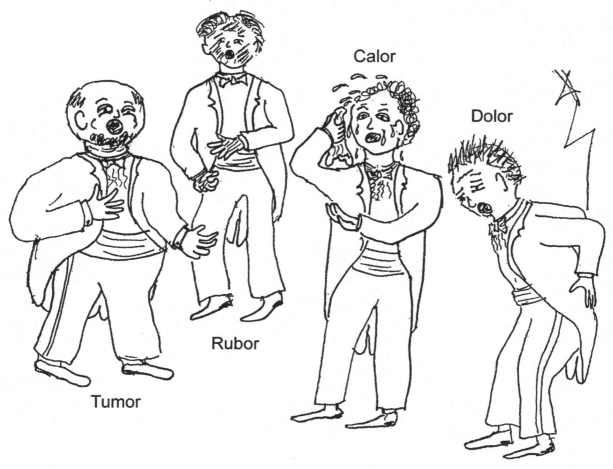

Calor

Dolor

Rubor

Tumor

Figure 1-9

2. **Steroids**: Prevent the formation of arachidonic acid by inhibiting phospholipases.
3. **COX2 inhibitors**: Block COX2 (a specific isozyme of the COX family) in the cyclooxygenase pathway.

TISSUE REPAIR
Purpose of Repair

Repair follows acute and chronic inflammation. **Granulation tissue** is the hallmark of the reparative process. It contains inflammatory cells (mostly chronic), as well as the new incoming fibroblasts and myofibroblasts. These components lay down collagen and form new blood vessels.

At this point I must mention a *common mistake* made by medical students. Granulation tissue is *NOT* the same as a granuloma. *Granulomatous inflammation* is a form of chronic inflammation, as discussed above. *Granulation tissue* is formed as part of the wound healing process.

Pathogenesis of Repair

Replacement of damaged cells and stroma by cells and connective tissue involves multiple components, collectively referred to as **granulation tissue**. Important factors in repair include: endothelial cell proliferation; formation of new, small blood vessels (**angiogenesis**); migration of fibroblasts and myofibroblasts.

New blood vessels form as off shoots of pre-existing blood vessels under the control of growth factors. Then, fibroblasts migrate to the site and proliferate. They form the majority of the connective tissue cell population and lay down the extracellular matrix (collagen). Specialized fibroblasts, called **myofibroblasts**, have smooth muscle properties and are responsible for wound contracture. After granulation tissue has formed, scarring begins. The connective tissue framework is remodeled by metalloproteinases (enzymes) to form a dense collagen. This collagenous architecture

BAND AND MATURE NEUTROPHILS

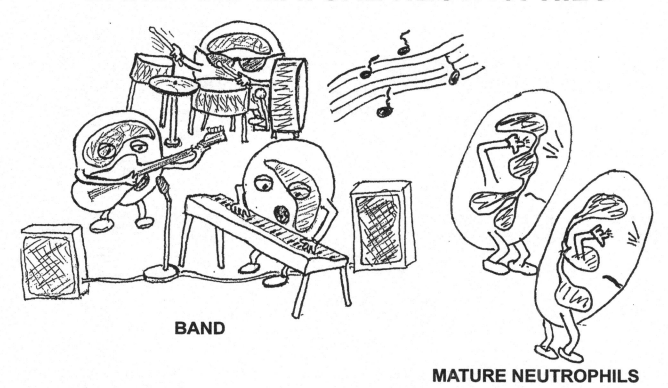

BAND

MATURE NEUTROPHILS

Figure 1-10

offers strength to the tissue, and its formation is the goal of scar formation.

The entire process from injury to scar formation is evident in wound healing. With limited cell loss and smaller defects, the reparative process involves healing by **primary intention**. When a larger tissue defect exists, healing occurs via **secondary intention**.

Primary intention is wound repair following surgical approximation of wound edges via stapling or suturing. Scab formation occurs when clotted blood fills the gap between the edges of the wound.

With **secondary intention** the wound edges are not directly opposed to aid in the repair process. In comparison with primary intention, healing by secondary intention takes longer, contains more granulation tissue, and has less wound contraction.

Timeline of Repair

With primary intention, neutrophils begin migrating toward the center of the scab 24 hours after wound edge approximation. Within 48 hours, the epithelial cells have extended to join the midline beneath the scab. By 72 hours, macrophages have replaced the neutrophils, and granulation tissue has begun to form. Granulation tissue fills the wound and collagen deposition begins within a

week. During the following week, the swelling, leukocytes, and granulation tissue begin to retreat. Vascular regression continues as the scar matures. Tissue strength returns within several months.

Fig. 1-11. Microscopic changes during wound repair.

With secondary intention, the wound is large, and a vigorous inflammatory reaction produces an excessive amount of granulation tissue. Therefore, the healing process is prolonged in comparison to healing by primary intent.

Chemical Mediators of Repair

Granulation tissue needs a signal to know when and where to form. The most important chemical mediators include:

1. **Platelet-derived growth factor (PDGF)**: Chemoattractant for PMNs and macrophages; induces proliferation of endothelium, smooth muscle cells, and fibroblasts.
2. **Tissue growth factor beta (TFG-b)**: Chemoattractant for PMNs and macrophages; induces proliferation of endothelium, smooth muscle cells, and fibroblasts.

WOUND REPAIR

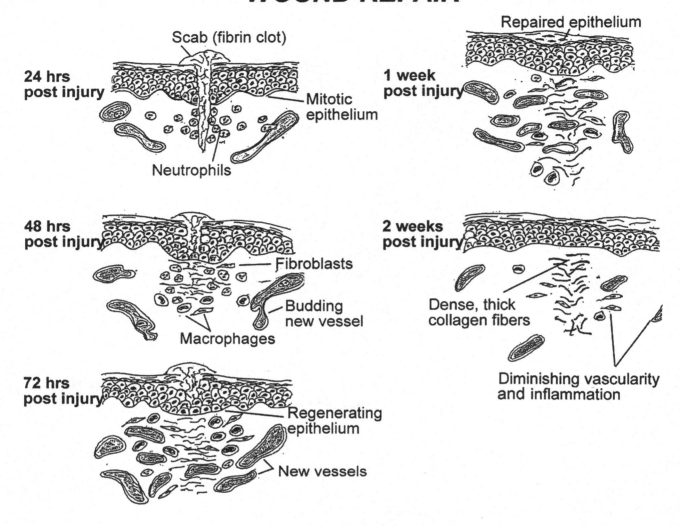

Figure 1-11

3. **Fibroblast growth factor (FGF):** Induces angiogenesis.
4. **Vascular endothelial growth factor (VEGF):** Induces angiogenesis; induces migration and proliferation of endothelial cells.

Microscopic Appearance of Repair

Since repair begins in the early phases of inflammation, many neutrophils are initially present. However, as granulation tissue formation progresses, the morphologic picture of inflammation progresses to include lymphocytes with numerous, small blood vessels in a collagenous background. The timeline of repair is an important factor in the histologic appearance of the healing tissue. The quantity and composition of the leukocytes, blood vessels, and connective tissue will change with time. Finally, the width and depth of the wound may look different in those healing by primary intention versus those healing by secondary intention.

2

Neoplasia

DEFINITIONS

Neoplasia, the Latin for "new growth," is an abnormal, uncontrolled growth of tissue, functioning autonomously and outside of regulation by surrounding tissues. Neoplasms contain two distinct components: the proliferating neoplastic cells of the parent tissue, called the *parenchyma,* and the supportive connective tissue and blood vessels known as the *stroma.* They can be either benign or malignant based on their biologic behavior. The term **cancer** refers only to malignant neoplasms.

Neoplasms derive their name from their tissue of origin. Some classic benign tumors generally have the suffix "-oma." Important exceptions include seminoma, melanoma, lymphoma, and mesothelioma, which are always malignant. Different types of benign neoplasms include:

Teratoma: These are derived from totipotent cells, containing tissue from all *3 germ cell layers*; they can be benign (more common) or malignant.

Fig. 2-1. Teratoma, receiving a Tarot card reading. Teratomas are benign neoplasms that typically involve tissues from all three germ layers.

Choristoma: This is an ectopic rest of normal tissue.

Hamartoma: These are disorganized masses of *mature tissue* with characteristic differentiation of normal surrounding tissue.

Adenoma: These tumors of benign epithelial cell origin form glandular patterns or are derived from *glandular tissue.*

Malignant tumors are divided into categories based on the type of tissue. Those of mesenchymal (connective tissue) origin are called *sarcomas,* while those of epithelial origin are known as *carcinomas.* One important subset of carcinomas is the *adenocarcinomas,* cancers derived from glandular or ductal epithelium.

Fig. 2-2. Adenocarcinoma. Well-differentiated carcinomas are better behaved than poorly differentiated ones, which carry a poor prognosis.

To complicate matters, many early cancer researchers liked to name tumors after themselves, such as Wilm's tumor or Burkitt's lymphoma. Generally speaking, though, the nature of a tumor can usually be gleaned from its suffix.

BENIGN VERSUS MALIGNANT TUMORS

Benign and malignant tumors are distinguished from one another in several key ways:

Differentiation versus Anaplasia

Differentiation is the degree to which neoplastic cells resemble normal cells of the tissue of origin. Well-differentiated cells closely resemble tissue of origin, while poorly differentiated cells are primitive and barely recognizable. (*Slide 2.1*) Benign tumors are generally well differentiated, and malignant tumors range from well differentiated to poorly differentiated. Cells that lack any evidence of differentiation are called **anaplastic.** Anaplasia is marked by:

Pleomorphism, the variation in size and shape of cells and/or nuclei.

Hyperchromatism, the extremely dark staining of nuclei due to an increase in DNA.

Increased nuclear-to-cytoplasm (N-C) ratio, in which the nucleus takes up more space in the cell when compared to non-neoplastic cells.

Clumpy chromatin, DNA of a cell grouped in clumps with clear areas interspersed, which denotes increased rate of transcription and cell activity.

Large nucleoli, which can be singular or multiple.

Increased mitoses, although the presence of mitotic figures does not necessarily indicate malignancy, since many normal tissues have a rapid turnover time; atypical

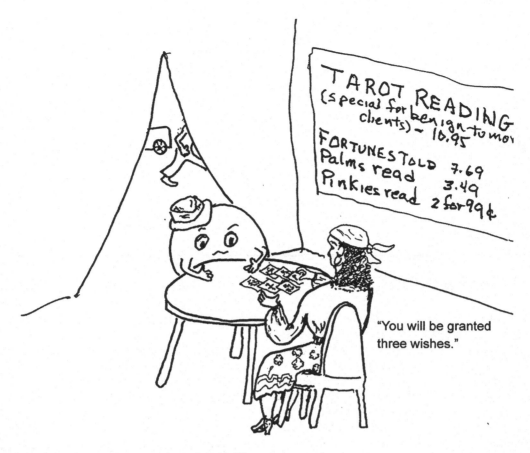

TAROT READING
(special for benign tumor clients) - 10.95
FORTUNES TOLD 7.69
Palms read 3.49
Pinkies read 2 for 99¢

"You will be granted three wishes."

Figure 2-1

mitoses (tripolar, multipolar) have a much stronger association with malignancy.

Loss of polarity of cell layers or nuclei.

Central necrosis, caused especially in malignant tumors when they outgrow their blood supply (*Slide 2.2*).

All of the above should not be confused with *dysplasia*, which is a premalignant lesion. Dysplastic tissue shows disordered and immature growth with accompanying genetic and functional alterations that have the potential to become malignant without treatment. Unlike malignancy, dysplasia is often reversible if the causative stimulus is removed.

Another premalignant lesion is *carcinoma-in-situ*, a severe dysplasia involving the entire thickness of an epithelial layer. It is not malignant because it has not yet broken through the basement membrane of the epithelial tissue. (*Slide 2.3*)

Fig. 2-3. The progression from normal to dysplasia to carcinoma in situ.

Rate of Growth

Benign tumors generally grow slowly over a period of years, while malignant tumors generally grow more rapidly than benign tumors.

Local Invasion

Fig. 2-4. Benign tumors generally remain localized to their site of origin. They may compress surrounding tissue, but they do not invade or metastasize. They also expand slowly, often with a rim of surrounding compressed fibrous tissue (**fibrous capsule**), all of which results in a freely movable mass on palpation. (*Slide 2.4*) On the other hand, malignant tumors by definition eventually invade surrounding tissue, causing a poorly demarcated, often "fixed" and immovable mass on palpation with irregular borders. (*Slide 2.5*) Aside from metastasis, tissue invasion is the most reliable feature of malignancy.

Metastasis

When tumor implants are far removed from (not directly continuous with) the primary neoplasm, **metastasis** has occurred. **The presence of a metastatic lesion unequivocally denotes malignancy.** Invasion into blood vessels, lymphatics, and body cavities allows travel of malignant cells to distal tissues, with implantation and continued growth at a new site. Generally, the larger and more poorly differentiated the neoplasm, the greater the chance

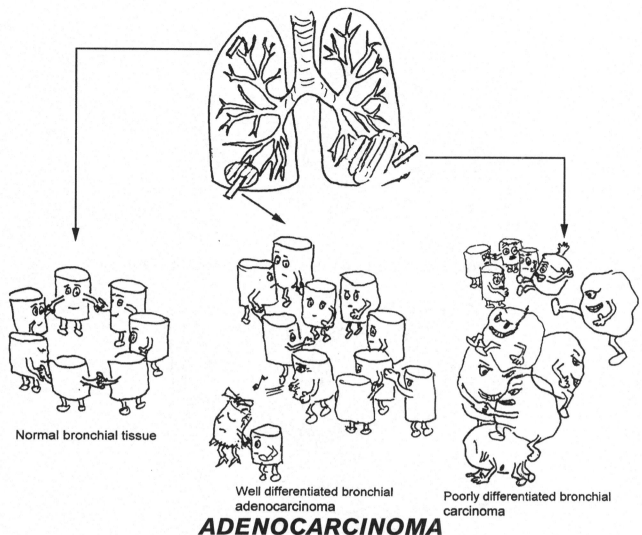

Normal bronchial tissue

Well differentiated bronchial adenocarcinoma

Poorly differentiated bronchial carcinoma

ADENOCARCINOMA

Figure 2-2

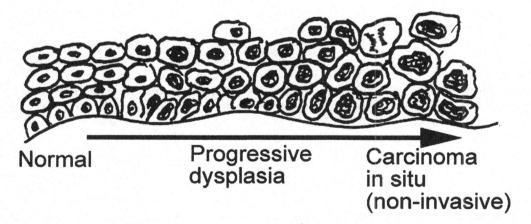

Normal

Progressive dysplasia

Carcinoma in situ (non-invasive)

PROGRESSION TO CARCINOMA IN SITU

Figure 2-3

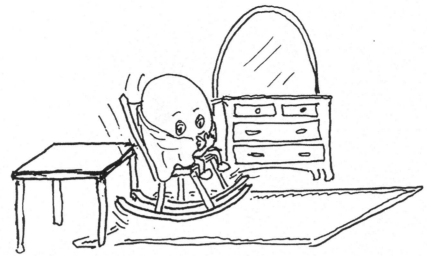

Benign, confined, well-demarcated, movable tumor

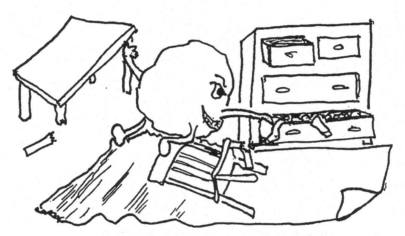

Malignant, infiltrating, attached to surroundings

Figure 2-4

of metastasis. Metastasis denotes a much reduced chance of cure (poorer prognosis). The three pathways of metastasis include:

1. **Seeding of body cavities**: This is typically seen in the peritoneal cavity, most commonly with ovarian cancer. The metastatic cells may grow as nodular implants on organ surfaces and cavity walls. The shedding of malignant cells from these implants is the basis for performing cytology of effusions in known cancer patients (lung, abdomen).
2. **Lymphatic spread**: This is the most common route of metastasis for carcinomas. The involvement of lymph nodes (*Slide 2.6*) generally follows stepwise fashion, following natural routes of lymphatic drainage, i.e., distal to proximal. Due to numerous bypass channels, the cancer may not involve all nodes in a chain, which forms the basis for extensive lymph node dissection in breast carcinoma, for example. Enlarged regional nodes may represent reactive hyperplasia, an immune response directed at tumor cells.
3. **Hematogenous spread**: This is most commonly used by sarcomas. Tumor spread may be venous (more common) or arterial.

EPIDEMIOLOGY

Cancer is the *second most common* cause of overall death in the United States, following heart disease. The **most common** cancers in males (descending order) are **prostate**, lung, and colorectal; and in females (descending order) are **breast**, lung, and colorectal. The **most common causes of death by cancer** in males (descending order) are **lung**, prostate, and colorectal; and in females (descending order) are **lung**, breast, and colorectal.

Geographic and Environmental Factors

There are striking differences in cancer types in different regions of the world, related to differences in environment and culture. For example, the death rate for gastric carcinoma is 7 to 8 times higher in Japan than the United States, likely due to diet, and the death rate for skin cancer is 6 times higher in New Zealand than Iceland, which is related in part to profound differences in sun exposure.

In addition, a large number of occupational carcinogens, such as benzene, have been implicated as causes of specific cancers. Smoking tobacco is implicated in numerous cancers, including cancer of the mouth, esophagus, pharynx, larynx, pancreas, and bladder. Alcohol abuse is associated with cancer of the mouth, pharynx, larynx, esophagus, and liver.

Age

In general, cancer incidence and risk increases with age, especially over age 55. Many cancers generally occur within a specific age range, some almost exclusively limited to one area of life. For example, common childhood solid neoplasms include neuroblastoma, Wilm's tumor, and rhabdomyosarcoma, all of which are quite rare outside of childhood.

Heredity

The possible role of heredity in many cancers is thought to be predominantly sporadic or environmental in nature; while there is an increased risk or predisposition to a cancer in offspring, it is usually not inevitable. However, several well characterized inherited cancer syndromes, arising from a mutant gene or defective product, significantly increase the chance of cancer in offspring:

1. **Familial retinoblastoma**: Children have an extremely high risk of developing retinoblastoma, usually bilateral. The "two hit" loss of a tumor-suppressor gene (see later sections) is responsible for this disease.
2. **Familial adenomatous polyposis (FAP)**: An autosomal dominant inheritance with development of numerous (>100) adenomatous polyps in the colon. 100% of patients develop carcinoma of colon by age 50, secondary to progression of at least one adenoma to carcinoma.
3. **Multiple endocrine neoplasia syndromes (MEN)**: Types I, IIa, IIb; develop multiple benign or malignant neoplasms.
4. **Neurofibromatosis types 1 and 2,**
5. **Von Hippel-Lindau syndrome**: Autosomal recessive inheritance of defective DNA repair genes (e.g.,

in xeroderma pigmentosum, Bloom syndrome, ataxia-telangiectasia, and Fanconi anemia) can lead to a number of inherited cancers.

Acquired Preneoplastic Disorders

A number of "precancerous" lesions have been identified, associated with an increased risk of progression to cancer. These are generally caused by prolonged or repeated environmental insults, resulting in repeated damage and regrowth. Several examples include:

1. Endometrial hyperplasia leads to endometrial carcinoma.
2. Cervical dysplasia leads to cervical carcinoma.
3. Actinic keratosis of skin leads to squamous cell carcinoma.
4. Barrett's metaplasia of esophagus leads to esophageal adenocarcinoma.

Treatment in the form of excision or ablation is generally recommended to reduce risk of transformation, but varies with the preneoplastic condition. These lesions do not always lead to cancer; the removal of the predisposing event, which led to the metaplasia, may result in a return to normal.

MOLECULAR ASPECTS OF CANCER
General Principles

Nonlethal DNA damage is the underlying cause of carcinogenesis. Causes range from environmental agents (chemicals, radiation, viruses) to inherited gene abnormalities. Tumor development results from clonal expansion of a single progenitor cell that has undergone genetic damage and subsequently replicates (tumors are initially monoclonal). Four classes of genes described below are involved in regulating cell cycle and division and are the principle targets involved in development of cancer.

Oncogenes

Fig. 2-5. Proto-oncogenes, oncogenes, and suppressor genes. Proto-oncogenes are essential for normal cellular growth and differentiation. Oncogenes ("cancer-causing genes") are derived from mutations in *proto-oncogenes*, and result in aberrant growth and differentiation. Suppressor genes keep cell growth in check, suppressing abnormal cellular growth and are thus good for the cell.

Oncogenes encode oncoproteins, which resemble normal products of proto-oncogenes, but are devoid of important regulatory elements and do not depend on growth factors or other external signals. Proto-oncogenes become oncogenic by retroviral transduction, a process where a viral genome creates an abnormal cellular protein (**v-oncs**) or by in situ alterations that convert them

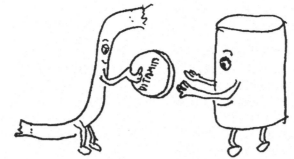

Proto-oncogene: product essential for healthy growth and differentiation

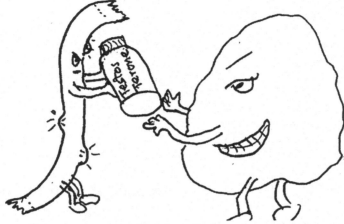

Oncogene: product results in exaggerated or aberrant growth and differentiation

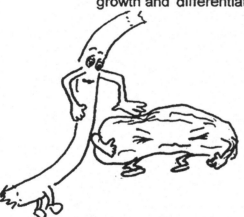

Suppressor gene: Actively counteracts growth stimulus as appropriate

Figure 2-5

into cellular oncogenes (**c-oncs**). V-oncs and c-oncs can both result in similar neoplastic changes; however, the mechanism of neoplastic change differs between v-oncs and c-oncs. Some viral genes can cause transformation to malignant phenotype by insertion near a proto-oncogene, either inducing a structural change in the resultant protein and converting it to a cellular oncogene (c-onc) or by altering/promoting expression of a normal cellular gene (*insertional mutagenesis*). Types of oncogenes include:

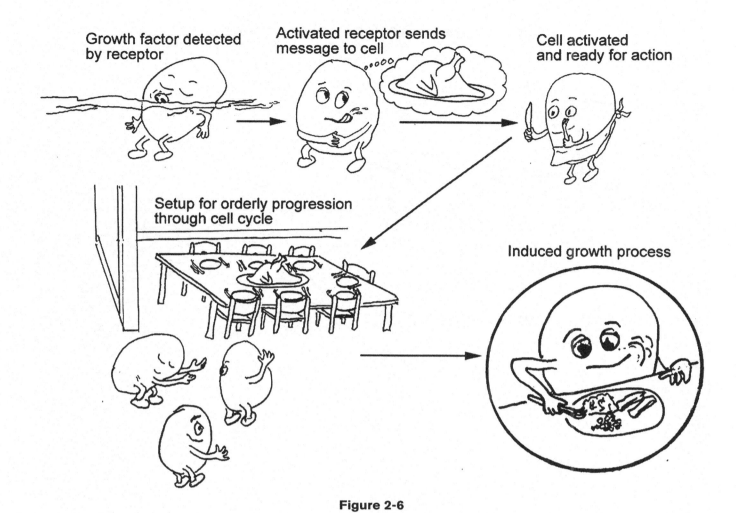

Growth factor detected by receptor

Activated receptor sends message to cell

Cell activated and ready for action

Setup for orderly progression through cell cycle

Induced growth process

Figure 2-6

1. **Growth factors**: These stimulate proliferation of cells. Mutations can render the cell prone to oncogenesis, but are not sufficient alone to induce transformation. Examples include platelet derived growth factor (PDGF) and fibroblast growth factors (FGF).

Fig. 2-6. Growth factor influence on cells.

2. **Growth factor receptors**: These are usually transmembrane proteins with an extracellular ligand-binding site and internal tyrosine kinase domain. They become persistently activated despite lack of growth factor stimulation. The result is a continuous delivery of mitogenic signals to the cell. Examples of this class include the epithelial growth factor (EGF) receptor family: *erb*-B1, *erb*-B2, *erb*-B3.

3. **Signal-transducing proteins**: Proteins in this category initiate a cascade of intracellular messengers, ultimately activating nuclear transcription factors. Mutant forms become persistently activated, similar to growth factor receptors, leading to continuous activation of the intracellular signal cascade. The activation of the intracellular signal cascade will then chronically activate the cell, hence promoting cellular growth and mitosis. Examples include *abl*, known for its role in the famous "Philadelphia chromosome" of chronic myelogenous leukemia, and *ras*, the single **most common** abnormality of dominant oncogenes.

4. **Nuclear transcription factors**: Proteins that contain specific sequences that allow the binding of DNA and are the endpoint of signal transduction pathways. They control the transcription of growth-related genes. Oncogenic transcription factors are also persistently expressed or overexpressed, resulting in unrelenting transcription of growth genes. Examples include **myc, N-myc, myb, jun**, and **fos**.

5. **Cyclins and cyclin-dependent kinases (CDK)**: These are involved in the orderly progression of cells through phases of the cell cycle, controlling entry of quiescent cells into the cell cycle and allowing time for DNA repair to occur before genome replication. Mutations that dysregulate activity of cyclins and CDKs favor cell proliferation and increased likelihood of replicating damaged DNA.

Oncogenes derive from proto-oncogenes by:

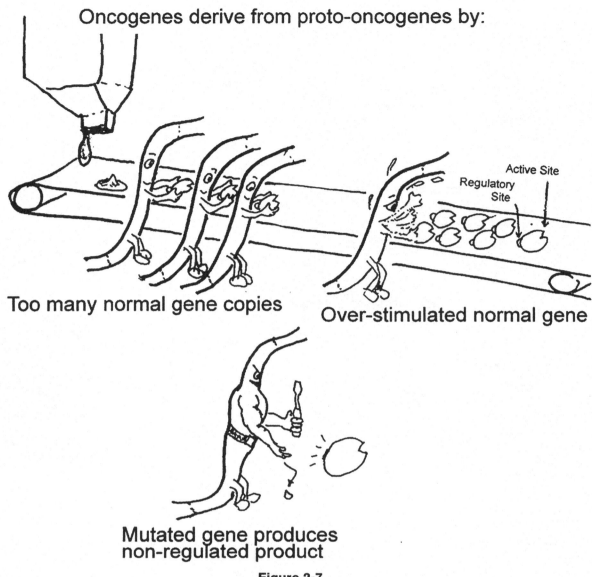

Too many normal gene copies

Over-stimulated normal gene

Active Site
Regulatory Site

Mutated gene produces non-regulated product

Figure 2-7

Fig. 2-7. Summary— how Proto-oncogenes can become oncogenes; the conveyor belt. Proto-oncogenes are transformed into oncogenes by a change in the number of gene copies made, a change in regulation of gene expression (enhanced production of structurally normal growth factors), or altered structure of the gene (synthesis of abnormal gene product with aberrant function). The primary causes of this transformation include point mutations and chromosomal rearrangements, such as translocations and inversions.

Tumor-suppressor Genes

These genes regulate cell growth through the interactions of their products with the products of growth-stimulating genes. Disruption of **both** copies is necessary for dysregulation of cell growth. The funda-mental theory that describes the role of tumor-suppressor oncogenesis is the **Knudson "two-hit" hypothesis**. The prototype of this process is familial retinoblastoma. Under this schema, the first hit is an inherited mutation in *Rb*, the tumor-suppressor gene. The second hit occurs when a sporadic, somatic mutation is acquired in retinal cells that already carry one mutated **Rb** gene. Loss of both alleles of **Rb** gene leads to the development of retinoblastoma.

A term often used to explain this progression is **loss of heterozygosity** (LOH). Patients with a known germline mutation in one allele of a tumor suppressor gene are therefore heterozygous at that locus. A mutation or loss of the other allele (to become homozygous at that locus) is called loss of heterozygosity and denotes a greatly increased risk of development of cancer.

Types of tumor-suppressor genes include:

1. **Nuclear transcription and cell cycle progression regulators**: Examples include the aforementioned Rb, which is expressed in every cell type so far examined; p53, another famous and widespread gene; and others such as BRCA-1 and BRCA-2, which are associated with the development of hereditary breast cancer. Mutations of these genes lead to loss of the cellular regulation mechanisms.

2. **Signal transduction regulators**: Examples include APC, involved in familial adenomatous polyposis, and **NF-1**, which results in development of numerous benign neurofibromas (neurofibromatosis type 1). Mutations in these genes lead to promotion of abnormal cellular growth.

3. **Cell surface receptors**: These molecules are expressed on the cell surface and regulate cell growth and behavior. They include receptors for growth inhibitory factors and proteins that regulate cellular adhesions. Examples include the **TGF-beta** family, which when mutated results in the loss of a growth inhibitory pathway; **cadherins**, which when mutated result in decreased cell-cell adhesion, allowing easier tissue invasion or metastasis; and **NF-2**, which causes neurofibromatosis type 2.

4. **Apoptosis regulators**: These normally prevent or induce programmed cell death (apoptosis). **bcl-2** is the classic example and is involved in follicular (B-cell) lymphoma. When overexpressed, **bcl-2** prevents apoptosis, allowing cells to survive for long periods of time, a key aspect of malignancy. **p53** and **c-myc** also serve as regulators of apoptosis and are commonly mutated in many cancers.

5. **DNA repair regulators**: Dietary carcinogens, sunlight, ionizing radiation, and everyday replication errors all damage DNA, which is normally repaired by certain enzymes. Inherited mutations of DNA repair proteins greatly increase the risk of developing cancer. For example, **hereditary nonpolyposis colon cancer (HNPCC) syndrome** (distinct from FAP) is a familial cancer of the cecum and proximal colon. A defect in genes involved in DNA mismatch repair allows errors to accumulate slowly during normal cell replication, eventually involving proto-oncogenes and tumor suppressor genes.

6. **Abnormal presence of telomerase**: Normal cells are arrested in a nondividing state (**cellular senescence**) after a fixed number of divisions, due to the shortening in somatic cells of telomeres, the ends of chromosomes. Germ cells, however, have the enzyme *telomerase*, which prevents telomere shortening. Cancer cells may use abnormally present telomerase to become immortalized.

Fig. 2-8. The multistep ("multihit") process by which normal cell becomes a cancerous cell, both henotypically and genotypically. Multiple, stepwise mutations are required for transformation and tumor progression, for example the ability to grow without contact inhibition, the ability to invade surrounding tissue, and the ability to metastasize. All cancers exhibit numerous genetic mutations of the kind described above.

BIOLOGY OF TUMOR GROWTH

A biologic sequence of events follows the molecular events, allowing malignant cells to evade host control, and host defenses, and invade with translocation to distant tissues (metastasis). The sequence involves **tumor growth, angiogenesis, development of heterogeneity**, and eventual **invasion and metastasis**.

Fig. 2-9. "Seeding" of a tumor via lymph node or bloodstream metastasis. Seeding via the blood stream allows for distant metastasis.

Tumor Growth

By the time a solid tumor is clinically detectable (1 gram), its population has doubled over 30 times (10^9 cells)! Tumors begin with an early growth phase, in which the majority of malignant cells are dividing. With continued growth, more cells begin to leave the cell cycle due to lack of sufficient nutrients, outgrowing the blood supply, causing necrosis and reversion to G_0. By the time of clinical detection, the majority of the cells are not in the replicative pool. Many chemotherapeutic drugs kill only cells involved in cell division and so are much more effective in fast-growing tumors, which have a large fraction of malignant cells dividing. Slow-growing tumors require surgery and/or radiation therapy first in order to shift other cells into the cell cycle, which then allows chemotherapy to be effective.

Tumor Angiogenesis

Without the ability to induce the growth of blood vessels within the malignant tissue, tumors will outgrow their blood supply. This is seen in many fast-growing tumors as *central areas of necrosis*. Cancers require a blood supply for nutrients and oxygen, as well as a path of entry for metastasis. To solve this problem, tumors release factors capable of stimulating and enhancing angiogenesis. Ironically, invading inflammatory cells, attempting to fight the tumor, also release angiogenic factors. The most important of these factors are vascular endothelial growth factor (**VEGF**) and basic fibroblast growth factor (**bFGF**). Angiogenesis is induced late in tumor progression, as mutations switch to an "angiogenic phenotype." Because most tumors rely on angiogenesis, regardless of their tissue of origin or instigating genetic defect, blocking

PROGRESSIVE TUMORIGENESIS BY
SEQUENTIAL GENETIC CHANGE

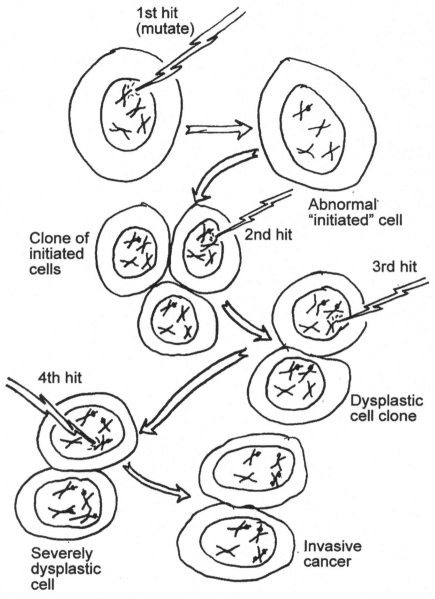

Figure 2-8

angiogenesis is an important current focus for new chemotherapeutic agents.

Tumor Heterogeneity

Though initially monoclonal, genetic instability and progressive mutations during replication produce sub-clones of cells with more "malignant" phenotypes. This results in the incremental acquisition of properties that improve the ability of the tumor to survive in the host. It may develop accelerated growth, the ability to

"hide" from the immune system, the ability to invade and metastasize, and increased or decreased response to hormones. Some subclones develop vulnerable attributes, such as increased susceptibility to chemo-therapeutics or surface antigens that increase immuno-susceptibility.

Mechanisms of Invasion and Metastasis

Invasion and metastasis are very complex processes. Metastasizing cells must possess the proper collection

PROGRESS OF NEOPLASIA IN THE HOST

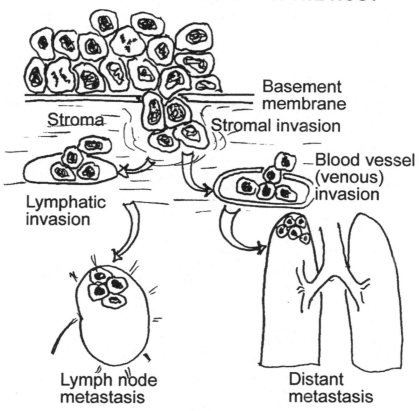

Figure 2-9

of numerous genetic attributes to be successful. This involves enzymes and proteins that allow cells to break into the bloodstream, escape destruction in the bloodstream, attach to distant tissue, exit the bloodstream, and reestablish their own blood supply for growth.

In order to detach from other tumor cells, a given cell must down-regulate **cadherins** and **catenins** involved in cell-cell interaction and adhesion. Next, invasion of surrounding extracellular matrix (ECM) is accomplished by attaching to matrix components (collagen, laminin, fibronectin) via **integrins** (normal cell components). The matrix is destroyed, creating a pathway for migration using proteolytic enzymes. Migration occurs through the basement membrane and ECM in a fashion similar to the diapedesis of neutrophils.

Once the cells penetrate the basement membrane and enter the blood or lymph, the biggest obstacle is evasion of the immune system. Tumor cells aggregate in clumps and may be coated with platelets to improve survival and the ability to implant. The cells then must attach to a vessel at a distant site, break through that basement membrane, and then survive in a "new" environment of a different organ. Interestingly, different tumors commonly metastasize to predictable, specific sites (e.g., prostate cancer to bone), which is possibly related to specific adhesion molecules expressed by the endothelium of the target organ or to the specific environmental requirements for growth.

CARCINOGENIC AGENTS AND CELL DAMAGE
Chemical Carcinogenesis

Numerous chemicals damage DNA, and so they have the potential to cause cancer. They often do so at a specific site related to area of greatest contact (e.g., skin, lungs) or site of greatest concentration (e.g., liver).

Carcinogenesis is divided into two phases: **initiation** and **promotion**. Initiation results from exposure of cells to a significant dose of a carcinogenic agent, which causes genetic damage that will likely give rise to a tumor. Initiation causes **permanent DNA damage** (mutation), and the damage still results in a tumor even if contact with the promoting agent is delayed for a prolonged amount of time. Promotion, on the other hand, involves agents that are **nontumorigenic** themselves, but can induce tumorigenesis when applied to initiated cells (cells with mutations induced by contact with initiating agent). Promoters

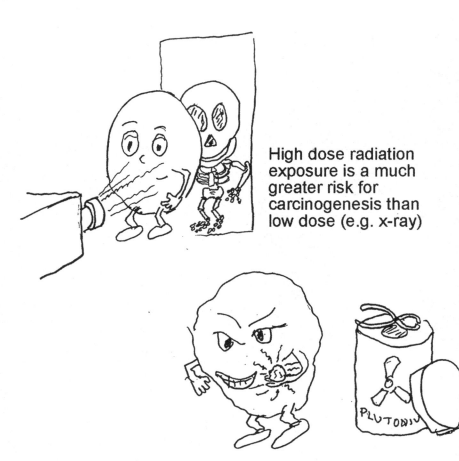

High dose radiation exposure is a much greater risk for carcinogenesis than low dose (e.g. x-ray)

Figure 2-10

stimulate cell replication, which renders cells susceptible to additional mutations. Another key difference between initiation and promotion is that changes induced by promoters are **reversible**, if they are removed before they cause damage to DNA, and alone do not affect DNA. Initiators are usually reactive **electrophiles** that covalently alter DNA, RNA, and cell proteins. Promoters are usually inflammatory or proliferative agents like drugs, hormones, infections, phenols, and tobacco.

Radiation Carcinogenesis

Radiation also has carcinogenic properties. The most important types are UV rays and ionizing radiation. UV rays increase susceptibility to squamous cell carcinoma, basal cell carcinoma, and malignant melanoma. The incidence is greater in high sunlight areas (Australia, the equator). **UV-B** is the most dangerous; it induces mutations, inactivates enzymes, and kills cells. Specifically, UV-B forms pyrimidine dimers in DNA, which are normally repaired by the nucleotide excision repair system. It is postulated that the system is overwhelmed in excessive sun exposure, and this leads to non-repaired DNA damage, with eventual progression to cancer. **Xeroderma pigmentosum**, for example, is an autosomal recessive disease caused by a faulty DNA repair system. This results in extreme photosensitivity with greatly increased risk of cancer in sun-exposed skin.

Ionizing radiation includes electromagnetic (x-rays, gamma rays) and particulate (alpha and beta particles, protons) radiation, all of which are carcinogenic. This is most evident in survivors of the atomic bomb, who developed leukemia or solid tumors years after exposure in greatly increased incidence. Skin, bone, and the GI tract are relatively resistant to the carcinogenic effects of radiation, though the GI tract is vulnerable to cell-killing effects. However, exposed patients are very susceptible to developing **leukemias**, or other common cancers such as thyroid, breast, lung, and salivary gland cancers.

The risk of cancer relates to cumulative dose, whether delivered all at once or repeatedly over time. Routine x-ray studies (chest, pelvis, etc.) involve very low doses with extremely low risk for carcinogenesis.

Fig. 2-10. Routine x-ray versus plutonium.

Viral and Microbial Carcinogenesis

Viruses and other microbes appear to be causative agents in a variety of cancers. The viruses implicated are generally DNA viruses, which integrate

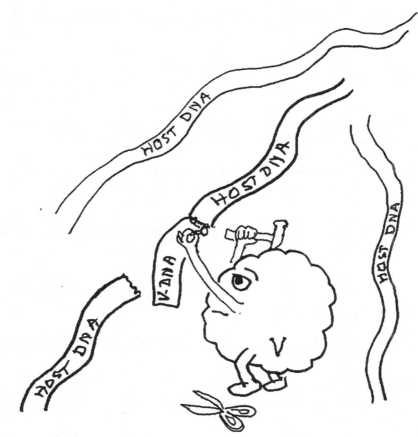

Figure 2-11

Viruses contributing to carcinogenesis integrate their DNA into the host genome.

their DNA into the host DNA; this insertion may alter an important region of host DNA, triggering carcinogenesis.

Fig. 2-11. Integration of viral DNA into the host genome. It copies its way into cells and then induces oncogenes to promote cell growth and replication.

Important cancer-causing microbes include:

1. **Human papillomavirus (HPV):** There are over 70 genetically distinct types identified. Types **1, 2, 4, 7** are associated with benign squamous papillomas (warts). Other types are sexually transmitted. HPV types **6** and **11** cause genital warts and have low malignant potential, but HPV types **16, 18, 31, 33, 35, 51** are found in the vast majority of invasive squamous cell carcinomas of the cervix and in severe cervical dysplasia. They are also involved in squamous cell carcinoma of the anogenital region (severe in AIDS and other immunosuppressed patients) and in oral and laryngeal papillomas and carcinomas. The malignant strains insert their

DNA into the host genome, while the benign strains do not.

2. **Epstein-Barr Virus (EBV):** This virus is implicated in nasopharyngeal carcinoma, B-cell lymphomas in chronically immunosuppressed patients, the **African** form of Burkitt lymphoma, and some cases of Hodgkin disease. In African Burkitt lymphoma, the virus causes a characteristic **(8;14) translocation.**

3. **Hepatitis B virus:** Patients infected with Hep B face an increased risk for hepatocellular carcinoma. The virus is endemic in the Far East and Africa, which have the highest incidence of liver cancer. Hep B causes chronic hepatocellular injury by direct effects and the inflammatory response with resultant regenerative hyperplasia; this increased proliferation increases the risk of mutation caused by environmental agents. The virus also encodes a protein that disrupts growth control of infected cells. Hepatitis C virus also causes a chronic infection that is strongly associated with development of liver cancer.

4. **Human T-cell Leukemia Virus Type 1 (HTLV-1):** This an **RNA virus** associated with T-cell leukemia/lymphoma. It is endemic in parts of Japan and Caribbean area, but sporadic elsewhere. After invading CD4+ T-cells, it causes leukemia in a small percentage of those infected, after a latency period of 2-3 decades. The infection stimulates proliferation of T-cells, increasing risk for secondary mutations, with an eventual monoclonal neoplastic population.

5. *Helicobacter pylori:* This is the **bacterial** agent associated with gastric and duodenal ulcers, gastric lymphomas, and rarely gastric carcinoma. A chronic infection encourages a polyclonal population of B cells through T-cell stimulation. Eventually, a monoclonal B-cell population develops, but it is still T-cell dependent. Proliferation often resolves with treatment of *H. pylori* with antibiotics.

IMMUNE RESPONSE TO CANCER
Host Response

Cancer cells often contain antigens that are recognized by the immune system as non-self, and subsequently the immune system attempts to destroy those cells. The host employs both a cell-mediated response using **cytotoxic T-cells**, **natural killer cells**, and **macrophages**, and a **humoral response** using antibodies and complement. The host immune system likely destroys most malignant cells before progression to frank neoplasm. This is suggested by the increased incidence of cancer in immunosuppressed hosts and the fact that humans encounter a large number of carcinogens daily, including air pollution, chemicals, natural toxins; even first- and second-hand cigarette smoke takes years of exposure before the development of cancer occurs.

Fig. 2-12. The host's natural immune response to combat tumors.

Tumor Avoidance of Host Response

Tumors, then, attempt to evade the immune system using several mechanisms including:
1. **Natural selection**: This is the selective growth of most "fit" tumor cell subclones; those lacking antigens that stimulate immune system continue the life cycle, while immunogenic subclones are eliminated.
2. **Down-regulation of histocompatibility antigens:** Without MHC class I molecules, no antigen are presented for recognition by cytotoxic T-cells.
3. **Immunosuppression**: Tumor products may suppress the immune system.
4. **Apoptosis of cytotoxic T-cells**: The expression of **Fas ligand** by tumor cells is recognized by T-cells and stimulates T-cell autodestruction.

5. **Lack of co-stimulating factors**: Tumor cells may not express receptors or release factors necessary to stimulate T-cell activation.

CLINICAL FEATURES OF TUMORS
Effects of Tumor on Host

Both benign and malignant tumors cause many deleterious effects on the host. Among them:
1. **Impingement on adjacent structures**: Masses may compress nerves, blood vessels, lymphatics, and normal tissue, with resultant compromise of function.
2. **Hormone synthesis**: For example, overproduction of parathyroid hormone by parathyroid adenoma, with resultant effects of hypercalcemia. Hormonal effects are more commonly seen with **benign** adenomas of endocrine organs, because endocrine carcinomas are often too undifferentiated to produce hormones.
3. **Bleeding and secondary infection**: For example, an ulcerating gastric carcinoma with secondary anemia and a superinfection.
4. **Acute symptomatology**: For example, a leiomyoma with infarction and central necrosis, producing pain.
5. **Cachexia** is the wasting syndrome seen in advanced cancer patients. It involves loss of fat and muscle with associated weakness, anemia, and loss of appetite. Cachexia is caused by factors released by a tumor or host response to a tumor, **not** by increased nutritional demands of a tumor. **Tumor necrosis factor (TNF-alpha)** is likely responsible in part; it is released by macrophages and some tumor cells.
6. **Paraneoplastic Syndromes** are symptom complexes in cancer patients that are not attributable to local tumor effects or overproduction of factors normally produced by the tissue of origin of the tumor. For example, hypercalcemia in a patient with lung cancer is a paraneoplastic syndrome, while hypercalcemia in a patient with a parathyroid adenoma is **not**.

Endocrinopathies are caused by ectopic hormone production; tumor cells produce a hormone or a related peptide not found in the tissue of cancer origin. Cushing syndrome is the most common example. It is caused by ectopic secretion of ACTH, often by small cell carcinoma of the lung. Another example is the secretion of parathyroid hormone-related peptide (PTHrP), which is often produced by squamous cell carcinoma of the lung.

Other syndromes affect the neuromusculature, such as dermatomyositis, acanthosis nigricans, and peripheral neuropathies. Others affect the bone, joint, and soft tissue, such as hypertrophic osteoarthropathy. Others affect the vascular and hematologic systems, such as migratory thrombophlebitis (*Trousseau's syndrome*: seen with pancreatic cancer) and disseminated intravascular coagulation, which is life-threatening.

HOST IMMUNE RESPONSE AGAINST TUMORS

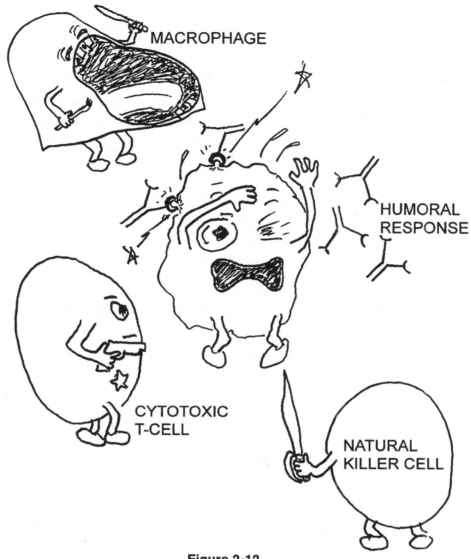

MACROPHAGE

HUMORAL RESPONSE

CYTOTOXIC T-CELL

NATURAL KILLER CELL

Figure 2-12

Grading and Staging

Grading and staging are used to determine the severity of malignancy and to estimate the prognosis.

Grade

Grade is the **level of differentiation** of a tumor. The degrees vary with tumor type and are based on the histopathological assessment of the extent of differentiation in tumor cells using standard cell characteristics (keratin production in squamous cell carcinoma, for example) and growth rate (frequency of mitoses). A tumor is usually classified as well-, moderately-, or poorly-differentiated. There is a rough correlation between grade and biologic behavior: anaplastic tumors tend to be more aggressive; well-differentiated tumors tend to be less invasive and metastasize less frequently.

Stage

Stage is the extent of spread of cancer in a patient. It is determined by the extent of local spread of tumor, tumor size, involvement of regional lymph nodes, and metastasis to distant sites. A combination of pathologic and surgical information determines the staging and is used in the TNM system.

T: primary tumor; refers to size
N: nodes; refers to number of lymph nodes involved
— surgeon resects regional lymph nodes, evaluated by pathology to detect cancer

M: metastases; generally presence or absence of different combinations assigned to stage of tumor, which are determined by clinical studies

Staging provides essential information, because staging at the time of diagnosis often determines the course of treatment and predicts prognosis and survival duration.

LABORATORY DIAGNOSIS OF CANCER

Finally, a variety of remarkable technologies exist to aid in the diagnosis of cancer.

Histology and Cytology

Histological characterization of a tumor involves examination of a specimen under a microscope after sectioning, fixation, and mounting on a slide. It is routinely performed on excised tumors and biopsy specimens to assess margins of neoplasm to ensure adequate resection, assess lymph nodes for metastases, and assess for microinvasion of blood vessels. The frozen section evaluation is performed with the patient still on the operating table; quick freeze of the specimen to evaluate resection margins or lymph nodes allows the surgeon to plan further immediate treatment.

Cytologic evaluation involves examining individual cells instead of tissues. Fine-needle aspiration of cells from a lesion using a small-bore needle allows for a less invasive method to determine whether the lesion is benign or malignant. (*Slide 2.7*) The Papanicolaou smear is a similar method for evaluating the cervix for dysplasia and cancer. Cells are scraped from the cervix and smeared on a slide, which is then stained and viewed under a microscope (*Slide 2.8*).

Immunohistochemistry

Use of monoclonal antibodies to cell products or surface markers allows identification of undifferentiated tumors, aids in determining the site of origin of metastatic tumors, and allows categorization of leukemias and lymphomas. In addition, the detection of molecules with prognostic or therapeutic significance is possible; for example, the detection of estrogen and progesterone molecules in breast cancer affects treatment and prognosis.

Molecular Diagnosis

Molecular diagnosis is a rapidly growing method of tumor diagnosis and characterization of tumors. It detects gene rearrangements specific to some tumors and can detect mutations in genes associated with increased risk for cancer, for example **Rb** mutation in hereditary retinoblastoma, **APC** in familial adenomatous polyposis.

Flow Cytometry

Flow cytometry is the rapid determination of multiple markers expressed by a cell, as well as DNA content of a tumor using fluorescently labeled antibodies against cell surface markers. It is most useful in leukemia and lymphoma, classifying tumor by antigens (**CD markers**) expressed on the surface. It also provides information on tumor ploidy, which is helpful for prognosis since aneuploidy is associated with poor outcomes.

Tumor Markers

Finally, serologic quantitation of tumor markers can be used to evaluate tumor status. They are **not specific enough** to use for primary diagnosis, but determining levels before treatment and after can help to evaluate response and monitor for recurrence. Examples include carcinoembryonic antigen (CEA), which is normally produced by embryologic tissues of the GI tract and can be elevated in many cancers, including colon, pancreas, and stomach cancer, and alpha-fetoprotein (AFP), which is elevated in hepatocellular cancer and some germ cell tumors of testis.

3

Molecular Pathology

OVERVIEW

Genetic disorders are much more common than many of us realize. The estimated lifetime incidence of genetic disease is 67 per 100 people. This statistic includes "conventional" genetic disorders like cystic fibrosis and Down syndrome, along with heart disease and cancer, which result from a combination of genetic and environmental factors. Now that the Human Genome Project is complete, we know increasingly more about the genetic complexities that make us human. First, we know that less than 2% of our genome codes for recognizable proteins. Moreover, 50% of the remaining genetic code translates into repetitive sequences that, as of yet, have unknown functions. Second, we've discovered that the human genome is fairly short—only about 30,000 genes long! This number is much smaller than the early estimates of 80,000 to 140,000 genes. Also, 99.9% of nucleotide bases are identical in all people. Therefore, only 0.1% of the genetic code makes us unique human beings. This may seem infinitely tiny, but 0.1% of the human genome translates into approximately 3 million base pairs (that's nearly 1 million codons—a **codon**, the functional unit of the genetic code, is a triplet of nucleotide bases). In this chapter, we will address basic molecular pathology, common examples of genetic disorders, and the rapidly growing field of diagnostic molecular genetics.

BASIC TERMINOLOGY

Normal human cells are **diploid (2N)**, containing 22 pairs of somatic chromosomes and 1 pair of sex chromosomes—46 chromosomes in total. The normal human genetic profile is written as **46,XX** for females or **46,XY** for males. The normal **haploid (1N)** number is 23.

Aneuploidy refers to an abnormal chromosome number that is not divisible by 23. Aneuploidy most commonly occurs due to **nondisjunction** during meiosis I, when two chromosomes fail to separate, leaving a cell with one too many **(trisomy)** or too few **(monosomy)** chromosomes. Aneuploidy also can be caused by **anaphase lag**, where one chromosome "lags behind" very early during mitotic or meiotic division and is lost.

Fig. 3-1. Aneuploidy, showing nondisjunction with anaphase lag of chromosomes during meiosis.

NONDISJUNCTION

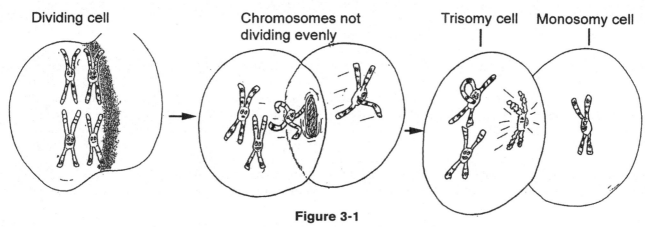

Dividing cell   Chromosomes not dividing evenly   Trisomy cell   Monosomy cell

Figure 3-1

BALANCED TRANSLOCATION

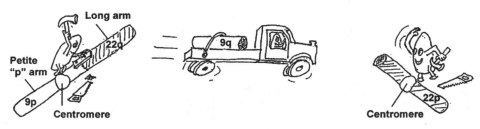

Figure 3-2

Nondisjunction and anaphase lag often result in a **mosaic** genotype. A mosaic genotype is one in which there are two different cell populations in one organism. Thus, in the example above, anaphase lag will create two different cell populations, one which is lacking a set of chromosomes, and one that has an extra pair of chromosomes. This phenomenon generally causes a milder disease phenotype than pure monosomy or trisomy. Another example of a mosaic variant is **Turner syndrome (45,X or XO)**, where a cleavage error in the ovum causes one daughter cell to receive three sex chromosomes and the other to receive only one (45,X/47,XXX). Thus, all future cells from this point on will either be 45,X or 47,XXX. The 45,X cells will express Turner syndrome, while the 47,XXX cells will have a clinically silent phenotype. In comparison, somatic chromosomes also can show mosaicism, but this is far less common than with sex chromosomes.

Polyploidy is a chromosome number that is more than two times greater than the normal haploid number. Examples include **triploidy** (69 chromosomes), **tetraploidy** (92 chromosomes), and so on. In humans, this condition is generally incompatible with life.

Inversion is an abnormal chromosome breakage, where the broken piece is reinserted upside down.

Translocation is the exchange of genetic material between **nonhomologous** chromosomes (not to be confused with "crossing over" between **homologous** chromosomes, a normal part of meiosis I). A translocation may be **balanced**, where the exchanged chromosome segments are equal and the results are clinically silent, or **unbalanced**, where the exchanged segments are unequal and genetic material is lost.

Fig. 3-2. Balanced translocation, in which there is an equal trade between nonhomologous chromosomes (here, chromosomes 9 and 22)

A **Robertsonian translocation** (also known as **centric fusion**) is a unique type of translocation where the "p" (short) arms of two acrocentric chromosomes are lost because the "q" (long) arms fuse together with a common centromere (loosing the "p" arms). Recall that **"acrocentric"** means the centromere is located very close to one end of the chromosome, making the *p* arms very **petite**. Robertsonian translocations are significant because they are common, occurring in 1 out of 1000 individuals, and they produce abnormal offspring, including children with a form of **Down syndrome**.

Fig. 3-3. Normal transcription and translation of three codons.

Deletions and **insertions** in the genetic material usually occur in part of the nucleotide sequence, although they may involve a whole chromosome. If the base pair alteration is not a multiple of three, a **frameshift mutation** can occur, causing the resulting codons to be read incorrectly all along the line. On the other hand, if the inserted or deleted base pairs are a multiple of three, this results in a gene product that is only locally abnormal since the rest of the chain remains normal.

Fig. 3-4. Abnormal transcription and translation:

A. Deletion of a single base, causing a frameshift mutation.
B. Addition of a single base, causing a frameshift mutation.
C. Deletion of a triplet, causing a loss of codon.
D. Insertion of a triplet, causing an addition of one codon.

Trinucleotide repeats are a special category of insertions because they involve amplification and insertion of a triplet nucleotide sequence. Every normal person has small trinucleotide repeats in his or her DNA, but larger amounts of a repeated sequence will result in genetic disorders such as **fragile-X syndrome** or **Huntington disease**.

More common than insertions or deletions are **point mutations**, where a single base is substituted for another. Point mutations within coding sequences may result in **missense mutations**, which alter the meaning of the genetic code. A good example of this is **sickle cell disease**, in which the base **valine** is substituted for **glutamate** on chromosome 6. The aberrant protein product of this rearrangement compromises the integrity of the red blood cell wall, causing the cell to sickle.

Nonsense mutations are point mutations that result in a **stop codon**, which terminates the amino acid chain and truncates the resulting peptide. **Beta-thalassemia** is due to a nonsense mutation in the beta-globin gene, resulting in abnormal hemoglobin and severe anemia.

Point mutations also may result in **silent mutations,** where a base substitution does not alter the gene product. Silent mutations occur fairly often, since the genetic code is **degenerate**, meaning that different codons will translate into the same amino acid. This phenomenon also is referred to as the "**wobble**" within the genetic code.

Sex Chromosome Definitions

Fig. 3-5. Barr bodies. These are clumps of X chromatin present in the nuclei of somatic cells of every normal female.

Each Barr body represents an inactivated X chromosome, which can be visualized in the interphase ("resting") nucleus of the female somatic cell as a dark spot touching the nuclear membrane. Very early in development, half of the female cells will inactivate the paternal X, and the other half will inactivate the maternal component. Thus, all normal women are, in fact, mosaics. This process is called **Lyonization** (or, more simply, X inactivation), named for Mary Frances Lyon, the geneticist who discovered it in 1961, along with Murray Llewellyn Barr—the Barr body's namesake!

In contrast, normal men (XY) and individuals with **Turner syndrome (45,X or XO)** do not have Barr bodies. Females with more than two X chromosomes (i.e., XXX and upward) will have multiple Barr bodies. Males with **Klinefelter syndrome (XXY)** also have a Barr body, which can be useful for the diagnosis.

Regarding normal male development, a Y chromosome is absolutely essential for growth and maturation. The **sex-determining region of the Y chromosome (SRY)** is located on the distal short arm and controls development of the testes. Currently, SRY is the only gene proven to dictate maleness in a developing embryo. However, other clusters of so-called "male-specific Y" genes are under investigation for their speculated roles in spermatogenesis.

CHROMOSOMAL ABNORMALITIES
Disorders of the Somatic Chromosomes

Down syndrome is the most common chromosomal disorder, accounting for about 1 in 700 live births each year in the United States. The most common cause (95%) of Down syndrome is **trisomy 21**, where the affected individual has three copies of chromosome 21 and 47 total chromosomes (47,XY, +21). As discussed earlier, all trisomies are most often caused by nondisjunction during meiosis I. Advanced maternal age has great influence on the incidence of trisomy 21, since nondisjunction occurs more frequently in the ova of women 35 or older. Recall that females are born with all of their eggs—they do not constantly produce germ cells as males do. As eggs "wait" to be ovulated for many decades, the chance for mutation grows!

Down syndrome also may be caused by a Robertsonian translocation between chromosome 21 and another large, acrocentric chromosome—often chromosome 14 (written in shorthand as 46,XY,t(14;21)). Note that the Robertsonian variants still have 46 chromosomes. Unfortunately, Robertsonian translocations usually are heritable, carried by the mother as a mutation in her germ cells (a "**germline mutation**"). The mother herself is not affected by the mutation, but many

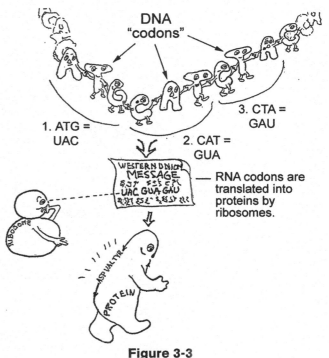

NORMAL TRANSCRIPTION AND TRANSLATION
OF THREE CODONS

DNA
"codons"

1. ATG = UAC

2. CAT = GUA

3. CTA = GAU

WESTERN UNION MESSAGE
UAC GUA GAU

— RNA codons are translated into proteins by ribosomes.

Figure 3-3

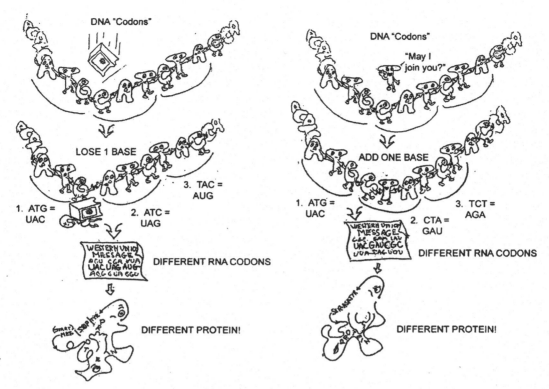

A. DELETION OF A SINGLE BASE (FRAMESHIFT MUTATION)   B. ADDITION OF A SINGLE BASE (FRAMESHIFT MUTATION)

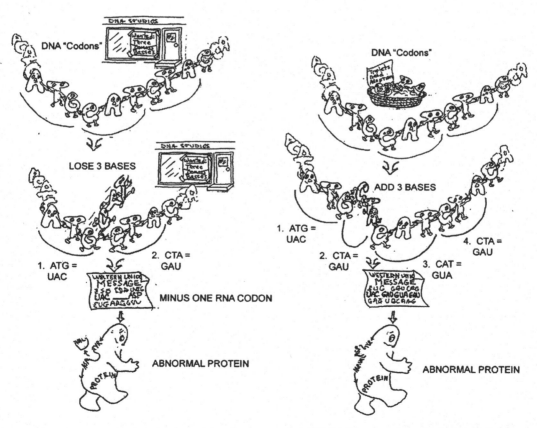

C. DELETION OF A TRIPLET (LOSS OF CODON)   D. INSERTION OF A TRIPLET (ADDITION OF ONE CODON)

Figure 3-4.

THE INFAMOUS "BARR BODY"

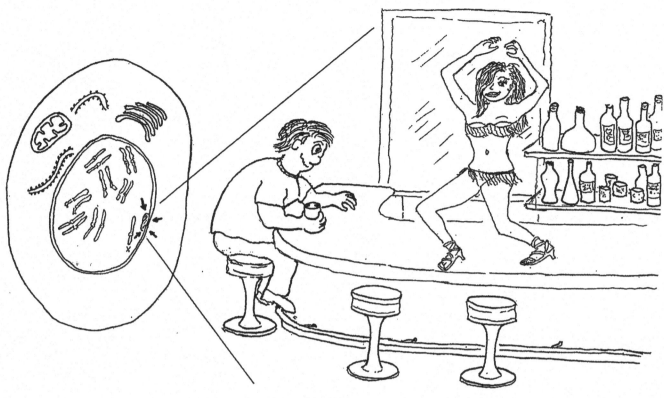

Figure 3-5

or all of her offspring will be affected. As a rule, if a young woman gives birth to a child with Down syndrome, or a family history of the disease is suspected, genetic counseling is in order.

Just 1% of the remaining Down syndrome population is comprised of **mosaics**. Mentioned earlier, mosaic individuals have one cell line with the normal complement of chromosomes (46,XX) and another with trisomy 21 (47,XX, +21). These individuals have a much milder, more variable phenotype.

Fig. 3-6. Somatic chromosome disorders:

3-6A. Down syndrome. Common clinical features include mental retardation, oblique palpebral fissures and epicanthal folds (sometimes called a "**Mongolian slant**"), increased neck skin, simian creases on the palms, a gap between the first and second toes, congenital heart defects, intestinal stenosis, and esophageal atresia. Down syndrome patients also are predisposed to acute leukemia, immunodeficiency disorders, and premature Alzheimer's disease.

3-6B. Edwards syndrome. This is caused by **trisomy 18**, resulting in mental retardation, renal malformations, congenital heart disease, and classic deformities, including micrognathia (small lower jaw), prominent occiput, low-set ears, short neck, overlapping fingers, and rocker-bottom feet.

3-6C. Patau syndrome. This is caused by **trisomy 13**. Mental retardation, congenital heart disease, renal defects, microcephaly (small head), microphthalmia (small eyes), cleft lip and palate, polydactyly (extra digits), and rocker-bottom feet are hallmarks of this severe disorder.

Unlike individuals with Down syndrome, patients with Edwards or Patau often die within weeks or months of birth. These unfortunate neonates have a wide range of severe birth defects that are incompatible with survival beyond the first year of life.

3-6D. Cri du chat ("cry of the cat") syndrome. This takes its name from the unusual catlike cry exhibited by babies born **without the short arm of chromosome 5 (5p-)**. This deletion is most commonly due to a sporadic mutation. Other features of this syndrome include severe mental retardation, microcephaly, low

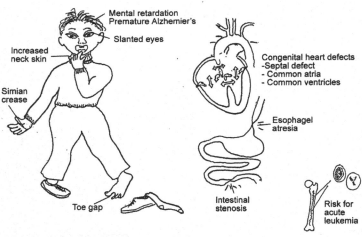

A. Down syndrome (trisomy 21)

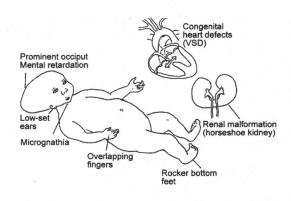

B. Edwards syndrome (trisomy 18)

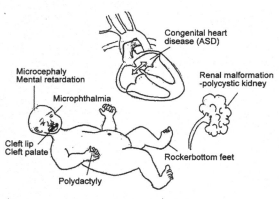

C. Patau syndrome (trisomy 13)

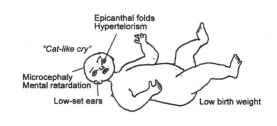

D. Cri du chat syndrome (missing 5p)

Figure 3-6

birth weight, hypertelorism (wide-set eyes), epicanthal folds, low-set ears, and round face.

Disorders of the Sex Chromosomes

Fig. 3-7. Sex chromosome disorders:

3-7A. Turner syndrome (45,X or XO). This results from **complete or partial monosomy of the X chromosome,** causing female hypogonadism. As a result, Turner syndrome is the most common cause of primary amenorrhea (inherent lack of menstruation), because the ovaries never completely develop. In their place, primitive gonadal streaks remain. Decreased estrogen production leads to immature genitalia and deficient breast development. Additional findings include short stature, webbed neck, and shield-shaped chest with widely spaced nipples. Aortic coarctation also is common in Turner syndrome patients. Fortunately, and in contrast to most other chromosomal anomalies, Turner syndrome does not cause mental retardation.

3-7B. Klinefelter syndrome (47,XXY). This condition occurs when a genetic male (XY) receives **an additional X chromosome** due to maternal nondisjunction during meiosis. The primary finding in Klinefelter syndrome is male hypogonadism, including atrophic testes and a small penis. Secondary sex characteristics, including deep voice, facial hair, and male distribution of pubic hair are lacking, while gynecomastia is common. Patients also exhibit tall stature due to delayed fusion of the epiphysis (a.k.a. "growth plate"). Although it can occur, mental retardation is not pronounced. Klinefelter syndrome usually is not diagnosed until after puberty, because the phenotypic manifestations involve secondary sex characteristics. This syndrome is the principal cause of male infertility.

XYY syndrome (47,XYY) results in tall stature, severe acne, and mild mental retardation. For the sake of comparison, **XXX (47,XXX) syndrome** usually is asymptomatic.

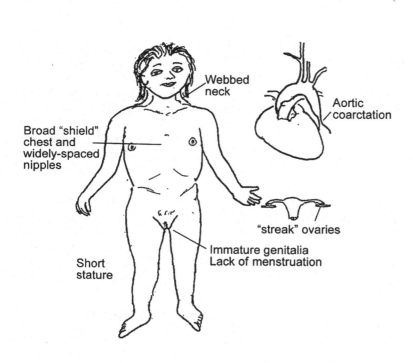

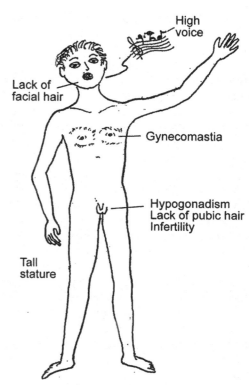

A. Turner syndrome (45, X or XO)

B. Klinefelter syndrome (47, XXY)

Figure 3-7

PATTERNS OF INHERITANCE
Autosomal Inheritance

Autosomal dominant phenotypes are expressed when only one chromosome of a pair contains an aberrant gene, whether or not the other chromosome is affected. Thus, a dominant phenotype is expressed in both heterozygotes and homozygotes. If an individual with an autosomal dominant disorder has children with an unaffected partner, 50% of the offspring should inherit the gene and thus be affected.

Autosomal recessive phenotypes, on the other hand, are expressed only when **both chromosomes** have the mutant allele. Accordingly, just those individuals who are homozygous for the trait will express it. Typically, 25% of children born to two affected parents will express the abnormal phenotype.

Sex-linked Inheritance

In an **X-linked recessive** pattern, the female parent commonly is an unaffected heterozygous carrier, and the male parent has a normal genotype. Consequently, the deviant X chromosome will be inherited by 50% of the male children (recall that boys receive an "X" from their mothers and a "Y" from their fathers), and half of the female children will be carriers like their mother. Alternatively, the male parent may carry the abnormal X chromosome. In the latter instance, male children will not inherit the mutant allele, but 100% of female children will be carriers. A good example of an X-linked disease pattern is the bleeding disorder **hemophilia**. England's Queen Victoria was a type A hemophilia carrier; consequently, many male children born within her bloodline inherited the disease and suffered from severe complications, but no female children were affected. Both forms of hemophilia (A and B) are explained more thoroughly in the hematopathology chapter.

X-linked dominant inheritance occurs very infrequently. In such situations, all heterozygous females and hemizygous males will express the disorder.

Y-linked inheritance, while not especially significant in the inheritance of serious disorders, has been implicated in rare cases of male infertility due to problems in sperm production.

Uncharacteristic Patterns of Inheritance

Mitochondrial inheritance is controlled by maternally transmitted mitochondrial DNA (mtDNA). Such mutations cause rare disorders like **Leber's Hereditary Optic Neuropathy (LHON)** and **Mitochondrial Epilepsy with Ragged-Red Fibers (MERRF)** and are exclusively inherited from the female parent. For example, if a woman has a mutation in her mtDNA, she will pass it on to all of her children. However, an affected man cannot transmit his mtDNA, so his children will remain unaffected.

Genomic imprinting is an unusual phenomenon that creates variability in the expression of a gene but does not change the DNA sequence. Since imprinting "breaks the rules" of normal Mendelian inheritance, it can be a difficult concept to understand. According to Mendelian theory, a gene is equally likely to be **transmitted** by either parent. However, Mendelian principles do not address the effect of an individual parent's sex on the **expression** of certain traits in the offspring. Currently, we know that some genetic disorders depend on whether or not the mutant allele was inherited from the mother or the father.

Each of us receives two copies of our genes, one from our mother and one from our father. **Imprinting** selectively inactivates either the maternal or paternal gene. Thus, an imprinted gene is "silenced." For example, **maternal imprinting** means that the maternal gene is inactivated and only the paternal component is expressed. **Paternal imprinting,** on the other hand, means that the maternal allele is expressed, while the paternal gene is silenced.

Fig. 3-8. Genomic imprinting. Genomic imprinting is best exemplified by two specific genetic disorders:

(A) Prader-Willi syndrome (PWS) is due to a deletion in the long arm of chromosome 15 (15q11-15q13) inherited from the child's father, and is characterized by obesity, excessive eating, small hands and feet, hypogonadism, short stature, and mental retardation.

(B) **Angelman syndrome (AS)** is due to a deletion in the long arm of chromosome 15 (15q11-15q13) **inherited from the child's mother,** and is characterized by spasticity, seizures, ataxia, severe mental retardation, short stature, and inappropriate laughter ("**happy puppet syndrome**").

In Angelman syndrome, the defective gene is maternal, and the paternal gene is the one that is imprinted, or silenced. Therefore, the only genetic material expressed on 15q11-15q13 is from the remaining maternal DNA. Unfortunately, in order to have a normal phenotype, both maternal and paternal copies of chromosome 15 must be present. **To remember that PWS is paternally imprinted, think of the phrase, "Proud poppa of a Prader-Willi patient"—kind of like a bumper sticker. Learn the phrase "Mommy's little angel" to recall that AS is maternally imprinted.** The stark contrast between these two disorders shows that the parental source of a genetic defect can have a major influence on the expression of a mutant phenotype.

In some cases, a patient with PWS or AS may have a "normal" cytogenetic profile (i.e., the patient's karyotype and other studies do not show a deletion on chromosome 15). In these instances, **uniparental disomy** is to blame. Uniparental disomy is defined as the inheritance of both chromosomes in a pair from only one parent. The net effect of this phenomenon is similar to imprinting, since only one parent's genetic material is expressed. Thus, PWS and AS also can be caused by uniparental disomy involving chromosome 15. Uniparental disomy has been implicated in many other disorders, including the rare **Beckwith-Wiedemann syndrome**, where affected children have severe hypoglycemia and an increased risk of kidney, adrenal, and liver cancers.

Multifactorial inheritance is responsible for many, if not the majority of, genetic disorders. These defects are the result of small genetic variations combined with environmental factors to cause disease. Common examples include Alzheimer's disease, cardiovascular disease, diabetes mellitus, and many types of cancer.

MENDELIAN DISORDERS

Please note: the next segment is meant to be an overview of some of the more important genetic disorders. Other disorders may be explained in system-specific chapters elsewhere in this text. Where appropriate, specific references are included.

Autosomal Dominant Disorders

Fig. 3-9. Marfan syndrome. This is an autosomal dominant connective tissue disorder caused by a mutation in the FBN-1 gene on chromosome 15q21, which codes for the protein fibrillin. Fibrillin is responsible for maintaining the integrity of many load-bearing structures in the body, including the aorta, ciliary muscle of the eye (which keeps the eyelid up), bone, and skin.

Physical manifestations of Marfan syndrome include extremely tall stature, arachnodactyly (spider-like fingers), pectus excavatum (concave chest), joint laxity, ectopia lentis (dislocated ocular lens), mitral valve prolapse, aortic regurgitation, and striae (aka "stretch marks") on the skin. It is thought that Abraham Lincoln had Marfan syndrome—recall that he was noted for being very tall and thin! Unfortunately, the cardiac abnormalities often are life threatening, and aortic root dissection is a common cause of death in these patients.

Other autosomal dominant disorders involving connective tissues defects include **Ehlers-Danlos syndrome** (hyperelasticity of the skin), **osteogenesis imperfecta** ("brittle bone disease"), and **achondroplasia** (dwarfism).

Adult Polycystic Kidney Disease (APKD) is the most commonly inherited renal disorder, present in approximately 1 in 600 adults and accounting for

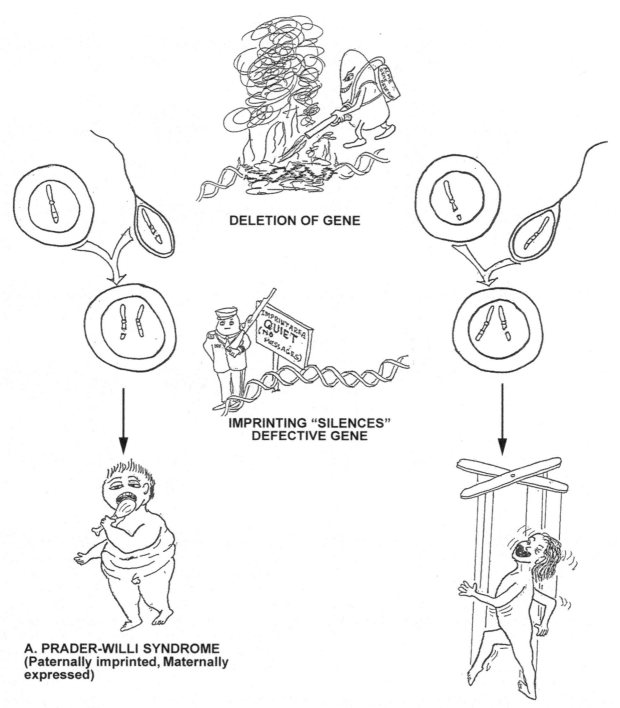

DELETION OF GENE

**IMPRINTING "SILENCES"
DEFECTIVE GENE**

**A. PRADER-WILLI SYNDROME
(Paternally imprinted, Maternally
expressed)**

**B. ANGELMAN ("HAPPY PUPPET") SYNDROME
(Maternally imprinted, Paternally expressed)**

Figure 3-8

nearly 80% of patients with end-stage renal disease in the United States. APKD is characterized by numerous large cysts in both kidneys that destroy the renal parenchyma and result in urinary tract infections, obstruction, renal hypertension, ischemia, and chronic renal failure. Studies have shown that the disorder is caused by **mutations on chromosomes 16p13.3 and 4q21**. APKD can become clinically significant at any age, but it most commonly is detectable between the ages of 30 and 50. In addition to renal cysts, patients

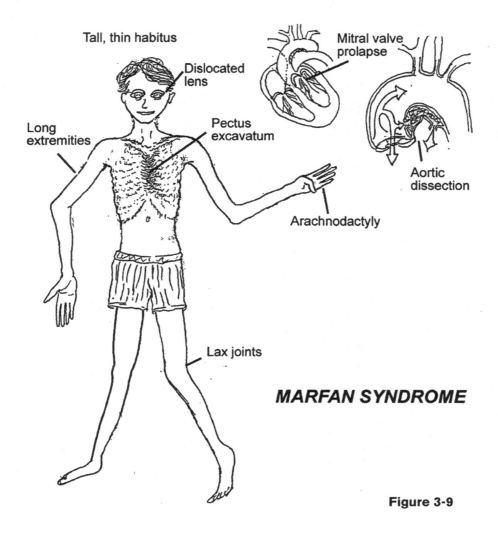

Tall, thin habitus

Dislocated lens

Long extremities

Pectus excavatum

Mitral valve prolapse

Aortic dissection

Arachnodactyly

Lax joints

MARFAN SYNDROME

Figure 3-9

also tend to develop cysts in other organs, diverticular disease of the colon, and Berry aneurysms in the Circle of Willis. This disorder is discussed in far greater detail in the renal pathology chapter.

Familial hypercholesterolemia (FH) is due to a **mutation in the low-density lipoprotein (LDL) receptor**. The mutated receptor reduces cholesterol uptake and metabolism by the liver. Consequently, LDL cholesterol remains in the blood, resulting in hypercholesterolemia, which progresses to early atherosclerosis and cardiovascular disease. Development of multiple xanthomas (lipid-filled yellow lesions on the skin and tendons) often is an early clinical sign of FH. Since this is a dominant disorder, both heterozygotes and homozygotes are affected. However, homozygotes tend to have more significant pathology, manifesting signs of disease as early as birth. Environmental factors (i.e., diet, exercise, and compliance with medication) also play a large role in the disease course and mortality.

Hereditary breast and ovarian cancer occurs when a **mutation is present in one of two different tumor suppressor genes, BRCA1 or BRCA2.** Tumor suppres-

sor genes normally play an important role in preventing malignancies by regulating DNA repair in the cell cycle. Familial cases of breast and ovarian cancer conform to the **"two-hit hypothesis,"** in which *both copies of a BRCA gene (either BRCA1 or BRCA2)* must be damaged to cause malignancy. Usually, one defective BRCA gene is inherited as a dominant mutation, and the other copy becomes inactivated later in life due to environmental causes or sporadic mutation.

In general, patients with hereditary breast and ovarian cancers have similar prognoses, when untreated, to those with sporadic cancers; however, the inherited cancers usually are higher grade and estrogen-receptor negative, making them more challenging to treat. Aside from breast and ovarian malignancies, women with BRCA1 mutations have increased risk for colon cancer, and their first-degree male relatives are more likely to develop prostate cancer. BRCA2 patients also have a greater risk for pancreatic, biliary, prostate, and male breast cancers. Please refer to the breast pathology chapter for further information about these and other forms of breast cancer.

Familial adenomatous polyposis (FAP) is caused by a **mutation in the adenomatous polyposis coli (APC) gene on chromosome 5q21**, another tumor suppressor gene. As in **BRCA** mutations, both copies of the **APC** gene must be inactivated to develop the disease. Generally, one defective copy is inherited, and the other copy becomes damaged after birth. FAP presents early in life (7 to 40 years of age) as hundreds to thousands of adenomatous polyps of the colon that inevitably progress to carcinoma. Accordingly, 93% of FAP patients develop colorectal cancer by the age of 50. Due to the aggressive nature of this disease, prophylactic removal of the entire colon is recommended, often as early as the second decade of life. APC gene mutations also can give rise to other disorders, such as **Gardner syndrome** (a combination of colon polyps, osteomas, and soft tissue tumors) and **Turcot syndrome** (colon polyps associated with tumors of the central nervous system).

Neurofibromatosis type 1 (NF-1, von Recklinghausen's disease) is manifested as multiple neurofibromas throughout the body, café au lait spots (light brown flat lesions) on the skin, and Lisch nodules (pigmented hamartomas) in the iris. Other associated abnormalities include skeletal disorders (especially scoliosis and bone cysts) and increased risk for specific tumors, such as Wilms' tumor, pheochromocytoma, rhabdomyosarcoma, meningioma, and optic glioma. **The neurofibromatosis type 1 gene has been mapped to chromosome 17q11.2. To remember that neurofibromatosis type 1 is due to a mutation on chromosome 17, note that there are 17 letters in "von Recklinghausen."**

Neurofibromatosis type 2 (NF-2), on the other hand, is due to a **mutation on chromosome 22q12.** This disorder commonly presents as bilateral acoustic schwannomas, multiple meningiomas, and café au lait spots. Ependymomas of the spinal cord also are common in these patients. **Notice that NF-2 is due to a mutation on chromosome 22. Remember "2 on 22" to help recall this disorder.**

Tuberous sclerosis is caused by a **mutation in the *TSC2* gene on chromosome 16p13.3** and is characterized by development of hamartomas and other benign tuberous lesions in the cerebral cortex. Other associated abnormalities include cardiac rhabdomyomas, angiomyolipomas, and cysts in multiple organs. Clinically, these patients present with seizures, mental retardation, and skin lesions. Most commonly, the skin lesions consist of ashen-leaf spots (hypopigmented areas), shagreen patches (leathery thickening), and adenoma sebaceum (perivascular fibromas that look like red spots around the nose). This disorder also may be caused by a mutation in the *TSC1* gene on chromosome 9q34, but much less frequently.

Individuals with **Von Hippel-Lindau (VHL) disease** develop cavernous hemangiomas of the cerebellum, brainstem, and/or retina, along with adenomas and cysts in multiple organs. The genetic cause of this disease has been **localized to the short arm of chromosome 3 (3p25-26)**, where a mutation deactivates a tumor suppressor gene. These patients also have a very elevated risk for sporadic renal cell carcinoma.

Osler-Weber-Rendu syndrome (hereditary hemorrhagic telangiectasia) results from an extremely rare mutation that compromises the normal growth of human vascular endothelial cells, causing multiple arteriovenous malformations (AVMs), aneurysms, and telangiectasias on the skin and mucous membranes. Often, these vascular lesions will hemorrhage, resulting in severe epistaxis (nosebleeds), GI bleeds, and hematuria (bloody urine). **Two genetic loci have been implicated in this disorder: chromosome 9q33-34 and chromosome 12q.** Osler-Weber-Rendu syndrome is seen more frequently in certain isolated populations, especially Mormon families in Utah.

Acute intermittent porphyria (AIP) is due to a defect in one of the enzymes needed to synthesize heme—porphobilinogen deaminase. Patients with AIP experience sudden attacks of abdominal pain, weakness, seizures, neurologic and autonomic dysfunction, and/or psychiatric disturbances. Episodes often are idiopathic, but they may be precipitated by infections, fasting, or drugs (especially sulfonamides or barbiturates). **The genetic defect in AIP is found on chromosome 11q24.1-24.2.** Other autosomal dominant disorders involving the hematopoietic system (i.e., von Willebrand disease and hereditary spherocytosis) are discussed in the hematopathology chapter.

Autosomal Recessive Disorders

Cystic fibrosis (CF, mucoviscidosis) is a metabolic disorder caused by a mutation in a transmembrane chloride channel, leading to malfunction of the exocrine glands, abnormal viscosity of mucous, and elevated concentrations of sodium chloride in sweat and tears. In fact, to diagnose CF, a **sweat chloride test** is the current preferred method. **The mutation in CF has been mapped to the long arm of chromosome 7 (7q31.2)**, affecting the cystic fibrosis transmembrane conductance regulator (**CFTR**) gene. The severe metabolic defect in CF is manifested by tissue-specific problems, including

1. **Chronic pulmonary disease:** Ranging from rhinitis and asthma to chronic bronchitis, bronchiectasis, and cor pulmonale (right-sided heart failure due to pulmonary dysfunction), the devastating pulmonary complications of CF are due to retention of thick mucous in the respiratory system. Secondary infections also are typical, usually due to *Pseudomonas aeruginosa*, *Staphylococcus aureus*, and *Hemophilus influenzae* species.

2. **Male infertility: Congenital bilateral absence of the vas deferens and/or azoospermia** (lack of sperm cells) is present in nearly 95% of male CF patients who survive into adulthood. In very mild cases of CF, male infertility may be the only clinical symptom.
3. **Meconium ileus:** Often the first symptom of CF, meconium ileus is a small bowel obstruction in the newborn caused by thick, viscous fecal material.
4. **Pancreatic insufficiency:** Accumulations of mucous in the exocrine pancreas can plug ductal structures and result in atrophy, fibrosis, and enzymatic deficiency. The decline in pancreatic enzymes leads to malabsorption and steatorrhea (fatty stool). Recurrent pancreatitis also is common in CF patients.
5. **Hepatic cirrhosis:** Following the same pathophysiologic model as in the pancreas, mucinous secretions obstruct the bile canaliculi, causing ductular proliferation, portal inflammation, and nodular cirrhosis of the liver.

Xeroderma pigmentosum (XP) results from a defect in DNA repair that causes abnormal sensitivity to UV irradiation. Patients with XP are unable to excise UV-damaged nucleotides from their DNA, resulting in accumulations of mutations in cells. Multiple genes are involved in DNA excision repair, and a mutation in any one of them can cause XP. Usually clinically detectable between 1 and 2 years of age, XP first presents with easy sunburning, photosensitivity, and freckling. Continued UV damage causes premature wrinkling, premalignant lesions, and malignant neoplasms. Approximately 45% of XP patients develop basal cell and/or squamous cell carcinomas, while 5% develop melanomas. Ocular defects, such as conjunctivitis, photophobia, blepharitis (chronic inflammation of the eyelids), ectropion (sagging of the lower eyelid and lashes), and ocular cancer, also are prevalent among patients with this disorder.

Fig. 3-10. Congenital adrenal hyperplasia (CAH). This is a group of inherited metabolic disorders, each distinguished by a deficiency or lack of a specific enzyme involved in steroidogenesis (the synthesis of cortical steroids). In affected individuals, the disease begins early in gestation, manifesting at birth. CAH presents as adrenal hyperplasia, virilization (ambiguous or male external genitalia in a newborn female), and salt wasting (mild to severe loss of body sodium due to impaired glucocorticoid secretion). Deficiency in 21-hydroxylase (which normally converts progesterone to 11-deoxycortisone) accounts for over 90% of CAH cases and is due to a mutation in the CYP21 gene on the short arm of chromosome 6. When 21-hydroxylase is not present, steroid synthesis is shunted into alternate pathways, leading to elevated production of androgens (testosterone, etc.), which

accounts for virilization of female patients and abnormal development in males. Indeed, a 21-hydroxylase deficiency should be suspected immediately in any newborn with ambiguous genitalia. The salt-wasting syndrome presents shortly after birth as hypotension and unbalanced electrolytes, which could lead to cardiovascular collapse if not treated. Deficiencies in 11-hydroxylase and/or 17-hydroxylase cause other forms of CAH with similar signs and symptoms.

The remaining autosomal recessive disorders presented in this chapter will be listed in table form for simplicity's sake. Please refer to **Table 3.1.**

X-linked Recessive Disorders

Duchenne muscular dystrophy (DMD) is an X-linked recessive disorder that presents in early childhood (usually age 6 or younger) as progressive muscle weakness and degeneration. This myopathy usually affects hip girdle and neck muscles first, eventually advancing to affect the trunk and distal limbs. Pseudohypertrophy of the calf muscles (replacement by fat and connective tissue) and the Gowers' sign (difficulty rising from the floor due to hip girdle instability) usually are present by age 5.

Fig. 3-11. Gowers' sign in Duchenne muscular dystrophy. The child must "climb" his own limbs in order to stand up.

By preteen years, most patients with DMD are confined to a wheelchair. Death often occurs by age 18, most frequently due to pneumonia and respiratory failure. **DMD is due to mutations within the gene encoding dystrophin**, a stabilizing intracellular protein present in all types of muscle and some neurons.

Other important X-linked recessive disorders are listed in **Table 3.2.**

Trinucleotide Repeat Disorders

While they may vary in inheritance pattern, these unique disorders deserve special mention due to their unusual insertion mutations.

Huntington disease (HD) is an autosomal dominant disorder characterized by degeneration of the caudate, putamen, and cerebral cortex, resulting in movement disorders (chorea, dystonia, etc.), personality changes, and severe dementia. In this case, the genetic defect is an expansion of **CAG** repeats within the *HD* gene on **chromosome 4p**. This gene encodes **huntington**, a protein of unknown function. As mentioned earlier, every person has a certain number of trinucleotide repeats in his or her DNA that is considered "normal." Unaffected

CONGENITAL ADRENAL HYPERPLASIA

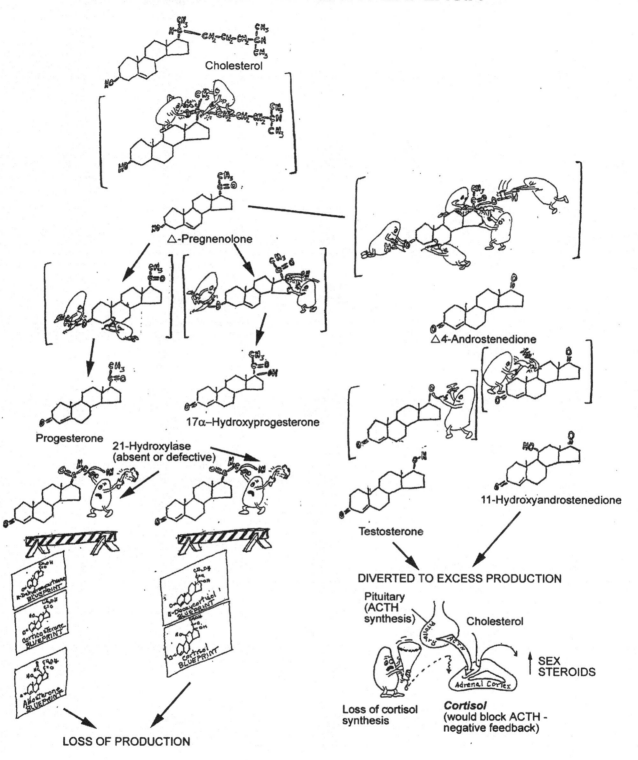

Figure 3-10

Table 3-1. Autosomal Recessive Disorders

Disease	Defect	Accumulated substance	Signs/symptoms	Notes
Phenylketonuria	Phenylalanine hydroxylase deficiency	Phenylalanine and its degradation products in urine and serum	Progressive cerebral demyelization, seizures, hyperactivity, blonde/blue eyed, mousy body odor	Phenylalanine is neurotoxic in these patients, and the disease may be managed with a phenylalanine-free diet.
Homocystinuria	Cystathionine beta synthase deficiency	Homocysteine in urine	Pectus excavatum, near-sightedness, ectopia lentis, tall/thin, arachnodactyly, hypercoagulability, pes cavus (arched feet)	Do not confuse with the clinically similar Marfans syndrome. Patients may respond to supplementary vitamin B6 and low methionine diet
Galactosemia	Galactose-1-phosphate uridyl transferase deficiency	Galactose-1-phosphate in multiple tissues	Failure to thrive, mental retardation, cirrhosis, liver failure, cataracts	This disorder may be managed by removal of galactose from the diet.
Wilson's disease (hepatolenticular degeneration)	ATP7B gene mutation on chromosome 13	Copper in liver and brain	Hepatitis, psychiatric problems, neurological degeneration	Kayser-Fleischer rings in the iris may be seen upon slit lamp evaluation
Hereditary hemochromatosis	HFE gene mutation on chromosome 6	Iron in multiple organs	Cirrhosis, diabetes, cardiomegaly, arthritis, skin pigmentation	This disease is managed by regular phlebotomy treatments.
Alkaptonuria	Homogentisic oxidase deficiency	Homogentisic acid in tissue and urine	Ochronosis (dark pigmentation of tissue and cartilage), severe arthritis	
Tay-Sach's disease (amaurotic familial idiocy)	Hexosamidase A deficiency	GM2 ganglioside in neurons	CNS degeneration, blindness, cherry red spots in the macula, death before age 4	Often seen in Ashkenazi Jews.
Gaucher disease	Glucocerbrosidase deficiency	Glucocerebroside in phagocytic cells	Hepatosplenomegaly, bony erosion, anemia in type 1, CNS defects and death in type 2	Gaucher cells are "wrinkled paper" histiocytes.
Niemann-Pick disease	Sphingomyelinase deficiency	Sphingomyelin	Hepatosplenomegaly, fever, anemia, neurologic degeneration, and death by age 3. May also see cherry red spot on macula.	"Foamy" histiocytes containing sphingomyelin
Hurler's syndrome	Alpha-L-iduronidase deficiency	Heparan sulfate, dermatan sulfate in heart, liver, brain	Gargoyle facies, dwarfism, progressive deterioration and mental retardation, corneal clouding, death by age 10	
Von Gierke's disease (hepatorenal glycogenosis)	Glucose-6-phosphatase deficiency	Glycogen in liver and kidney	Hepatomegaly, severe hypoglycemia	
Pompe's disease	Alpha-1, 4-glucosidasedeficiency	Glycogen in heart, liver, skeletal muscles	Splenomegaly, cardiomegaly, hypotonia, cardio respiratory failure by age 3	
Cori's disease	Amylo-1, 6-glucosidase (debranching enzyme) deficiency	Glycogen in heart, liver, skeletal muscles	Hepatomegaly, hypoglycemia, stunted growth	
McArdle's disease	Muscle phosphorylase deficiency	Glycogen	Muscle weakness, severe cramping	

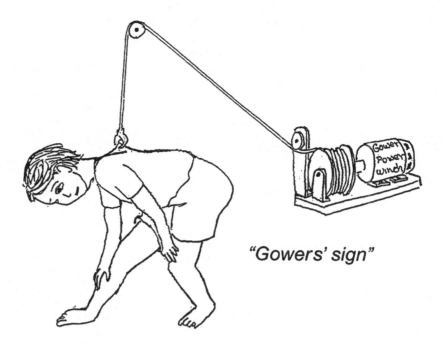

"Gowers' sign"

Figure 3-11

people have approximately 18 or 19 CAG repeats in their *HD* gene, while HD patients have 40 or more repeats (the average is 46). HD typically has an adult onset, with half of affected individuals showing symptoms by the age of 40. Early onset disease may occur in childhood or adolescence, but only in some families where the gene is paternally transmitted. This phenomenon, called **"anticipation,"** causes HD to develop earlier and earlier in subsequent generations due to the instability of the CAG repeat.

Friedreich ataxia is an autosomal recessive spinocerebellar ataxia characterized by uncoordinated movements, diminished tendon reflexes, loss of position and vibratory sense, scoliosis, foot deformities (especially pes cavus), and speech problems. This disorder is due to an expansion of **AAG** repeats within **frataxin**, a mitochondrial protein on **chromosome 9q13** that aids in iron metabolism. While normal individuals have a repeat length ranging from 7 to 34 copies, Friedreich ataxia patients have a repeat expansion between 100 and 1200 copies.

Myotonic dystrophy, another autosomal recessive disorder, manifests as myotonia (inability to relax the muscles), hypogonadism, brainwave abnormalities, cataracts, and balding. This disorder has a wide range of phenotypes, and severe cases may be a cause of mental retardation. In myotonic dystrophy, an expanded repeat of **CTG** is present in the *DMPK* gene on **chromosome 19**. Unaffected people have 5 to 30 triplets in this region, but individuals with the disease may have more than 2000 copies.

Fragile-X syndrome is the most common **heritable form** of mental retardation, second only to Down syndrome among **all genetic causes** of mental retardation. As the name implies, fragile X syndrome has an *X-linked* inheritance pattern. In male patients with this defect, a "fragile site" on the **X chromosome (Xq27.3)** does not condense properly during mitosis, causing a mutation in the *FMR-1* gene. Eventually, it was discovered that this mutation is due to an expansion of 200 to 4000 **CGG repeats** within the X chromosome (carrier females have 55 to 200 repeats; the normal population has even fewer). When the patient's karyotype is examined, the X chromosome appears "broken" at this point. Males with fragile-X syndrome also express characteristic physical findings, including a long face with a large jaw, large ears, and macro-orchidism (large testicles).

DIAGNOSIS OF GENETIC DISORDERS
Indications for Chromosomal Studies

1. **Developmental problems:** Failure to thrive, delayed growth, abnormal facial features, mental retardation, ambiguous genitalia, and/or other "birth defects" are definite indications for gene studies, unless a different nonchromosomal diagnosis already is confirmed.
2. **Family history:** Any suspected or confirmed chromosomal abnormality in a first-degree blood relative is a sign that chromosomal analysis could be useful.
3. **Fertility problems, multiple miscarriages, stillbirth, or neonatal death:** Problems in any one of these areas may indicate a need for gene studies. The incidence of chromosomal abnormalities in stillborn babies and neonatal deaths is nearly 10% each. At least 6% of miscarriages also are due to genetic defects. In these instances, chromosomal studies are essential for proper genetic counseling.

Table 3-2. X-linked Recessive Disorders

Disease	Defect	Accumulated substance	Signs/symptoms	Notes
Hunter's disease	L-iduronosulfate sulfatase deficiency	Heparan sulfate, dermatan sulfate in multiple tissues	Hepatosplenomegaly, micrognathia, retinal degeneration, mental retardation, joint difficulties, cardiomyopathy	Similar to but less severe than Hurler's syndrome
Fabry's disease (a.k.a. angiokeratoma corporis diffusum universale)	Alpha-galactosidase A	Ceramide trihexoside	Angiokeratomas (dilation of superficial dermal vessels), extremity pain, cardiovascular and CNS involvement, early death due to renal failure	
Lesch-Nyhan syndrome	Hypoxanthine-guanine phosphoribosyltransferase (HGPRT) deficiency	Uric acid in multiple tissues, especially joints, kidney, bladder, ureter	Early hypotonia and developmental delay, mental retardation, choreoathetosis, gout, orange crystals present in diaper, self-injurious behavior	

THE KARYOTYPE SPREAD

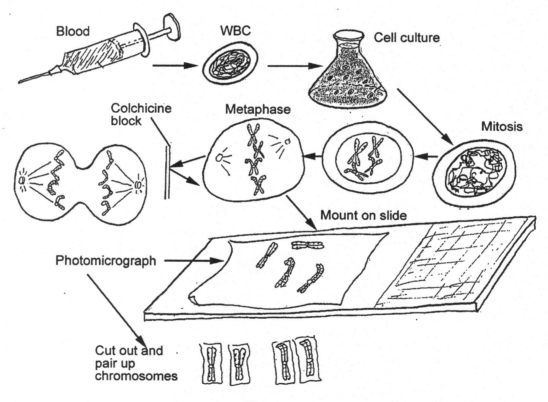

Figure 3-12

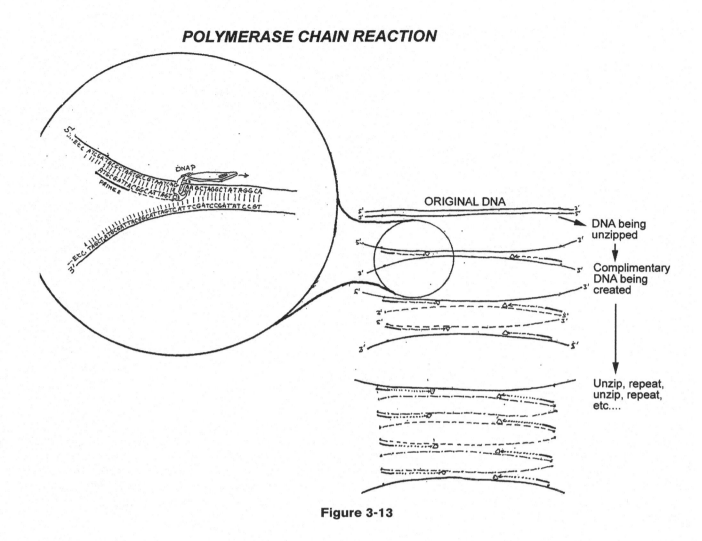

Figure 3-13

4. **Cancer**: Cancer is due to some sort of genetic anomaly in nearly all cases. Chromosomal analysis of the cancerous tissue may aid in diagnosis, prognosis, and treatment.
5. **Advanced maternal age in pregnancy**: After the age of 35, any pregnancy is considered "high risk." Genetic counseling and fetal chromosome analysis are considered standard of care in these situations.

Diagnostic Methods

Fig. 3-12. Karyotype analysis. Human chromosomes are best analyzed during metaphase, when the chromosome pairs are condensed and separated. To prepare a chromosome spread, a blood sample is obtained from the patient and mixed with heparin (an anticoagulant) to prevent clotting. The white blood cells are separated (remember that mature red blood cells do not have a nucleus...no nucleus means no DNA!) and grown in culture medium. Later, the dividing cells are arrested in metaphase with a mitotic spindle inhibitor, collected,

and lysed to release the chromosomes. The chromosomes then are fixed, spread on slides, and stained for viewing. To make a karyotype, a photomicrograph is taken of the chromosome spread, and the chromosomes are cut out and arranged in pairs.

Fig. 3-13. Polymerase Chain Reaction (PCR). PCR allows a short stretch of DNA (called the "target sequence") to be amplified more than a million-fold and sequenced or tested. An alternative to cloning, PCR is both rapid and exquisitely sensitive, allowing billions of specific gene copies to be made in less than a day. The steps involved in PCR are quite complex and are not relevant to this discussion. PCR is an extraordinary tool that has solved both the problems of quantity and quality of genetic material available for testing.

Fig. 3-14. Fluorescence In Situ Hybridization (FISH). Commonly used in both gene mapping and chromosome analysis, FISH uses a gene probe to locate specific

FLUORESCENCE IN SITU HYBRIDIZATION (FISH)

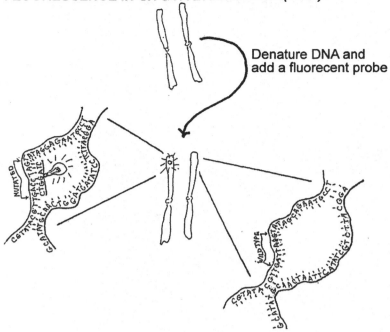

Figure 3-14

defects within a patient's chromosomes. The "probe" used in this case is a short nucleotide sequence complementary to the mutation in question. The patient's DNA is denatured and separated into single strands. Subsequently, the probe should bind the mutation sequence if it is present. Finally, a chromosome spread is prepared in order to view the results. The gene probe is labeled with a fluorescent dye, so if the test is positive, the mutated chromosome segment will glow. FISH has been invaluable in diagnosing countless genetic disorders. The only downside to this procedure is that a *specific* mutation must be suspected. FISH is not useful in diagnosing unknown genetic diseases.

4

Cardiovascular Pathology

OVERVIEW

Heart disease and vascular disorders are the leading causes of morbidity and mortality in industrialized nations. Cardiovascular disease leads to serious and catastrophic physiological changes that either cause the heart to fail as an effective pump or damage the ability of vasculature to adequately circulate blood throughout the body. Heart disease alone is responsible for nearly 40% of all adult deaths in the United States, which is more that twice the number of all cancers combined. Due to the high prevalence of cardiovascular disease, it is essential to have a strong comprehension of the various disease processes in this aspect of pathology.

ANATOMY OF NORMAL VASCULATURE

Arteries are categorized into subgroups depending on their size and functional ability to withstand pressure.

Fig. 4-1. Kinds of blood vessels. Large elastic arteries have thick walls that are able to withstand higher degrees of pressure and expand during systole. Medium sized muscular arteries (distributing arteries) distribute blood from large elastic arteries to various organs. Small arteries (arterioles) are less than two millimeters in diameter and carry oxygenated blood predominantly within tissues and into capillary beds. Capillaries are seven to eight micrometers in diameter, which is approximately the size of a red blood cell. Capillaries merge into venules.

Due to their relatively small lumen, arterioles are the main point of blood flow resistance, which decreases both the velocity of blood and the pressure exerted upon the arteriolar wall. This results in a change from a pulsatile to a steady blood flow leading into the capillary beds. Capillary beds are the site of substance exchange across a semi-permeable membrane. Venules have a lower pressure than capillaries and interstitial tissue, allowing fluid to flow freely into the venules. Venules then return blood to veins that have a relatively large caliber lumen and thin wall, which allows for a larger capacity and accounts for nearly two thirds of the total systemic blood volume. The force of gravity is overcome by valves within veins that prevent reversed flow of blood returning to the heart.

HISTOLOGY OF NORMAL ARTERIES

Arterial walls are composed of three layers: the **intima**, **media** and **adventitia**, in order from internal to external. The intima is separated from the media by the **internal elastic lamina**, and the media is separated from the adventitia by the **external elastic lamina**. The cell layer of the intima that is adjacent to the lumen, known as the endothelium. Small vessels located in the adventitia known as the vasa vasorum nourish the walls of blood vessels.

HISTOLOGY OF THE NORMAL HEART

The heart is composed of three layers: the **endocardium**, **myocardium**, and **epicardium**, in order from internal to external. The myocardium is comprised of specialized striated muscle cells known as **cardiac myocytes**. The normal heart weighs approximately 250 – 300 grams in females and 300 - 350 grams in males. The normal free wall of the right and left ventricle measures 0.3 to 0.5 centimeters (right) and 1.3 to 1.5 centimeters (left) in thickness. The heart is comprised of four chambers: the right atrium and ventricle and the left atrium and ventricle. It also houses four valves: the tricuspid valve, the pulmonary valve, the mitral (bicuspid) valve, and the aortic valve.

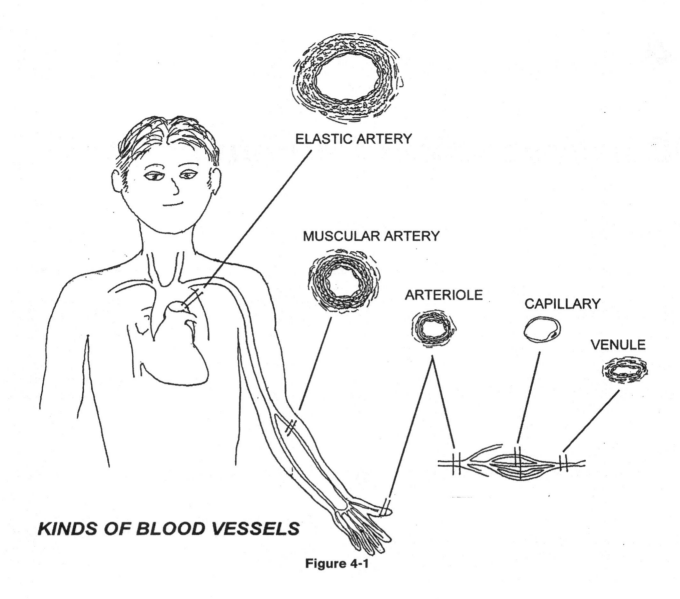

ELASTIC ARTERY

MUSCULAR ARTERY

ARTERIOLE

CAPILLARY

VENULE

KINDS OF BLOOD VESSELS

Figure 4-1

PATHOLOGY OF THE VASCULAR SYSTEM
Hypertension

Hypertension is an abnormally elevated blood pressure greater than 140 mm Hg systolic or 90 mm Hg diastolic. Hypertension predisposes to other significant pathology such as **coronary heart disease, congestive heart failure (CHF), left ventricular hypertrophy, renal failure (nephrosclerosis), cerebrovascular accidents (CVA), aortic dissection, and retinal changes.**

Essential Hypertension

Essential hypertension is the most common cause (nearly 90% of cases) of hypertension and is of unknown etiology. There are several factors that influence the development of essential hypertension, such as genetics, increasing age, obesity, physical inactivity, diabetes, stress, smoking, and significant intake of dietary sodium. All of these factors are related by their tendency to increase either cardiac output or total peripheral resistance. There is often also a significant family history in patients with essential hypertension, which is more common and severe in patients of African decent.

Fig. 4-2. Risk factors for essential hypertension.

Secondary Hypertension

Secondary hypertension is an elevated blood pressure due to a known cause such as renal disease, endocrine disorders, e.g., primary aldosteronism (Conn's syndrome), acromegaly, Cushing's syndrome, pheochromocytoma or hyperthyroidism, congenital anomalies (e.g., coarctation of the aorta), central nervous system disorders (e.g., brain tumors), drugs (e.g., amphetamines and steroids), or toxemia of pregnancy.

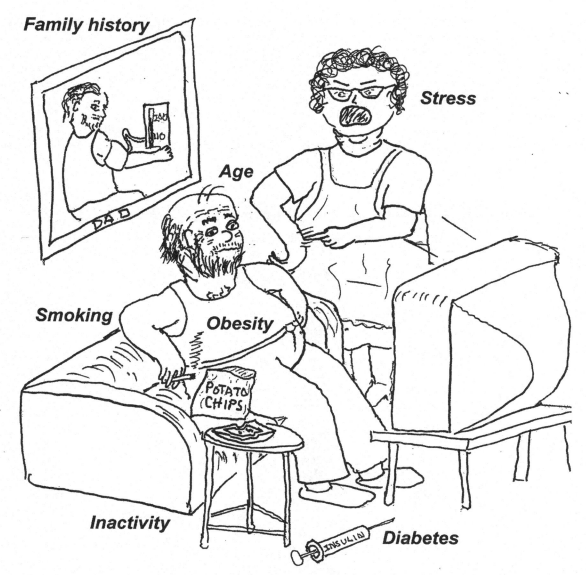

RISK FACTORS FOR ESSENTIAL HYPERTENSION
Figure 4-2

Renal disease is the most common cause of secondary hypertension and is due to either a disorder of the renal parenchyma or unilateral renal artery stenosis. The renal artery can become stenotic as a result of atherosclerotic disease or fibromuscular dysplasia, causing atrophy of the kidney. Hypertension ensues due to the subsequent activation of the renin-angiotension system via the release of renin from the juxtaglomerular (JG) complex in the kidney. Angiotensin II acts as a vasoconstrictor and promotes the release of aldosterone, which enhances sodium and water retention.

Malignant Hypertension

Malignant hypertension is an accelerated and severe complication of essential or secondary hypertension. It is typically characterized by a diastolic blood pressure of greater than 120 mm Hg. Malignant hypertension occurs in only approximately 5% of all patients with hypertension and is more common in young men of African heritage. Clinically, patients may present with microangiopathic hemolytic anemia, retinal hemorrhages, papilledema and left ventricular hypertrophy/failure. **Malignant nephrosclerosis** may also occur and is characterized by a "flea-bitten" appearance of the cortical surface of the kidney, due to the rupture of arterioles and glomeruli.

Atherosclerosis

Atherosclerosis is the formation of **fibrinous plaques** (atheromas), within the intima layer of large elastic arteries and medium muscular arteries, resulting in stenosis. Atherosclerosis is the most common cause of morbidity and mortality due to vascular disease. Subsequently, cardiac ischemia is the most common cause of death in industrialized nations. The most frequent sites for plaque formation are the abdominal aorta, the coronary arteries, cerebral arteries (Circle of Willis), large arteries of the lower extremities, mesenteric arteries, renal arteries, and carotid arteries. **Risk factors** for the development of atherosclerosis include: **hypertension, hyperlipidemia, increased low density lipoprotein (LDL) and/or decreased high density lipoprotein (HDL), smoking, increased age, family history, and diabetes mellitus.** Atherosclerosis also has a higher prevalence in men and postmenopausal women.

The formation of a plaque can be due to multiple mechanisms such as the infiltration of lipid and protein into the intima, aggravation of the intimal surface by

PATHOGENESIS OF ATHEROSCLEROSIS

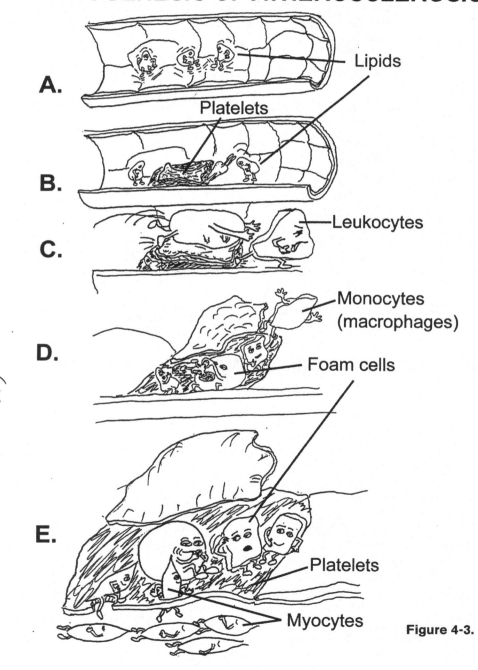

A.
— Lipids

Platelets

B.

C.
— Leukocytes

D.
— Monocytes (macrophages)

— Foam cells

E.

— Platelets

— Myocytes

Figure 4-3.

mural thrombi, independent smooth muscle migration and proliferation within the intima, or direct injury to the endothelium. Injury to the endothelium may be due to mechanical injury, hypercholesterolemia, immune disorders, toxins or infectious agents such as viruses. Endothelial injury in most patients with hyperlipidemia is due to increased levels of circulating lipid.

Fig. 4-3. The pathogenesis of atherosclerosis.
A. Injury to the vascular endothelium by lipids
B. Lipids and platelets adhere to the damaged endothelial surface in aggregates and gain access to the intima (subepithelium).
C. Leukocytes and platelets start to release platelet-derived growth factors and other mitogens, which will cause smooth muscle cells to migrate into the intima from the media and proliferate throughout the atherosclerotic process.
D. Occupation of the intima by macrophages (monocytes) and lipids leads to phagocytosis of lipids by the macrophages, which become "foam cells."
E. Fatty streak with foam cells, platelets, and myocytes (smooth muscle cells) starts to grow up by proliferation of the smooth muscle cells, as well as increased numbers of foam cells and platelets, forming an atherosclerotic plaque. (*Slide 4.1*)

As the lesion develops into an atheroma, a central core is formed. The central core can become necrotic and is typically comprised of foam cells, cholesterol, and perhaps calcium. A fibrous cap develops over the central core with components such as fibrin, smooth muscle, foam cells, extracellular matrix material, and various proteins. Plaques may become complicated by calcification, hemorrhage, and ulceration.

Atherosclerosis often results in many catastrophic sequelae, such as ischemic heart disease and myocardial infarction, stroke, aneurysms, ischemic bowl disease, peripheral vascular disease, and renal ischemia. Embolization and thrombosis involving the fibrinous cap of the atheroma may occur as well.

Arteriolosclerosis

Arteriolosclerosis is thickening of the vascular walls of small arteries and arterioles, resulting in stenosis. Arteriolosclerosis is commonly a result of chronic hypertension or diabetes mellitus. It occurs frequently in the renal arterioles. Arteriolosclerosis is divided into two subtypes: hyaline arteriosclerosis and hyperplastic arteriolosclerosis. **Hyaline arteriolosclerosis** results from hyaline deposition in arteriolar walls and may cause benign nephrosclerosis due to subsequent hypertension. **Hyperplastic arteriolosclerosis** is a concentric and laminated thickening of arteriolar walls, which gives an "**onion skin**" appearance of the small artery or arteriole when cut on cross section.

In the presence of malignant hypertension, both **necrotizing arteriolitis** and **malignant nephrosclerosis** are possible complications. Necrotizing arteriolitis involves deposits of fibrin and acute necrosis of the vessel walls (fibrinoid necrosis), which may lead to a more advanced stage, malignant nephrosclerosis.

Necrotizing arteriolitis involves deposits of fibrin and acute necrosis of the vessel walls. Malignant nephrosclerosis is associated with fibrinoid necrosis of the renal arterioles.

Varicose Veins

Varicose veins are prominent and tortuous superficial veins of the lower extremities. Superficial veins of the lower extremities often become dilated due to an increase in venous pressure that can result from obesity, pregnancy, or thrombophlebitis. Persons who tend to stand for long periods of time can be predisposed to this condition. Varicose veins are often a cosmetic problem, but they can be painful and cause ulceration of the overlying skin. Otherwise, they are benign and can be removed by sclerotherapy or surgery. Varicose veins have a tendency to thrombose. However, they **do not** give rise to pulmonary embolisms.

Deep Venous Thrombosis

Deep venous thrombosis is an occlusion of the venous system most commonly in the lower extremities. **Virchow's Triad** predisposes this condition, which includes: **blood stasis, hypercoagulability, and endothelial damage.** Blood stasis is the most common cause of thrombosis. **Approximately 95% of all pulmonary embolisms derive from deep leg vein thrombosis**; subsequently, the released emboli may travel to the lungs and cause chest pain, dyspnea, tachycardia, and possibly death. The risk of thrombosis of the deep leg veins also increases with pregnancy, cardiac failure, and prolonged bed rest. Patients with hypercoagulable states such as those with the **Factor V Leiden** gene mutation must also take special precautions to prevent thrombosis of deep veins and subsequent pulmonary embolism by not sitting for long periods of time and avoiding oral contraceptives, which have the potential to increase coagulability.

When thrombosis is accompanied by inflammation, this is termed **thrombophlebitis**.

Embolism

Emboli are circulating aggregate substances that occlude a vessel and may have many different origins such as: **thrombus, fat, air, bacterial vegetation, tumor, and amniotic fluid.** Fat emboli are encountered after long bone fractures and as a complication of liposuction. Emboli associated with amniotic fluid may cause disseminated intravascular coagulation (DIC) in the postpartum period.

Aneurysms

An aneurysm is a circumscribed, abnormal dilation of an artery, vein or heart chamber due to an acquired or congenital weakness in the wall of the vasculature or heart. Aneurysms may involve adjacent structures or rupture, resulting in hemorrhage.

Dissecting Aneurysm

A dissecting aneurysm is a longitudinal interluminal tear of vasculature or the heart. A dissecting aneurysm frequently occurs in the thoracic aorta. It **commonly results from cystic medial necrosis**, which destroys elastic and muscular tissue and essentially forms an additional lumen to which the blood gains access from the tear. If undiagnosed, the aneurysm may rupture into the pericardial sac, causing hemopericardium (cardiac tamponade) and possibly death. Patients present with severe chest pain and usually have a history of hypertension. **There is also an increased incidence of dissecting aortic aneurysms in patients with Marfan's syndrome.**

Atherosclerotic Aneurysm

An atherosclerotic aneurysm is an abnormal dilation of vasculature due to atherosclerotic disease, commonly in the abdominal aorta.

Arteriovenous Aneurysm (Fistula)

An arteriovenous aneurysm is an abnormal communication between an artery and a vein that results in ischemic changes and hypervolemia from the shunting of blood from the arterial to venous circulation. The shunting of blood causes the communicating vein to dilate from the elevation in venous pressure. The subsequent increase in blood return to the heart can cause high output cardiac failure if the fistula is not surgically repaired.

Syphilitic (Luetic) Aneurysm
and Syphilitic Heart Disease

Tertiary syphilis causes obliterative endarteritis of the vaso vasorum in the adventitia of arteries and medial necrosis of the aortic root, which results in subsequent dilation of the aorta and aortic valve insufficiency. An aneurysm of the ascending aorta or aortic arch may ensue. Grossly, the thoracic aorta develops a "tree-bark" appearance. Since primary syphilis is easily treated with a single dose of penicillin, this condition is rarely encountered clinically.

Berry Aneurysm

Berry aneurysms are small dilations of the cerebrovasculature due to a weakness in the media of arteries. Berry aneurysms are often found at the bifurcations of the Circle of Willis; **40% occur at the branch point of the anterior cerebral artery**. A rupture of a Berry aneurysm results in hemorrhage into the subarachnoid space, causing blood to mix with the cerebral spinal fluid. Most Berry aneurysm ruptures are fatal. They have a **higher incidence in patients with adult polycystic kidney disease and connective tissue disorders, such as Marfan's and Ehlers-Danlos syndrome.**

Benign Tumors of Blood Vessels

Hemangiomas (Angiomas)

Hemangiomas are benign proliferations of blood vessels that resemble a mass. They occur anywhere in the body, typically the skin and subcutaneous tissues. A hemangioma is usually a congenital anomaly, and it is the most common tumor of infancy.

Capillary hemangiomas (*Slide 4.2***)** are capillary structures that proliferate and become closely packed and intertwined. Capillary hemangiomas frequently occur in the skin and subcutaneous tissues, as well as lips, liver, spleen, and kidneys.

Cavernous hemangiomas (*Slide 4.3***)** are large vascular spaces that are filled with blood, typically in the skin, as well as the liver, pancreas, spleen, and brain. Cavernous hemangiomas **have a higher incidence in patients with Von Hippel-Lindau disease.**

Fig. 4-4. Cavernous hemangioma. These contain large vascular spaces.

Pyogenic granulomas are polypoid capillary hemangiomas that grow rapidly into red nodules attached by a stalk to the skin, gingival, or oral mucosal surface. Pyogenic granulomas often bleed easily and tend to ulcerate as well.

Hemangioblastoma

Hemangioblastomas are slow growing, benign cerebellar tumors composed of endothelial and stromal cells Together these form capillaries. Hemangioblastomas typically affect middle-aged individuals and have an **increased incidence in patients with Von Hippel-Lindau disease.** They are also known as angioblastomas or Lindau tumors.

Vascular Ectasias

Vascular ectasias are a category of prominent vascular lesions caused by a local dilation of preexisting vessels, usually on the skin or mucus membranes.

Nevus Flammeus is the most common form of ectasia and is characterized by a flat, light pink to dark purple "salmon patch" birthmark that commonly occurs on the head or neck and ultimately fades and regresses. Nevus Flammeus may also present as a "port-wine stain" birthmark, which will grow as the child ages. A

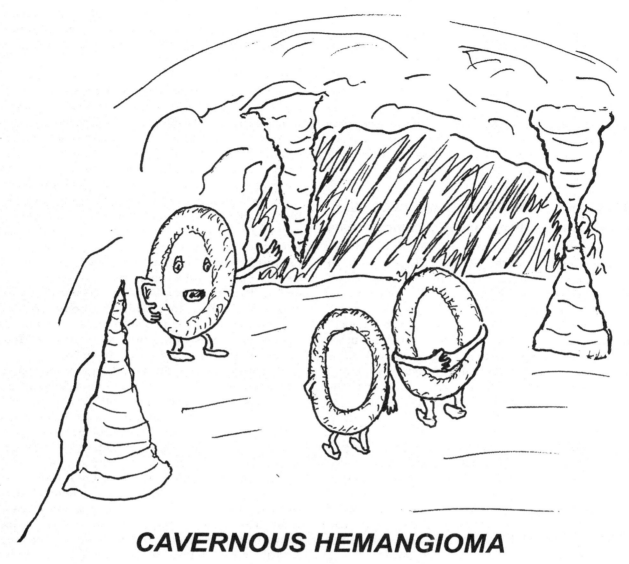

CAVERNOUS HEMANGIOMA

Figure 4-4.

"port-wine stain" may also be indicative of **Sturge-Weber syndrome** if the ectasia follows the distribution of the trigeminal nerve. Sturge-Weber syndrome is associated with mental retardation, seizures, hemiplegia and radio-opacities of the skull.

Spider angiomas are telangiectatic (dilated) arterioles in the skin with radiating capillary branches that grossly resemble the appearance of a spider. Spider angiomas are often a sign of hyperestrogenemia, as in liver disease or pregnancy (resolving after delivery).

Hereditary hemorrhagic telangiectasia (Osler-Weber-Rendu Syndrome) is an autosomal dominant disorder that causes the dilation of capillaries and venules, which become convoluted in a localized area and can cause epitaxis and/or gastrointestinal bleeding.

Glomangioma (Glomus Tumor)

Glomangiomas (*Slide 4.4*) are benign neoplasms composed of **glomus cells.**. Glomus cells are found in specialized arteriovenous anastomoses involved in thermoregulation, that occur in nodular masses in the skin. The most frequent sites of glomus tumors are the fingers and toes. These small usually purple nodules can be **very tender and painful**.

Bacillary Angiomatosis

Bacillary angiomatosis, a vascular proliferation caused by an opportunistic infection of immunocompromised patients, may involve tissues such as the skin, bone, and brain. The causative agents of bacillary angiomatosis tend to be the bacteria *Bartonella henselae* or *Bartonella quintana*. Treatment of bacillary angiomatosis includes a macrolide antibiotic, such as erythromycin.

Lymphangioma

Lymphangiomas are local proliferations of lymphatic vessels. A **simple lymphangioma** is a mass composed of small lymphatic channels that occurs in the subcutaneous tissues of the head, neck, and axilla. A **cavernous lymphangioma** (cystic hygroma) (*Slide 4.5*) is a cystic swelling containing serous fluid that occurs more commonly on the neck or in the axilla of children.

MALIGNANT TUMORS OF BLOOD VESSELS
Hemangioendothelioma and Hemangiosarcoma

Hemangioendotheliomas are neoplasms of blood vessels composed of endothelial cells. These can occur individually, in groups, or in the lining of congeries of vessels. In children, a hemangioendothelioma is usually benign and represents the growth stage of a hemangioma. However, in the elderly, hemangioendotheliomas may develop into a rare malignant tumor known as a **hemangiosarcoma (angiosarcoma)** (*Slide 4.6*), which is a poorly differentiated (anaplastic), rapidly growing, infiltrating tumor that can occur in the skin, musculoskeletal system, breast, or liver.

Kaposi's Sarcoma

Kaposi's sarcoma is an opportunistic (occurring in immunosuppressed individuals), multifocal, malignant neoplasm of the vasculature of the skin, lymph nodes, or viscera.

Histologically, Kaposi's sarcoma is a collection of spindle cells (specialized muscle cells) that form small vascular spaces with a few hemosiderin-laden macrophages and some red blood cells. (*Slide 4.7*)

Clinically, the cutaneous lesions present as red/purple or dark blue macules, plaques, or raised nodules. Kaposi's sarcoma usually occurs in men over the age of sixty (90% of cases) and it has an **increased incidence in Ashkenazic Jews and AIDS patients.** Kaposi's sarcoma accounts for up to 10% of all tumors in Africa, due to the relatively high prevalence of AIDS. **Kaposi's sarcoma also has a strong association with the herpes simplex-8 virus as well.**

Hemangiopericytoma

Hemangiopericytomas are rare neoplasms composed of round and spindle cells that are derived from pericytes. (Pericytes are the endothelial cells that line the normal vessels.) Hemangiopericytomas may recur, and up to 50% may metastasize to the lungs, bone, or liver.

Vasculidites

Vasculidites are a group of diseases characterized by an inflammation of blood or lymphatic vessels, often resulting in necrosis. They are typically caused by immune complexes, infectious pathogens, or physical/chemical injury.

Microscopic Polyangiitis

Microscopic (hypersensitivity; leukocytoclastic) vasculitis is an acute inflammation of small blood vessels. It may be limited to the skin, where the lesions present as multiple, palpable purpuric areas that arise in unison. If the mucus membranes, lung, brain, heart, gastrointestinal tract, kidneys, or muscle are involved, patients may present clinically with hemoptysis, hematuria, proteinuria, bowel pain/bleeding, and muscle pain/weakness. Glomerulonephritis and pulmonary capillaritis are common sequelae as well. Certain drugs, food, infections, systemic diseases, and malignancies can precipitate this condition. Pertinent laboratory studies often show an elevated erythrocyte sedimentation rate (ESR) and a **positive perinuclear pattern of the anti-neutrophil cytoplasmic antibody (P-ANCA).** Small-vessel vasculitis may also present in unique syndromes known as **Churg-Strauss syndrome, Henoch-Schonlein purpura**, and **serum sickness**.

Churg-Strauss syndrome (allergic granulomatosis and angiitis) is a variant of microscopic polyangiitis that is associated with eosinophilia, allergic rhinitis, and asthma. Vessels in the lung, heart, spleen, peripheral nerves, and skin are frequently involved.

Histology shows an infiltration of eosinophils within the vessels and perivascular tissues.

Henoch-Schönlein purpura is the development of hemorrhagic purpuric lesions due to a **leukoclastic vasculitis** of the dermis, with IgA deposition in vascular walls. This disorder most frequently affects children between the ages of three to eight years old. The purpura typically arises on the extensor surfaces of the arms and legs as well as the buttocks. Henoch-Schönlein purpura can present with multiple systemic symptoms as well, such as fever, joint pain/swelling, vomiting, colic pain, and **hematochezia** (blood in the stool). A rapidly progressive glomerulonephritis may also occur, resulting in a nephrotic syndrome, which is more severe in adult patients. Symptoms often follow an upper respiratory tract infection or after the application of a particular drug or the ingestion of a certain food item. The characteristics of Henoch-Schönlein purpura are similar to **Berger's disease (IgA nephropathy)** and may be a spectrum of the same disease.

Serum Sickness is an immune-complex-mediated (Type III hypersensitivity) systemic reaction occurring one to two weeks after the injection of a serum or protein product. Antibodies are produced to a foreign antigen and form antigen-antibody immune complexes, which are deposited in the membranes of the heart, joints, kidney, skin, serosal surfaces, and small blood vessels. Deposited immune complexes then fix complement. The subsequent complex-mediated acute inflammatory reaction involving neutrophils and macrophages ultimately leads to tissue damage. Patients with serum sickness may present with fever, edema, urticaria, lymphadenopathy, arthritis, and proteinuria. This condition is not commonly encountered clinically. It was historically caused by the administration of tetanus antitoxin derived from horse serum. Modern cases are often a manifestation of an adverse reaction to medications, such as antibiotics.

Polyarteritis Nodosa (Classic)

Polyarteritis nodosa is a segmental, necrotizing, transmural inflammation of medium and small arteries, due to immune complex deposition. Aneurysmal nodules are formed due to the destruction of the media and the internal elastic lamina. These nodules can cause microaneurysms and may resemble palpable purpura. Unlike the urticaria produced in hypersensitivity vasculites, **these lesions are at different stages of progression and there is little association with antineutrophil cytoplasmic antibodies (ANCA)**. Polyarteritis nodosa commonly affects young males. **Thirty percent of patients are hepatitis B antigen positive**. Many organs and organ systems can be involved by this vasculitis, such as the kidney, heart, liver, gastrointestinal tract, pancreas, testes, musculoskeletal system, nervous system, and skin.

Clinically, patients with polyarteritis nodosa can present with multiple symptoms, such as "cotton-wool" patches of the retina, fever, headache, malaise, myalgia, weight loss, nausea, abdominal pain, hematochezia, and hypertension. Ischemic heart disease can result as well. However, the largest contributors to mortality are renal involvement and hypertension. The treatment for polyarteritis nodosa includes corticosteroids, azathioprine, and/or cyclophosphamide.

Wegener's Granulomatosis

Wegener's granulomatosis is a focal necrotizing vasculitis of unknown etiology that predominantly affects medium and small vessels of the upper respiratory tract and kidneys. Wegener's granulomatosis may also be exclusively limited to the upper respiratory tract. Histologically, arteries and veins in Wegener's granulomatosis become necrotic and are infiltrated by neutrophils and subsequently other inflammatory cells, with some fibrosis. Granulomas with giant cells are also prominent. (*Slide 4.8*) Men are affected more commonly, at the average age of forty years.

Clinically, patients with Wegener's granulomatosis may present with dyspnea, cough, hemoptysis, chronic sinusitis, otitis media, mastoiditis, and a perforation of the nasal septum. **The cytoplasmic pattern of the antineutrophilic cytoplasmic antibody (C-ANCA) is positive in 90% of patients,** and a titer provides a good marker to track the progression of the disease. A chest x-ray may show large nodular densities; hematuria and red cell casts may be identified upon urinalysis.

The treatment for Wegener's granulomatosis includes cyclophosphamide, corticosteroids, and/or methotrexate.

Giant Cell (Temporal) Arteritis

Giant cell arteritis is an acute and chronic granulomatous inflammation of medium and small arteries, especially the arteries of the head, including the temporal artery. **Giant cell arteritis is the most common of the vasculitides.** It typically occurs in females over the age of fifty years. Other than the temporal artery, the vertebral and the ophthalmic arteries may also become involved. **Involvement of the ophthalmic artery may lead to blindness**.

Clinically, patients with temporal arteritis may present with unilateral headache, jaw pain on chewing, fatigue, malaise, visual impairment, palpable nodules along the involved artery, and **polymyalgia rheumatica** (proximal muscle pain, periarticular pain, and morning stiffness).

Histologically, sections from an involved vessel in temporal arteritis will show degeneration of the internal elastic membrane. (*Slide 4.9*)

Laboratory studies may also show an increased erythrocyte sedimentation rate (ESR), and patients typically respond well to steroids.

Takayasu's Arteritis

Takayasu's arteritis is a granulomatous vasculitis of large and medium arteries. Takayasu's arteritis causes thickening along the aortic arch and its branches. This produces a condition known as **aortic arch syndrome**, which is characterized by absent pulses in the carotid, radial, or ulnar arteries. Therefore, Takayasu's arteritis is also known as the **"pulseless disease."** Asian women under the age of forty years are more commonly affected.

Clinically, patients with Takayasu's arteritis may present with fever, malaise, myalgia, arthralgia, arthritis, night sweats, eye problems, and painful skin nodules. Blood pressure in the upper extremities may also fall, causing fingers to become cold and numb. Laboratory studies may show an increased erythrocyte sedimentation rate (ESR). The course of the disease tends to be variable.

Kawasaki Disease

Kawasaki disease is a self-limiting, acute necrotizing vasculitis of medium and small arteries, associated with fever. **Kawasaki disease affects predominantly children under the age of four years old** and is endemic in Japan. Clinically, children may present with a fever, conjunctival and oral mucosal erythema and erosion, "Strawberry tongue," edema of the hands and feet, erythema of the palms and soles, skin rash, and lymphadenitis. Approximately 20% of patients will develop cardiovascular sequelae including coronary aneurysms, which are fatal in 1% of cases.

Thromboangiitis Obliterans (Buerger's Disease)

Thromboangiitis Obliterans is a segmental, thrombosing, acute and chronic inflammation of medium and small peripheral arteries. The tibial and radial arteries are most frequently involved. The disease process can extend into veins and nerves of the extremities. **Buerger's disease occurs almost exclusively in smokers**, typically before the age of thirty-five years. It also has a relatively higher prevalence in the Jewish population. This is a painful ischemic disease that results in intermittent claudication, superficial nodular phlebitis, cold sensitivity, and possible gangrene. Patients should quit smoking as soon as possible!

Lymphomatoid Granulomatosis

Lymphomatoid Granulomatosis is a rare vasculitis due to an infiltration of atypical plasmacytoid and lymphocytoid cells. It may progress from a chronic disorder to a T-cell non-Hodgkin's lymphoma.

Raynaud's Disease and Raynaud's Phenomenon

Raynaud's disease involves intense recurrent vasospasm of small arteries, resulting in paroxysmal pallor or cyanosis of the digits precipitated by chilling or emotion. Raynaud's disease is typically a benign, chronic condition of otherwise healthy young women. The exact cause of Raynaud's disease is still under investigation. **Raynaud's phenomenon** is paroxysmal pallor or cyanosis of the extremities due to arterial insufficiency as a result of arterial stenosis.

Raynaud's phenomenon may be the first manifestation of an underlying disease state such as systemic lupus erythematosus (SLE), scleroderma, atherosclerosis, or Berger's disease (Thromboangiitis Obliterans).

PATHOLOGY OF THE HEART
Congestive Heart Failure

Congestive heart failure is a failure of the left ventricle, right ventricle, or both ventricles due to ischemic heart disease, hypertension, valvular disease, or myocardial disease. The failure of the heart to adequately pump blood can result in greater ventricular end-diastolic volumes and eventual cardiac dilation. A failure of the left ventricle may lead to an increase in pulmonary venous pressure. This will cause pulmonary congestion and edema, resulting in dyspnea and orthopnea.

A pleural effusion may also develop, due to pulmonary venous distention and transudation of fluid,

resulting in a hydrothorax (fluid in the thoracic cavity). Perfusion of the kidneys may be reduced as well, causing a stimulation of the renin-angiotensin system and subsequent aldosterone release, leading to retention of salt and water. In severe cases, cerebral anoxia may occur due to lack of perfusion of the brain. Microscopically, sections from the lung will show **hemosiderin-laden macrophages** ("heart failure cells").

Fig. 4-5. Signs and symptoms of congestive heart failure.

The most common cause of right heart failure is left heart failure. Pulmonary hypertension due to chronic lung disease may also lead to right-sided heart failure. Pitting edema of the ankles is usually an early sign of fluid retention. Transudation may lead to a characteristic rash known as **stasis dermatitis**. Typically, the degree of renal hypoxia is greater with right-sided heart failure than with left-sided heart failure alone. In addition to a hydrothorax, which may be a component of both right and left-sided heart failure, ascites (fluid in the abdominal cavity) may also be another manifestation of fluid retention.

The elevation in central venous pressure in CHF will also cause an increase in resistance to portal blood flow. Therefore, the liver and spleen become enlarged due to chronic passive congestion with blood. Grossly, the liver parenchyma will have a characteristic "nutmeg" appearance upon serial sectioning.

Ischemic Heart Disease

Ischemic heart disease is an insult of cardiac myocytes, due to a partial or complete occlusion of arterial blood flow to the myocardium. The most common cause of coronary vascular stenosis is atherosclerotic coronary artery disease. However, the acute symptoms of ischemic heart disease can be precipitated by a thrombus or vasospasm. Ischemic heart disease can be clinically silent, or it can present clinically as angina pectoris, myocardial infarction, or sudden cardiac death.

Angina Pectoris

Angina pectoris is severe constricting chest pain due to inadequate coronary perfusion of the myocardium. The pain radiates to the shoulder, neck, or jaw. Vasodilators such as nitroglycerin help relieve episodes of pain.

Stable angina, where pain frequently follows exertion and is relieved by rest, is the most common presentation of angina pectoris.

Unstable angina consists of prolonged or recurrent pain that occurs even at rest. It is due to a disruption of an atherosclerotic plaque with a thrombosis, embolization, or vasospasm. Unstable angina is an ominous sign of an impending myocardial infarction.

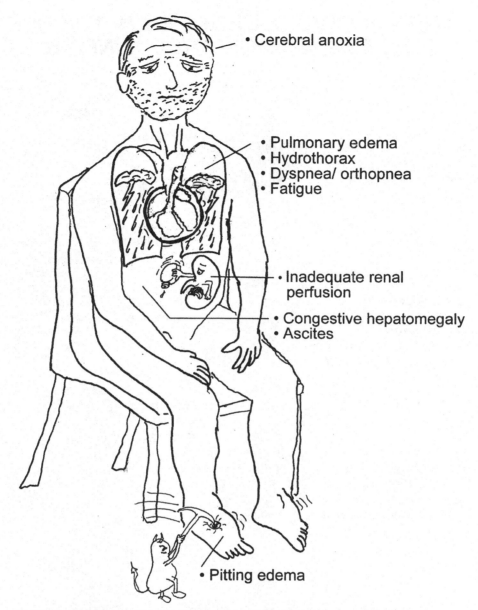

- Cerebral anoxia

- Pulmonary edema
- Hydrothorax
- Dyspnea/ orthopnea
- Fatigue

- Inadequate renal perfusion

- Congestive hepatomegaly
- Ascites

- Pitting edema

SIGNS & SYMPTOMS OF CONGESTIVE HEART FAILURE

Figure 4-5

Prinzmetal's angina is intermittent chest pain that occurs with physical activity or at rest and is caused by coronary artery vasospasm.

Myocardial Infarction

Myocardial infarction is a lack of oxygenation to an area of the heart, resulting in necrosis of cardiac myocytes. Myocardial infarction is the most significant cause of morbidity and mortality in the industrialized world. It is usually a result of underlying coronary artery disease. **The most frequently occluded coronary artery in myocardial infarction is the left ante-** rior **descending**, which supplies much of the left ventricle. (*Slide 4.10*)

Clinically, patients with myocardial infarction may present with severe retrosternal chest pain/tightening radiating to the left arm or jaw, shortness of breath, fatigue, and andrenergic symptoms.

Infarcts, in general, can be divided into two groups based upon the extent of perfusion to a particular tissue or organ:

- A **red (hemorrhagic) infarct** indicates an infarct took place, and then the area of infarct was reperfused

HISTOLOGICAL CHANGES IN THE HEART FOLLOWING MYOCARDIAL INFARCTION

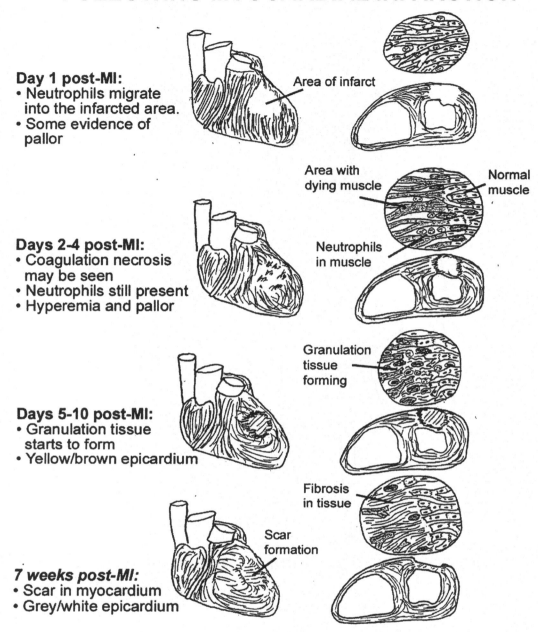

Day 1 post-MI:
• Neutrophils migrate into the infarcted area.
• Some evidence of pallor

Area of infarct

Area with dying muscle

Normal muscle

Days 2-4 post-MI:
• Coagulation necrosis may be seen
• Neutrophils still present
• Hyperemia and pallor

Neutrophils in muscle

Granulation tissue forming

Days 5-10 post-MI:
• Granulation tissue starts to form
• Yellow/brown epicardium

Fibrosis in tissue

Scar formation

7 weeks post-MI:
• Scar in myocardium
• Grey/white epicardium

Figure 4-6.

with blood due to collateral blood flow. These occur in tissues or organs with collateral circulation, such as the lungs or intestine.

• A **pale infarct** occurs in organs or tissues with a single vascular route of perfusion such as the heart, brain, kidney, or spleen.

Myocardial infarctions are typically given two histological classifications based upon the extent of necrosis. A **subendocardial infarct** designates that necrosis due to an ischemic event is limited to the interior third of the ventricular wall. A **transmural infarct** designates that myocardial necrosis involves the entire ventricular wall.

Myocardial infarctions follow a progression of changes from the onset of the ischemic event to eventual scarring, if the patient survives.

1. The **first day** after an ischemic event, changes in the myocardium may be very subtle. Grossly, the epicardium of the infarcted area may show some evidence of pallor. Microscopically, neutrophils begin to respond to chemotactic factors released into the blood stream due to coagulative necrosis and migrate into the myocardium. (*Slide 4.11*)
2. After **two to four days**, the epicardium may begin to display signs of hyperemia as well as pallor. Microscopically, the myocardium shows coagulative necrosis, dilated vessels, and acute inflammation as neutrophils continue to migrate. (*Slide 4.12*)
3. After **five to ten days**, the epicardium appears yellow/brown with some softening surrounded by a hyperemic boarder. Microscopically, granulation tissue begins to form around the periphery of the infarcted area and neutrophils and macrophages are abundant, later disappearing. (*Slide 4.13*)
4. After **seven weeks**, the epicardium appears gray/white and there is extensive fibrosis that forms a contracted scar within the myocardium. (*Slide 4.14*)

Fig. 4-6. Progressive histological changes in the heart following a myocardial infarction.

Multiple laboratory tests can be performed to diagnose a myocardial infarction as well as to determine the time line of the event. Based upon the relative serum concentrations of these protein markers, it may be possibly to determine the age of a myocardial infarction.

1. In the first six hours following a myocardial infarction, an **electrocardiogram (EKG)** is the best diagnostic test and will show ST elevation and Q wave changes.
2. **Cardiac Troponin I** is the most specific of the serum protein markers and will rise within the first four hours of an ischemic event and remain elevated for seven to ten days.
3. **Creatine kinase-myocardial bound (CK-MB)** is a good test to use within the first twenty-four hours post-infarct. CK-MB will reach its peak concentration about one day after a myocardial infarction and then quickly taper off to a baseline level in just over two days.
4. **Lactate dehydrogenase 1 (LDH1)** levels slowly rise and are elevated two to seven days following an ischemic event.
5. **Aspartate aminotransferase (AST)** is a nonspecific protein marker, which reaches its peak concentration in one to two days post-infarct. It is also found in liver and skeletal muscle cells.

Many sequelae may result from a myocardial infarction, such as:

1. The development of a **cardiac arrhythmia** occurs in approximately 90% of cases and is the most common complication and cause of death following a myocardial infarction. The incidence of arrhythmia is greatest two days post-infarct.
2. **Left ventricular failure** occurs in approximately 60% of cases, followed by pulmonary edema.
3. A **mural thrombus** may form on the endocardial surface of an infarcted area, resulting in a possible thromboembolism.
4. If there is a substantial infarct, **cardiogenic shock** may ensue, which also increases the risk of mortality.
5. Structures of the heart, such as the ventricular free wall, interventricular septum or papillary muscle may **rupture** four to ten days after a myocardial infarction. If a ventricular aneurysm occurs, cardiac tamponade may ensue.
6. **Fibrinous pericarditis** is a less common complication that occurs three to five days post-infarct. It presents clinically as a friction rub.
7. Finally, a form of fibrinous pericarditis known as **Dressler's syndrome** may develop several weeks after a myocardial infarction due to an autoimmune phenomenon.

Chronic Ischemic Heart Disease

Chronic ischemic heart disease is ischemic myocardial damage over many years that results in the progressive onset of **congestive heart failure (CHF)**. Microscopically, the myocardium may show hypertrophic myocytes and scars due to old myocardial infarcts.

Sudden Cardiac Death

Sudden cardiac death is an unexpected death due to cardiac causes that occur within one hour of the onset of symptoms if present. In the majority of cases, **the cause of sudden cardiac death is a lethal arrhythmia**.

Cardiomyopathies

Cardiomyopathies are diseases of the heart resulting from a primary abnormality of the myocardium. These diseases are non-inflammatory and are **not** associated with hypertension, coronary artery disease, valvular disease, or congenital heart disease. Cardiomyopathies typically cause left ventricular dysfunction, which is manifested by ventricular enlargement, ventricular arrhythmia, and ultimately heart failure.

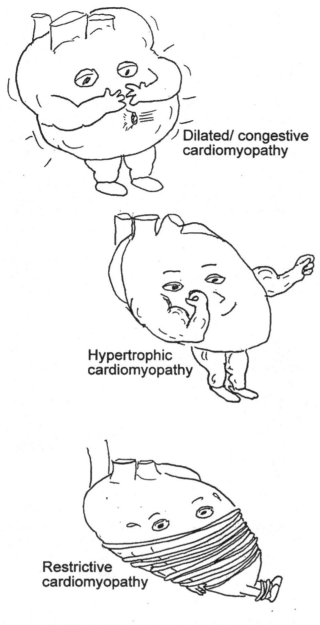

THE CARDIOMYOPATHIES

Figure 4-7

Dilated/Congestive Cardiomyopathy

Dilated cardiomyopathy is a dilatation of the ventricles and subsequently the atria due to both left and right-sided heart failure. This results in a "flabby" heart, progressive cardiac hypertrophy and systolic dysfunction. Dilated cardiomyopathy is the most common cardiomyopathy (90% of all cardiomyopathies). It can be due to a variety of causes. Alcohol abuse is a frequent cause of dilated cardiomyopathy. Coxsackie B virus, wet beriberi (thiamine deficiency), cocaine abuse,

Chaga's disease, doxorubicin toxicity, pregnancy, genetics, hemochromatosis, chronic anemia, and sarcoidosis all may cause dilated cardiomyopathy. Finally, dilated cardiomyopathy may be idiopathic.

The ejection fraction of patients with a dilated cardiomyopathy is less than 40%. On x-ray, their heart looks like a "balloon." Approximately 75% of patients with a dilated cardiomyopathy will die within five years post diagnosis without cardiac transplantation.

Arrythmogenic right ventricular cardiomyopathy is a variant of a dilated cardiomyopathy characterized by right-sided heart failure due to a loss of myocytes, fatty infiltration and interstitial fibrosis. The ventricular wall is thinned, resulting in various rhythm disturbances most notably ventricular tachycardia. Arrythmogenic right ventricular cardiomyopathy is often a familial disorder. The left ventricle can be involved, but less frequently.

Hypertrophic Cardiomyopathy

Hypertrophic cardiomyopathy is an asymmetric hypertrophy of the ventricular myocardium in which the ventricular free wall grows unproportionally to the ventricular septum. Hypertrophic cardiomyopathy causes reduced diastolic filling, but the ejection fraction remains in the normal range of 50-80%. In many cases, the anterior mitral leaflet moves toward the ventricular septum during systole causing a left ventricular flow outlet obstruction, which places the patient at high risk for syncope and sudden cardiac death. Grossly, the left ventricle appears thickened and the ventricular chamber resembles a "banana" on echocardiogram.

Histologically, there is a disarray of cardiac myofibrils in hypertrophic cardiomyopathy. Approximately 50% of cases are familial through the inheritance of an autosomal dominant trait. The condition can also be associated with Fredreich ataxia, storage diseases, or children of diabetic mothers, or it may be idiopathic. Hypertrophic cardiomyopathy is often found as the cause of sudden death in young athletes.

Restrictive/Obliterative Cardiomyopathy

Restrictive cardiomyopathy is a primary decrease in ventricular compliance due to an infiltrative process within the myocardium. This results in a stiffening of the heart that impairs ventricular filling during diastole. The causes of restrictive cardiomyopathy are amyloidosis, sarcoidosis, scleroderma, hemochromatosis, radiation, endocardial fibroelastosis, endomyocardial fibroelastosis (**Loffler's disease**), or idiopathic.

Fig. 4-7. Dilated, hypertrophic, and restrictive cardiomyopathies.

Myocarditis

Myocarditis is any inflammatory process that results in injury to cardiac myocytes. (*Slide 4.15*) The most common cause of myocarditis is a viral infection of the Coxsackie A or B virus or other enteroviruses. Cytomegalovirus (CMV), human immunodeficiency virus (HIV), enteric cytopathic human orphan virus (ECHO), and influenza virus are also involved in a few cases. Less common infectious agents include chlamydiae, rickettsiae, *Corynebacterium diphtheriae*, *Neisseria meningococcus*, *Borrelia burgdorferi*, trypanosoma, toxoplasmosis, candida, and trichinosis. Immune mediated reactions such as post-viral, rheumatic fever, systemic lupus erythematosus (SLE), drug hypersensitivity, and transplant rejection may also cause myocarditis. Other forms of myocarditis due to unknown mechanisms are sarcoidosis and giant cell myocarditis.

PERICARDIAL DISEASES
Acute Pericarditis

Acute pericarditis is an acute inflammation of the pericardium. It presents in five different variations: **fibrinous, serous, purulent, hemorrhagic, and caseous pericarditis.**

Fibrinous pericarditis is a noninfectious inflammatory process that produces a fibrin-rich exudate with serous fluid. This is the most common form of acute pericarditis. It is typically caused by uremia, myocardial infarction (**Dressler's syndrome**), rheumatic fever, chest radiation, systemic lupus erythematosus (SLE), trauma, and surgery.

Serous pericarditis is an acute noninfectious inflammatory process that produces a clear to straw-colored, protein-rich pericardial exudate, containing some inflammatory cells. Common causes of serous pericarditis are systemic lupus erythematosus (SLE), rheumatoid arthritis, uremia, scleroderma, tumors, and bacteria and viruses of the upper respiratory tract.

Purulent pericarditis is an infectious inflammatory process, which produces a purulent inflammatory exudates. Bacteria are the most commonly involved organisms.

Hemorrhagic pericarditis is an inflammatory process that produces an exudate composed of blood with a fibrinous or purulent effusion. The most common causes of hemorrhagic pericarditis are tumor invasion into the pericardium (e.g., melanoma) and bacterial infections (e.g., tuberculosis).

Caseous pericarditis is caseation within the pericardial sac due to tuberculosis or fungal organisms. Caseous pericarditis is the rarest form of acute pericarditis, but it is also one of the most severe if not treated.

Clinically, patients with acute pericarditis can present with pericardial pain, friction rub (fibrinous pericarditis), electrocardiogram (EKG) changes (diffuse ST elevations in all leads), pulsus paradoxus (pulse becomes weaker on inspiration and stronger on expiration), and distant heart sounds. Acute pericarditis can

resolve without scarring or lead to constrictive pericarditis or adhesive mediastinopericarditis.

Chronic (Constrictive) Pericarditis and Adhesive Mediastinopericarditis

Constrictive pericarditis is a proliferation of fibrous tissue in the pericardium that essentially obliterates the pericardial cavity and limits diastolic filling. Constrictive pericarditis often resembles right-sided heart failure or a restrictive cardiomyopathy clinically due to reduced cardiac output with decreased venous return. The most common causes of constrictive pericarditis are tuberculosis (caseous and hemorrhagic pericarditis) and staphylococcal infections (purulent pericarditis). Pericardectomy is the method of treatment in severe cases.

Adhesive mediastinopericarditis is an adherence of the external aspect of the pericardium to surrounding structures, with obliteration of the pericardial sac due to fibrosis. Adhesive mediastinopericarditis may follow suppurative pericarditis, caseous pericarditis, cardiac surgery or irradiation to the mediastinum. Systolic contraction pulls on all structures adhered to the pericardium, which can cause myocyte hypertrophy and dilation of the heart chambers, mimicking a dilated cardiomyopathy.

Cardiac Tamponade

Cardiac tamponade is a potentially fatal compression of the heart by a fluid in the pericardium, leading to a decrease in cardiac output and an equilibration of pressure in the heart chambers. Clinically, patients present with pulsus paradoxus. An electrocardiogram (EKG) will show electrical alterans (beat-to-beat alterations of the QRS complex height).

Two conditions that can result in cardiac tamponade are hydropericardium and hemopericardium. **Hydropericardium** is the accumulation of a serous transudate within the pericardial sac as a result of a condition that produces edema, such as congestive heart failure (CHF) or hypoproteinemia due to a nephrotic syndrome or liver disease. **Hemopericardium (*Slide 4.16*)** is the accumulation of blood within the pericardial sac caused by a dissecting ventricular or aortic aneurysm or direct trauma.

ENDOCARDITIS
Infective Endocarditis

Infective endocarditis is a bacterial or, rarely, fungal infection of the endocardium. Vegetations (*Slide 4.17*) composed of fibrin, inflammatory cells, and bacteria develop on valvular surfaces. These may cause ulceration or perforation of valve cusps and possibly a rupture of the chordae tendinae. **The mitral valve is the most frequently involved heart valve. However, the tricuspid valve is often involved in patients with a** history of intravenous (IV) drug use. These vegetations are soft, friable and easily detached from the endocardial surface and may result in embolization and subsequent hemorrhage. **Splinter hemorrhages** may be observed in the nail beds of patients.

Clinically, patients with infective endocarditis may present with a new murmur, anemia, fever, **Osler nodes** (tender raised nodules on the finger or toe pad), **Roth's spots** (round white spots on the retina, encircled by hemorrhage), and **Janeway lesions** (small erythematous lesions on the palm or sole). Other complications include glomerulonephritis and suppurative pericarditis. A continuous bacteremia will be present. Multiple positive blood cultures for infectious organisms are needed in order to make a diagnosis.

There are two types of infective endocarditis:

1. **Acute infective endocarditis** is a rapid infection caused by highly virulent organisms such as *Staphylococcus aureus* (50% of cases), which produce large vegetations on previously normal valves.
2. **Subacute infective endocarditis** is an infection by low virulence organisms such *as Streptococcus viridans* (>50% of cases) that produce small vegetations on abnormal or diseased valves. Often, valvular damage is a result of congenital heart disease or rheumatic fever. Subacute infective endocarditis has an insidious onset. It can be a complication of dental procedures due to bacteremia. Therefore, patients with a history of valvular damage are often given antibiotics such as amoxicillin or erythromycin prophylactically prior to dental work to prevent infection.

Marantic Endocarditis

Marantic (nonbacterial thrombotic) endocarditis is the formation of small, sterile deposits of fibrin, platelets, and blood along the line of closure of valve leaflets in a random pattern. It is secondary to a wasting disorder such as cancer. Hypercoagulable states, such as an increase in circulating mucin produced by mucinous adenocarcinoma of the pancreas, predispose to this condition. Other debilitating diseases associated with hypercoagulability and subsequent Marantic endocarditis are disseminated intravascular coagulation (DIC), promyelocytic leukemia, hyperestrogenism, extensive burns, and sepsis. Trauma to the endocardium is also a well-known predisposing condition.

Libman-Sacks Endocarditis

Libman-Sacks endocarditis is the formation of small, sterile, vegetations on either or both surfaces of the leaflets of the mitral or tricuspid in patients with systemic lupus erythematosus (SLE). The aortic valve is less commonly involved.

Carcinoid Heart Disease

Carcinoid heart disease is the formation of thick, fibrous endocardial plaques involving the mural endocardium and/or the cusps of the valves of the right side of the heart in patients with a carcinoid tumor. Plaques are formed in response to carcinoid secretory products, especially serotonin. **The left side of the heart is rarely involved** because vasoactive peptides and amines, including serotonin, are inactivated in the lungs by monoamine oxidase. Carcinoid heart disease typically results from carcinoid tumors outside the portal system of venous drainage such as in the lungs or ovary, because serotonin is rapidly metabolized in the liver. Therefore, carcinoid tumors of the gastrointestinal system do not often contribute to this disease unless there is hepatic metastasis.

RHEUMATIC FEVER AND RHEUMATIC HEART DISEASE

Rheumatic fever is an acute, immunologically mediated, multisystem, inflammatory disorder that usually occurs one to four weeks following a throat infection by group A, beta-hemolytic streptococci in children and young adults. However, only 3% of patients with a group A, beta hemolytic streptococcal throat infection actually progress to rheumatic fever. It is thought that streptococcal antigens elicit an immunological response not only to streptococcal organisms, but to heart and other tissues, due to cross-reactivity. Therefore, patients with rheumatic fever will usually have **elevated anti-streptolysin antibodies (ASO) titers** in addition to an elevated erythrocyte sedimentation rate (ESR).

Histologically, focal inflammatory lesions in rheumatic fever, especially in the heart, show **Aschoff bodies (*Slide 4.18*)**, characterized by fibrinoid degeneration surrounded by primarily T-cells and large macrophages known as **Anitschkow cells (caterpillar cells)**, which have chromatin that is slender and wavy. Giant cells, **Aschoff cells,** may be observed as well.

The **Jones criteria** is used to make a diagnosis of rheumatic fever, which requires a recent infection with group A, beta-hemolytic, streptococcus as well as two major criteria or the combination of one major and two minor criteria. The major criteria include:

• carditis
• mild migratory polyarthritis of large joints
• erythema marginatum
• subcutaneous nodules a
• Sydenham chorea (St. Vitus' dance).

Minor criteria include nonspecific signs such as fever and arthralgia.

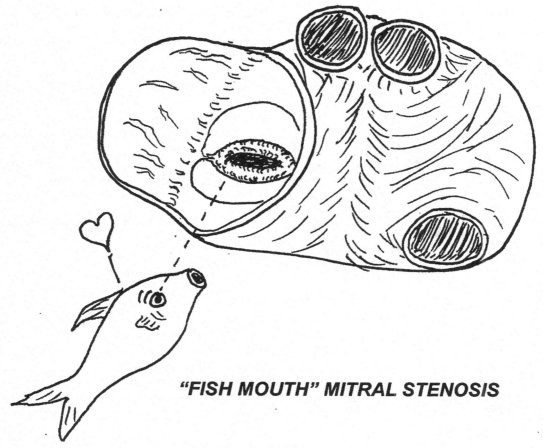

"FISH MOUTH" MITRAL STENOSIS

Figure 4-8.

Rheumatic heart disease is a late major manifestation, characterized by endocarditis with cardiac valvular damage and deforming fibrosis. **High-pressure valves, namely the mitral and aortic valves, are more commonly affected.** In 50% of cases, only the mitral valve is involved. During the acute phase of rheumatic heart disease, the leaflets become inflamed, and nonfriable veruccae are formed along the lines of valve closure due to fibrin deposition. Irregular thickenings known as **MacCallum plaques** are also formed in areas of high hemodynamic pressure.

In the chronic or healing phase, the valves and chordae tendinae become thickened and sometimes calcified with a fusion of the valve cusps. This gives the valve a "fish mouth" appearance and leads to mitral stenosis, which may require valvular replacement surgery.

Figure 4-8. "Fish mouth" appearance of mitral valve in severe mitral stenosis, in rheumatic heart disease. (Slide 4.19)

As with any type of valvular damage, **rheumatic heart disease can predispose to infective endocarditis.** Mural thrombi leading to systemic embolization may also occur due to blood stasis and endothelial damage. Fibrinous pericarditis and myocarditis can also be sequelae of rheumatic fever, leading to pericardial friction rubs, weak heart sounds, tachycardia, and arrhythmia.

The mortality rate from rheumatic fever is only 1%. Myocarditis is usually the cause of death in these cases. After an initial episode of rheumatic fever, there is an increased risk of developing the disease again with each subsequent pharyngeal infection of group A, beta hemolytic streptococci. Due to early diagnosis and improved treatment of pharyngeal infections, improving socioeconomical conditions, and a decrease in the virulence of group A streptococci, the incidence of rheumatic fever has greatly decreased in industrialized nations. However, it remains an important health issue in developing countries.

VALVULAR HEART DISEASE
Mitral Valve Stenosis

Mitral valve stenosis in the majority of cases results from rheumatic heart disease. It causes the pressure in the left atrium to be much greater than the left ventricle. **Mitral valve stenosis is manifested clinically by a**

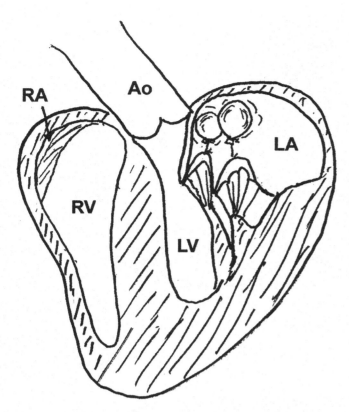

MITRAL VALVE PROLAPSE

Figure 4-9.

rumbling murmur that occurs late in diastole, following an opening snap.

Mitral Valve Prolapse

Mitral valve prolapse is a "floppy" cusp of the mitral valve that "balloons" into the atrium during systole due to a stretching of the posterior valve leaflet. It is a common valvular abnormality that affects approximately 3% of the total population, predominately women. Mitral valve prolapse also has a **higher incidence in patients with connective tissue disorders, such as Marfan's syndrome.** The underlying pathology of this condition is a myxomatous degeneration of the mitral valve.

Fig. 4-9. Mitral valve prolapse with ballooning of the valve into the atria. (LA, left atrium; LV, left ventricle; RV, right ventricle; RA, right atrium; Ao, aorta)

Mitral valve prolapse is manifested clinically by a late systolic murmur with a midsystolic click. It is typically an incidental finding, but it may predispose to bacterial endocarditis, arrhythmia, thrombus formation, and valvular insufficiency.

Mitral Valve Regurgitation (Insufficiency)

Mitral valve regurgitation is the leakage of blood back through the mitral valve from the left ventricle and into the atrium during systole. This condition is usually the result of rheumatic heart disease. Mitral valve insufficiency can also be caused by mitral valve prolapse, infective endocarditis, or papillary muscle damage following a myocardial infarction. In some patients with a dilated cardiomyopathy, stretching of the mitral valve ring may be sufficient to cause regurgitation. **Mitral valve regurgitation is manifested clinically by a holosystolic, high-pitched "blowing" murmur.**

Aortic Stenosis and Atresia

Aortic atresia is the congenital absence of the normal valvular orifice into the aorta. Aortic stenosis and atresia cause a narrowing and obstruction of the aortic valve that result in a much greater left ventricular pressure than aortic pressure during systole. **Aortic stenosis is manifested clinically by a crescendo-decrescendo systolic ejection murmur following an ejection click. The murmur radiates to the carotid arteries and apex of the heart.** It can also cause "pulsus parvus et tardus" in which pulses are weak as compared to heart sounds. There are three types of stenosis: supravalvular, valvular and subvalvular.

Valvular aortic stenosis (*Slide 4.20*) is a congenital or commonly acquired valvular abnormality. Congenital aortic stenosis occurs when the aortic cusps are hypoplastic, dysplastic, or abnormal in number. Severe cases may result in hypoplastic left heart syndrome. Acquired aortic stenosis is a result of valvular damage or calcification. When calcification of a previously normal aortic valve occurs as an age-related process, typically in patients seventy to eighty years old, the disease is known as **senile calcific aortic stenosis.** Bicuspid aortic valves have a higher predilection to become calcified in younger patients, typically fifty to sixty years old. Rheumatic heart disease can cause the aortic valve to become stenotic as well.

Subvalvular aortic stenosis is typically an isolated congenital abnormality characterized by a thickened ring/collar of fibrous tissue inferior to the aortic cusps.

Supravalvular aortic stenosis is a familial disorder that causes the aorta superior to the aortic cusps to become thickened, resulting in luminal constriction. Supravalvular aortic stenosis has an increased incidence in patients with hypercalcemia of infancy associated with **Williams' syndrome.**

Aortic Regurgitation (Insufficiency)

Aortic regurgitation is the leakage of blood from the aorta back through the aortic valve and into the left ventricle during diastole. The most common causes

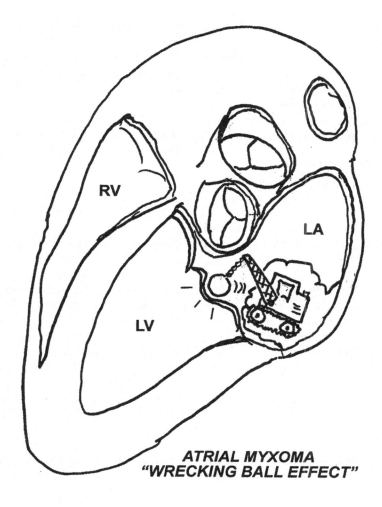

Figure 4-10

ATRIAL MYXOMA
"WRECKING BALL EFFECT"

of aortic regurgitation are a nondissecting aortic aneurysm, rheumatic heart disease, syphilitic aortitis, and ankylosing spondylitis. **Aortic regurgitation is manifested clinically by an immediate high-pitched "blowing" diastolic murmur and wide pulse pressures.**

Tricuspid Valve Dysfunction

Tricuspid valve dysfunction is rarely encountered. The tricuspid valve is involved in only 5% of all cases of rheumatic heart disease. However, **the tricuspid valve may be involved in a carcinoid syndrome and in bacterial endocarditis of intravenous (IV) drug abuse.** Tricuspid stenosis can be differentiated from mitral stenosis because the murmur it produces becomes louder upon inspiration.

Pulmonary Valve Dysfunction

Pulmonary valve dysfunction is commonly encountered in children afflicted with congenital malformations and as a part of a carcinoid syndrome in adults. The pulmonary valve is rarely involved in rheumatic heart disease.

CARDIAC NEOPLASMS

First, it should be known that primary tumors of the heart are very rare. The heart more commonly is involved in metastatic cancer than primary cancer.

Myxoma

A myxoma of the heart (*Slide 4.21*) is a benign neoplasm derived from primitive multipotential mesenchymal cells. Cardiac myxomas commonly arise in the atria, with an increased incidence on the septum of the left atrium near the fossa ovalis. A cardiac myxoma is characteristically a pedunculated mass (*Slide 4.22*) that is mobile and may have a "wrecking-ball" effect causing damage to the valve leaflets.

Fig. 4-10. The wrecking ball effect of an atrial myxoma.

Atrial myxoma may also cause a "ball-valve" obstruction of the mitral valve, embolization, and symptoms of fever/malaise. **Carney syndrome** is a familial cardiac myxoma syndrome that accounts for 10% of all cardiac myxomas. It incudes spotty pigmentation of the skin and endocrine overactivity.

Lipoma

A lipoma of the heart is a localized, encapsulated benign proliferation of adipose cells. Cardiac lipomas occur most often in the left ventricle, right atrium, or the atrial septum. They can cause "ball-valve" obstructions or arrhythmias. When a proliferation of adipose cells occurs in the atrial septum, it is known as **lipomatous hypertrophy**.

Papillary Fibroelastoma

Papillary fibroelastomas are benign projections of possibly organized thrombi from the ventricular surface of semilunar valves and the atrial surface of atrioventricular (A-V) valves. Similar lesions known as **Lambl excrescences** are often found on the aortic valves of older patients at autopsy as an incidental finding.

Rhabdomyoma

A rhabdomyoma is the most common tumor of the heart in children. It can obstruct a valve or heart chamber. Cardiac rhabdomyomas are thought to be hamartomas or malformations rather than true neoplasms because of their **increased incidence in patients with tuberous sclerosis**.

Histologically, the cells of rhabdomyoma are characteristically known as **spider cells**.

Sarcomas

Cardiac angiomyosarcomas and other sarcomas of the heart are similar to sarcomas found in other organs and tissues of the body.

Metastatic Cardiac Tumors

Metastatic cardiac tumors are more frequent than primary cardiac tumors. They commonly include lung cancer, breast cancer, melanoma, leukemia, and lymphoma.

CONGENITAL HEART DISEASE

Congenital heart disease is any defect of the heart that is present from birth. Many of these defects arise between the 3rd and 8th week of gestation, during cardiogenesis. There are many factors that contribute to congenital heart disease, such as chromosomal abnormalities, familial inheritance, environmental factors and prenatal infections, such as rubella. A maternal rubella infection, especially during the first trimester, can be extremely detrimental to the fetus. It can cause **congenital rubella syndrome**, which includes heart defects, microcephaly, deafness, and growth retardation. Therefore, it is essential to determine an expectant mother's immune status to rubella.

Left-to-Right Shunts (Late Cyanosis)

The left side of the heart has a relatively higher pressure than the right side. Therefore, left-to-right shunts result in the flow of oxygenated blood from the left side to the right side of the heart. The increase in blood flow to the right side of the heart can cause eventual pulmonary hypertension, which may produce an increase in the pressure of the right side resulting in a reversal of blood flow through the shunt. This condition is known as **Eisenmenger's syndrome**. Deoxygenated blood from the right side of the heart then mixes with oxygenated blood in the left side, producing late cyanosis.

Ventricular Septal Defect (VSD)

A ventricular septal defect is an endocardial cushion defect of the ventricular septum, resulting from an incomplete closure that allows communication between the ventricles. **Ventricular septal defect is the most common congenital heart defect** and can vary in size. Small defects may close spontaneously. However, larger defects require surgery because they may cause an excessive amount of blood to inappropriately enter the right ventricle due to the pressure gradient between the two ventricles. Approximately 90% of VSDs occur in the membranous septum. Defects of the muscular septum may be multiple, producing a "swiss-cheese septum." There is a higher incidence of endocardial cushion defects of the ventricular and atrial septums in patients with Down syndrome. A **ventricular septal defect is manifested clinically by a holosystolic murmur**.

Atrial Septal Defect (ASD)

An atrial septal defect is an endocardial cushion defect of the atrial septum resulting in an abnormal communication of blood between the atria. Approximately 90% of atrial septal defects occur in the septum secundum due to a defect in the fossa ovalis. Approximately 5% of atrial septal defects occur in the lower portion of the septum primum. Large defects of the septum primum may be associated with deformities of the atrioventricular (A-V) valves, as in **Lutembacher's syndrome**, which includes mitral stenosis with an ASD. A defect of the sinus venosus accounts for 5% of atrial septal defects; it occurs in the upper part of the septum near the entrance of the superior vena cava. **Atrial septal defects should never be confused with a patent foramen ovale**, which is normally present in 33% of the general population and is clinically insignificant unless the right atrial pressure becomes elevated. Symptoms of ASDs are usually delayed until adulthood. Heart failure, paradoxic embolism, and irreversible pulmonary vascular disease are possible sequelae.

Patent Ductus Arteriosus (PDA)

A patent ductus arteriosus is a failure of the closure of the fetal ductus arteriosus. The ductus arteriosus in the

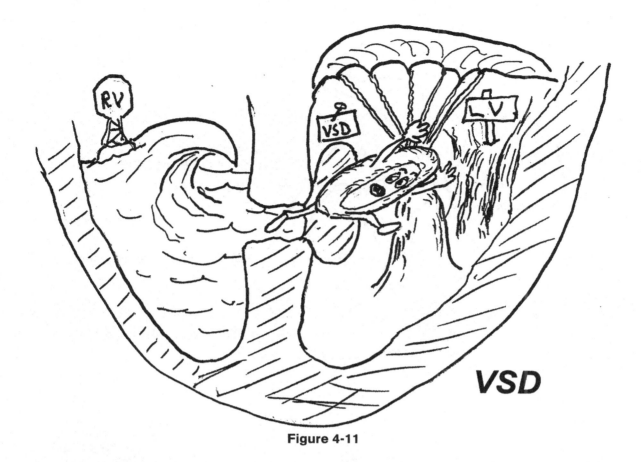

Figure 4-11

VSD

fetal circulation normally shunts blood from the pulmonary artery to the aorta. PDAs have a higher incidence in patients living in high altitudes, due to low oxygen tension. A patent ductus arteriosus may be maintained by prostaglandin synthesis or administration of prostaglandin E and closed with indomethacin treatment or by surgery. If a PDA is not properly closed, pulmonary hypertension, right ventricular hypertrophy, and late cyanosis can occur. **A patent ductus arteriosus is manifested clinically by a continuous machine-like heart murmur that is loudest at the second heart sound.**

Eisenmenger's Syndrome

Persistent left to right shunts (VSDs, ASDs and PDAs) can cause pulmonary hypertension due to increased right-sided heart pressure and subsequent increased pulmonary resistance from arteriolar thickening. The pressures on the right side may exceed the pressure on the left side of the heart, causing the shunt to reverse to a right to left flow. The mixture of oxygenated and deoxygenated blood results in late cyanosis and possible clubbing and polycythemia.

Fig. 4-11. A ventricular septal defect may be associated with a right-to-left shunt.

Right-to-Left Shunts (Early Cyanosis)

Right-to-left shunts allow deoxygenated blood from the right side of the heart to flow into the left side. The mixture of deoxygenated and oxygenated blood in the systemic circulation may produce early cyanosis.

Tetralogy of Fallot

In Tetralogy of Fallot there is an anterior-superior displacement of the infundibular septum, resulting in pulmonary stenosis, right ventricular hypertrophy, a ventricular septal defect, and an overriding aorta The subsequent increase in right ventricular pressure produces a right to left shunt and early cyanosis.

Fig. 4-12. Tetralogy of Fallot.

Tetralogy of Fallot is also the most common cause of early cyanosis. Patients will often suffer "cyanotic spells" and they may squat to lessen the right to left shunting and increase venous return. The hypertrophic right ventricle will also cause the heart to resemble a "boot" on x-rays. Complete surgical repair is possible for patients with classic Tetralogy of Fallot, but pulmonary atresia and dilated bronchioles may complicate some cases.

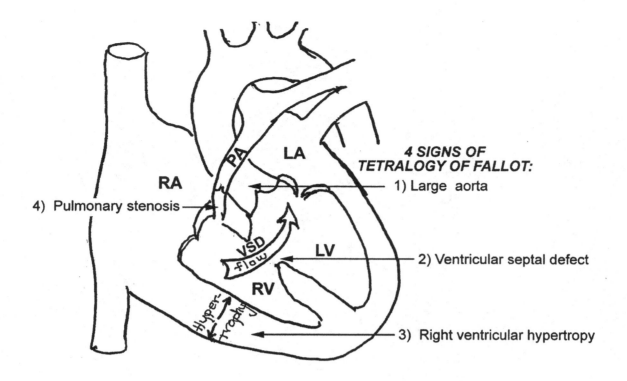

4 SIGNS OF TETRALOGY OF FALLOT:

1) Large aorta

2) Ventricular septal defect

3) Right ventricular hypertropy

4) Pulmonary stenosis

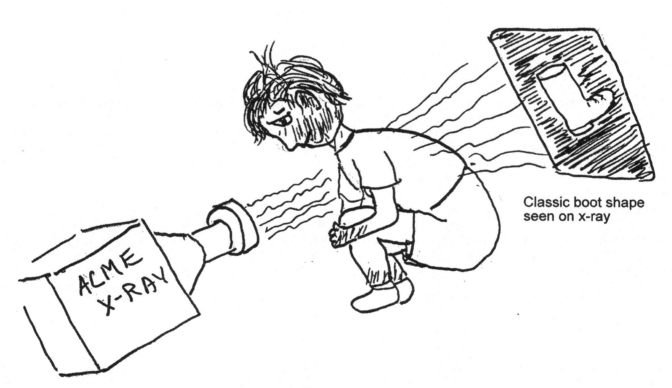

Classic boot shape seen on x-ray

Figure 4-12.

Transposition of the Great Vessels

In transposition of the great arteries, the aorta arises anteriorly from the right ventricle and the pulmonary artery arises posteriorly from the left ventricle. There is a higher incidence of transposition of the great vessels in children of diabetic mothers. Most infants will die within a few months after birth without surgical correction. A shunt, such as in a ventricular septal defect, atrial septal defect, or a patent ductus arteriosus, must be present to allow some oxygenation of blood in order to sustain life.

Truncus Arteriosus

A persistent truncus arteriosus arises from a failure of the separation of the embryonal truncus arteriosis, causing one large artery for both the pulmonary artery and the aorta. This structure receives blood from both the right and left ventricles, resulting in a mixture of deoxygenated and oxygenated blood that causes pulmonary hypertension and early cyanosis.

Coarctation of the Aorta

Coarctation of the aorta is a narrowing of the aorta, usually distal to the origin of the subclavian arteries. Coarctation of the aorta has a higher incidence in males. However, **females with Turner's syndrome are also at higher risk**. Approximately 50% of cases occur with a bicuspid aortic valve. Clinically, the extent of symptoms will vary depending upon the degree of stenosis.

Patients with aortic coarctation may present with notching of the ribs on x-ray due to overcompensation of collateral circulation and dilation of the intercostal arteries. Hypertension of the upper extremities and weak pulses in the lower extremities are also common. Therefore, it is essential to check femoral pulses during the physical exam.

Coarctation of the aorta is classified into an infantile and an adult type. The **infantile type** is preductal because it occurs proximal to the insertion of a patent ductus arteriosus. Children will not survive the neonatal period without surgical intervention because of the extent of deoxygenated blood entering the systemic circulation, resulting in early cyanosis. The **adult type** occurs beyond the insertion of a closed ductus arteriosus. The adult type is less severe, and children may go unrecognized until adulthood.

Hypoplastic Left Heart Syndrome

Hypoplastic left heart syndrome is an obstruction of the left ventricular outflow tract due to severe aortic stenosis or atresia that results in an underdevelopment of the left ventricle and ascending aorta. Fibroelastosis of the left ventricular endocardium can also cause the endocardium to become dense. The ductus arteriosus allows blood to reach the aorta and perfuse the coronary arteries. If the ductus is closed, this condition is not compatible with life, and children will often die within a week of birth.

5

Hematopathology

OVERVIEW

Hematopathology deals with the pathology of blood cells. This subject can be divided into two main categories:

1. **Myeloid**: from the bone marrow; commonly refers to red blood cells (RBCs), granulocytes (eosinophils, neutrophils, and basophils), monocyte/macrophages, and platelets
2. **Lymphoid**: from lymph nodal, thymic, and splenic tissue; commonly refers to B and T lymphocytes and natural killer cells

Although this division is beneficial for study purposes, it is important to remember that myeloid and lymphoid cells are intimately related and can cause pathologies with each other. For example, a patient with a lymphoid leukemia also can have anemia as a result of diseased white blood cells infiltrating the bone marrow.

NORMAL HEMATOPOIESIS

Hematopoiesis, the process of blood cell development, begins in the yolk sac within the first month of fetal development. As the fetus grows, the liver is the primary site of hematopoiesis, with some also occurring in the thymus, spleen, and lymph nodes. By the time the baby is born, the entire bone marrow is the principal source of hematopoiesis. Portions of the marrow (**red marrow**) of the adult humerus, femur, pelvis, skull, vertebrate, and ribs will continue to produce blood cells, while the remainder is replaced by fat (**yellow marrow**). If the marrow is compromised in any fashion, the body can compensate by making blood cells in the liver, spleen, and lymph nodes again, also known as **extramedullary hematopoiesis**.

Fig. 5-1. Blood cell differentiation from a pluipotent stem cell. All blood cells originate from "**pluripotent**" stem cells, meaning that they are capable of forming many different cell types. Stem cells give rise to a common myeloid stem cell that makes — you guessed it — the myeloid cells and a common lymphoid stem cell that makes the lymphoid cells. Once a stem cell develops into the precursors to a given blood cell, it is committed to only becoming that blood cell type.

MYELOID PATHOLOGY
Anemia

Anemia simply is a reduced number of red blood cells. Regardless of the cause, all severely anemic patients have similar findings: weakness, pallor of the skin, malaise (feeling ill), and dyspnea (shortness of breath) on exertion. The lack of adequate tissue oxygenation can result in **koilonychia** (brittle, concave "spoon-shaped" nails).

Anemia is diagnosed by the use of a peripheral blood smear and complete blood count (CBC). The peripheral blood smear allows one to evaluate the relative shapes and sizes of the blood cells and whether they contain pathologic inclusions. These RBC morphologies and inclusions are helpful in determining the etiology of an anemia

Fig. 5-2. Morphology of different RBCs and inclusions.

1. **Schistocytes** are fragments of RBCs, and are associated with microangiopathic hemolytic anemias. They are also known as "helmet cells."
2. **Target cells** are RBCs with a rim of pallor around a normochromatic core, and they look like targets! These are associated with thalassemia, liver disease, and hemoglobin C disease.
3. **Spherocytes** are hyperchromic sphere-shaped RBCs with no central pallor, which are associated

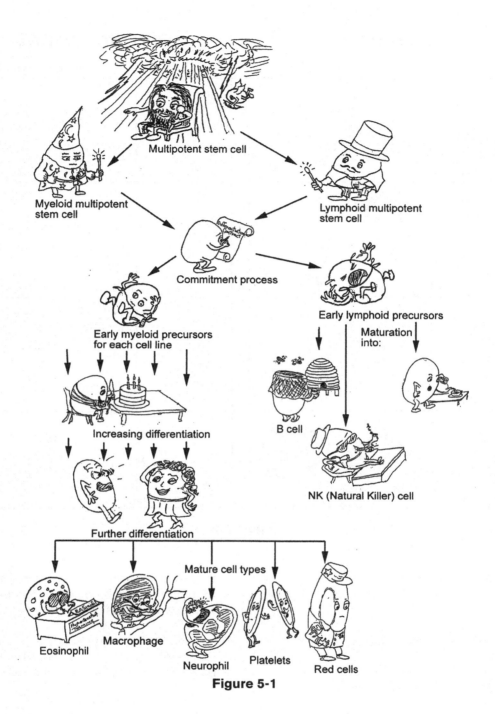

Multipotent stem cell

Myeloid multipotent stem cell

Lymphoid multipotent stem cell

Commitment process

Early myeloid precursors for each cell line

Early lymphoid precursors

Maturation into:

Increasing differentiation

B cell

NK (Natural Killer) cell

Further differentiation

Mature cell types

Eosinophil

Macrophage

Neurophil

Platelets

Red cells

Figure 5-1

with immune hemolytic anemia and hereditary spherocytosis.

4. **Sickle cells** are banana-shaped RBCs associated with sickle cell anemia.

5. **Howell-Jolly bodies** are characterized as a single, smooth, round remnant of nuclear DNA normally removed from immature RBCs by the spleen. They are associated with hemolytic anemia, megaloblastic anemia, and splenectomy. (*Slide 5.1*)

6. **Pappenheimer bodies** are multiple inclusions of iron in a cluster that are normally removed from immature RBCs by the spleen. They are associated with hemolytic anemia, thalassemia, and splenectomy.

7. **Basophilic stippling** consists of granules of RNA from precipitation of ribosomes uniformly distributed across the RBC. These are associated with lead poisoning and thalassemia.

RBC FORMS

TYPE	HOW IT IS NAMED
Helmet Cells	
Target Cells	
Spherocytes	
Sickle Cells	

RBC INCLUSIONS

TYPE	HOW IT IS NAMED
Howell-Jolly Bodies	
Pappenheimer (Pepperhammer) Bodies	
RBC Stippling (Coarse, e.g. lead poisoning)	
Heinz Bodies	

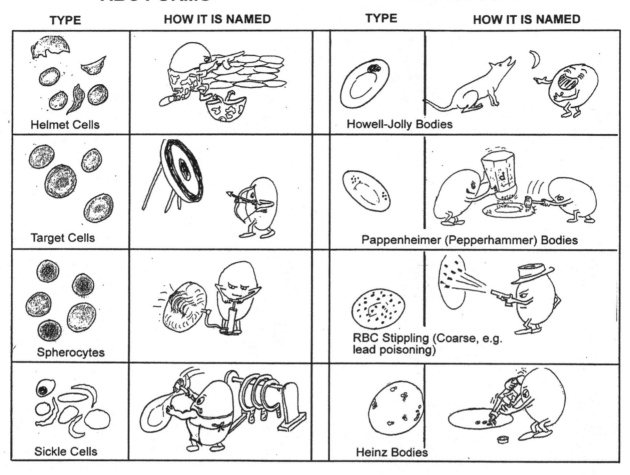

Figure 5-2

8. **Heinz bodies** are inclusions of denatured hemoglobin associated with thalassemia and G6PD deficiency.

The complete blood count (CBC) contains these important variables:

1. The RBC, white blood cell, and platelet count.
2. Hemoglobin concentration.
3. **Hematocrit**: the percentage of whole blood that is comprised of RBCs.
4. Mean Corpuscular Volume (**MCV**) is used to estimate the size of RBCs, because it is a measurement of the average volume taken up by an RBC. An MCV >100 mm^3 indicates a **macrocytic** anemia. An MCV <80 mm^3 indicates a **microcytic** anemia (an MCV between 80-100 mm^3 is **normocytic**).
5. Mean Corpuscular Hemoglobin (**MCH**) is the average weight of hemoglobin in an RBC.
6. Mean Corpuscular Hemoglobin Concentration (**MCHC**) equals the MCH divided by the MCV; and

it is used to determine whether the RBCs are pale from less hemoglobin (**hypochromic**) or strongly colored due to lots of hemoglobin (**hyperchromic**).

For memorization purposes, it is beneficial to classify the types of anemia into **macrocytic**, **microcytic**, and **normocytic** anemias based on the MCV.

Macrocytic (Megaloblastic) Anemias

Think **"Vitamin deficiencies make RBCs large, just like the bellies of malnourished children"** to remember the two major causes of macrocytic anemia: Vitamin B12 and folate deficiency. These anemias are also known as **"megaloblastic"** anemias because they are characterized by **large RBC precursors** (blasts) in the patient's bone marrow. Both vitamin B12 and folate are needed to synthesize the DNA base, thymidine. Remember that uracil is used rather than thymidine in RNA. Therefore, deficiencies in B12 and folate will affect DNA synthesis but not really RNA or protein synthesis. Thus, the cytoplasm of the cell grows more efficiently than the nucleus. All RBC precursors become enlarged, as well as the **neutrophils,** which are **characteristically hypersegmented** (having five or more nuclear lobes rather than two or three). In addition, the abnormal blood cells undergo apoptosis due to poor nuclear maturation, leading to **pancytopenia** (low levels of all blood cells).

Fig. 5-3. Hypersegmented neutrophils. Continual nuclear production without cell division. *Slide 5.2* shows RBC macrocytosis.

Vitamin B12 Deficiency and Pernicious Anemia: Vitamin B12 (cobalamin) is found in a diet that incorporates animal products. Therefore, strict vegetarians are at risk for a deficiency in Vitamin B12. Dietary deficiency is an important cause of Vitamin B12-related megaloblastic anemia, but pernicious anemia is the most common. Pernicious anemia is believed to be an immune-mediated atrophic gastritis caused by antibodies to either intrinsic factor or stomach parietal cells. Vitamin B12 binds with the parietal cell-produced intrinsic factor and is absorbed in the terminal ileum. Therefore, anti-intrinsic factor prevents the adequate absorption of cobalamin from the intestine. This factor is a specific marker for pernicious anemia. Patients also can be diagnosed by a positive Schilling test, in which their impaired cobalamin absorption is corrected by oral intrinsic factor.

Fig. 5-4. The Schilling test.

Pernicious anemia usually is insidious in its onset and occurs in patients in their fifth to eighth decades. Patients with pernicious anemia are at an increased risk of **gastric carcinoma** as a direct consequence of the gastritis.

There are two important biochemical pathways that utilize Vitamin B12. Methylated cobalamin serves as a cofactor for methionine synthase, which generates tetrahydrofolate that can be utilized to make thymidine bases for DNA synthesis. This pathway explains why both folate and Vitamin B12 deficiency cause similar megaloblastic anemias. However, cobalamin-deficient patients also have **neurologic symptoms** that folic acid deficient patients do **not.** This is possibly due to Vitamin B12's other action as a cofactor for methyl-malonyl mutase, the enzyme that produces succinyl CoA from methylmalonyl CoA. Excess methylmalonic acid may accumulate in neurons, resulting in myelin breakdown, particularly in the dorsolateral spinal tracts. This syndrome, characterized by impaired position and vibration sense in the lower limbs, ataxic gait, and hyperreflexia, is called **subacute combined degeneration (SACD).**

Vitamin B12-deficient patients also have **beefy red stomatitis** (very red inflamed tongue). Other possible

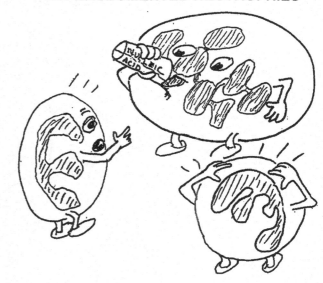

HYPERSEGMENTED NEUTROPHILS

Figure 5-3.

causes of vitamin B12 deficiency include increased need (as in pregnancy and cancer) and impaired absorption (as in ileal resection, inflammatory bowel disease, and *Diphyllobothrium latum,* a fish tape worm).

Folate Deficiency: Folate deficiency manifests similarly to Vitamin B12 deficiency; however, the neurologic symptoms are absent. Folic acid is introduced into the human diet mostly by uncooked leafy green vegetables. It is absorbed in the jejunum, where it can be stored for months. Folate deficiency usually is seen in chronic alcoholics and the elderly due to their poor diets. Other causes are related to intestinal malabsorption: sprue, Giardia lamblia, chemotherapeutic folic acid antagonists, etc. Of special note, it is important to identify whether a patient is Vitamin B12 deficient as well, because administering folic acid alone will mask the megaloblastic anemia without curing the neurologic symptoms of Vitamin B12 deficiency. SACD is irreversible!

Microcytic Anemias

Iron Deficiency and Chronic Blood Loss: Iron deficiency probably is the most common nutritional disorder in the world. Most iron is introduced in the body by digesting heme from animal products. The rate of absorption of iron in the duodenum then regulates body iron levels. Iron is utilized functionally in hemoglobin, myoglobin, and other enzymes. It also may be stored as hemosiderin or ferritin. Iron deficiency will not cause anemia until these stores of iron are depleted.

Iron deficiency anemia is characterized by a **hypochromic microcytic anemia,** because lack of iron,

SCHILLING TEST

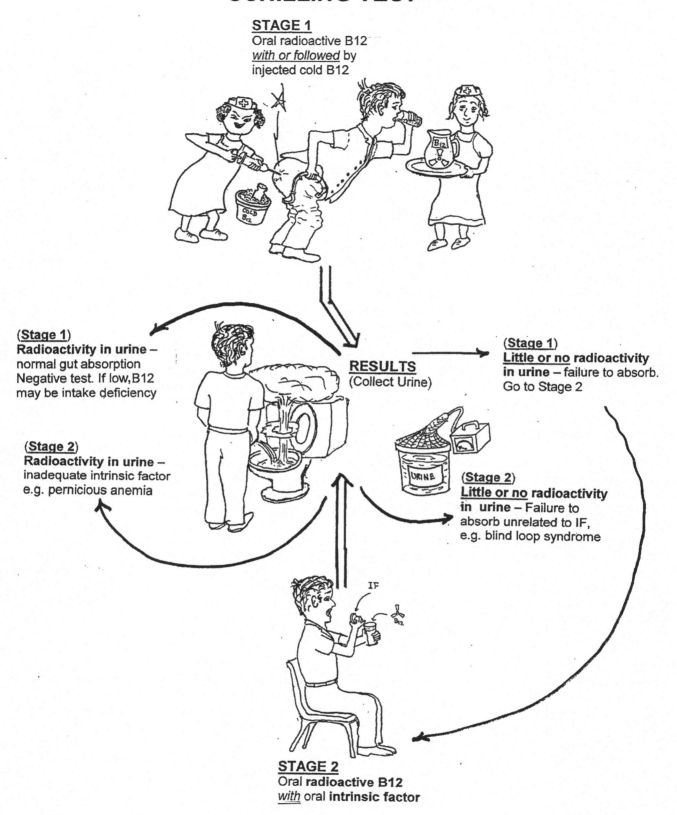

STAGE 1
Oral radioactive B12
with or followed by
injected cold B12

(Stage 1)
Radioactivity in urine –
normal gut absorption
Negative test. If low, B12
may be intake deficiency

(Stage 2)
Radioactivity in urine –
inadequate intrinsic factor
e.g. pernicious anemia

RESULTS
(Collect Urine)

(Stage 1)
Little or no radioactivity
in urine – failure to absorb.
Go to Stage 2

(Stage 2)
Little or no radioactivity
in urine – Failure to
absorb unrelated to IF,
e.g. blind loop syndrome

STAGE 2
Oral **radioactive B12**
with oral **intrinsic factor**

Figure 5-4

and thus hemoglobin, will decrease the size and pigmentation of the RBC. (*Slide 5.3*)

The patient's **hemoglobin, hematocrit, serum iron, and ferritin levels will also be decreased with an increased total plasma iron binding capacity.** (The total iron binding capacity increases because there are empty binding sites for iron on the transferrin molecules.) Severe iron deficiency can result in hair loss, atrophy of the tongue and gastric mucosa, intestinal malabsorption, and **Plummer-Vinson syndrome** (iron deficiency anemia, atrophic glossitis, and esophageal webs). Iron deficiency has four common causes:

1. **Dietary deficiency** commonly occurs in developing countries, but also can occur in infants in the western world due to inadequate amounts of iron in milk. The elderly, the indigent, and alcoholics are at risk as well.
2. **Impaired duodenal absorption** can occur in cases of chronic diarrhea or sprue.
3. **Increased need** for iron in young children and pregnant women is a cause.
4. **Chronic blood loss** is the **major** cause of iron deficiency anemia. Women of child-bearing age are likely to have iron deficiency just from menstruating. Any cause of external hemorrhage from the gastrointestinal or urogenital tract can cause anemia. For example, **peptic ulcer, colon cancer,** and **uterine cancer** commonly result in iron deficiency anemia. This is why iron deficiency anemia in adult men or postmenopausal women is due to gastrointestinal bleeding until proven otherwise. **Cancer must be ruled out in these patients!**

Thalassemias: Thalassemias are a group of genetic disorders that cause decreased production of one of the two globin chains in hemoglobin A (remember normal adult hemoglobin is comprised of a tetramer of two alpha and two beta globin chains, $alpha_2beta_2$). Patients will have symptoms related to **hypochromic microcytic anemia** because they produce inadequate amounts of normal hemoglobin. Additionally, excess unpaired globin chains will precipitate in the RBC, causing more problems. Peripheral blood smears will demonstrate **target cells, basophilic stippling, marked anisocytosis** (variations in RBC size), **and poikilocytosis** (variations in RBC shape). (*Slide 5.4*)

Thalassemia is most common in people from **Africa, Southeast Asia, India,** and the **Mediterranean.** The thalassemias are classified based on which globin chain is affected.

1. **Beta Thalassemia.** There are two genes that code for the beta globin chain of HbA. Beta thalassemia can be due to any of a variety of different defects in the beta globin genes—usually **point mutations.** The mutated gene product could either produce no beta globin chains ($beta^0$) or diminished numbers of the chain ($beta^+$). The severity of the patient's symptoms is based on heterozygosity of the gene. **Thalassemia major** occurs in various genotypic states ($beta^0/beta^0$, $beta^+/beta^+$ or $beta^0/beta^+$). Normal beta globin chains will precipitate in the RBC, causing cell membrane damage, leading to apoptosis of the RBC or destruction in the spleen (which causes **splenomegaly**). The resulting severe anemia will cause a compensatory increase in erythropoietin production of the kidney, which leads to **extramedullary hematopoiesis** and **bone marrow hyperplasia.**

The patient with beta thalassemia will have distorted long bones, facial bones, and cranial bones in a characteristic **"crew-cut" appearance.**

Fig. 5-5. Characteristic "crew cut" x-ray of beta thalassemia, and various RBC morphologies seen on a blood smear.

Thalassemia major manifests as severe anemia in babies that are **6-9 months old,** correlating to the time that HbF ($alpha_2gamma_2$) **production is exchanged for HbA.** In fact, the adult body will later compensate with an abnormal **increase in HbF,** since it does not use beta globin chains. Transfusions must be given to maintain life. The coupling of multiple transfusions and RBC destruction puts the patient at risk for **secondary hemochromatosis** (acquired excessive accumulations of iron) and cardiac disease. **Thalassemia minor** occurs in the heterozygous state ($beta^0$/ beta or $beta^+$/beta) and causes a mild anemia. The body compensates for inadequate HbA by producing **HbA$_2$ ($alpha_2delta_2$).** Thalassemia minor might provide **resistance to falciparum malaria.**

2. **Alpha Thalassemia.** Four genes code for the alpha globin chain of HbA. The severity of disease is based on how many of these genes are deleted. If one gene is deleted, then the person will have no obvious pathology and be a **silent carrier** of alpha thalassemia. Two gene deletions result in **alpha thalassemia trait,** in which the patient has mild anemia similar to beta thalassemia minor. Three gene deletions will result in **Hemoglobin H Disease.** In these patients, beta globin chains will form tetramers (called **HbH**) that have a higher affinity for oxygen than HbA, leading to hypoxia and a moderate anemia. Four gene deletions result in **hydrops fetalis** (generalized edema of the fetus). The gamma chains of fetal hemoglobin will form tetramers called **hemoglobin Barts (Hb Barts)** which have a very high affinity for oxygen so that no oxygen can be released to perfuse the tissues. Therefore, intrauterine death occurs.

BETA-THALASSEMIA

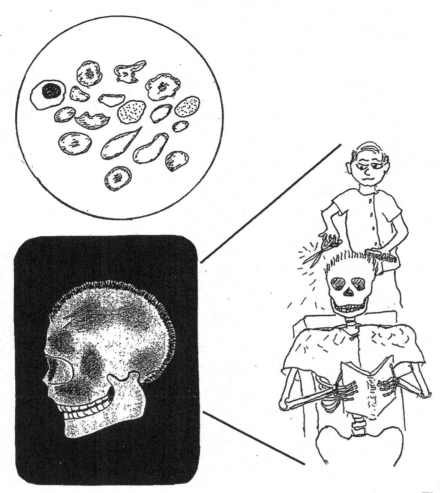

Figure 5-5

Normocytic Anemias

Acute Blood Loss: Acute blood loss is a sudden loss of RBCs and plasma in parallel; therefore, anemia due to this cause will at first not necessarily show a drop in hemoglobin or hematocrit. Until the body has time to compensate, while the patient is anemic, the blood smear may demonstrate a normocytic normochromic morphology. The symptoms of acute blood loss are more associated with sudden hypovolemia with resultant shock and death than typical anemic symptoms. If the patient bleeds internally, iron can be reabsorbed, but if the bleeding is external, iron deficiency anemia may result. As the kidneys compensate by producing erythropoietin to stimulate hematopoiesis, the anemia might become hyperchromic. There is an increase in reticulocytes (young, blue-staining RBCs).

Anemia of Chronic Disease: **Chronic infections, chronic immune disorders** (e.g., rheumatoid arthritis) and **cancer** have been associated with impaired RBC production, resulting in mild normocytic normochromic anemia. It is hypothesized that cytokines produced by these conditions inhibit erythropoietin and hematopoiesis. Anemia of chronic disease can **imitate iron deficiency anemia** with a hypochromic microcytic anemia and decreased serum iron levels. However, the **total plasma iron binding capacity is decreased, and the ferritin level is increased**.

Bone Marrow Failure: Since the bone marrow is the site of hematopoiesis, it is intuitive that bone marrow failure can cause anemia. Along with typical anemic symptoms, such patients also will have petechiae and ecchymoses from decreased platelet counts (**thrombocytopenia**) and greater susceptibility to infection from decreased granulocyte counts. There are several types of bone marrow failure:

1. **Aplastic anemia** is a type of bone marrow failure in which myeloid stem cells are suppressed, resulting

in **pancytopenia** and **hypocellular bone marrow**. Aplastic anemia is most likely to be idiopathic; however, when the cause is known, it is usually due to toxic exposure to radiation, pharmaceuticals (particularly chloramphenicol), and viral infection (like parvovirus). Removal of the offensive agent can reverse the pancytopenia, but aplastic anemia has an unpredictable prognosis.

2. **Fanconi anemia** is a special, rare form of aplastic anemia in which there is an autosomal recessive defect in DNA repair. Patients with Fanconi anemia have pancytopenia as well as hypoplasia of the kidney, spleen, and bone.

3. **Myelophthistic anemia** has the same consequences as aplastic anemia, but it is caused by replacement of the bone marrow by entities like malignant neoplasms, fibrosis, and granulomas.

4. **Pure red cell aplasia** is a rare form of bone marrow failure in which only the erythroid elements of the bone marrow are suppressed, while granulocytes and platelets develop naturally. This type of failure has been associated with neoplasia, particularly thymic tumors.

Hemolytic Anemias

Intrinsic Hemolytic Anemias: Hemolytic anemias are characterized by premature destruction of RBCs. If red cell destruction occurs within the vasculature, hemoglobin can be detected in the patient's blood and urine. The patient will be jaundiced from high levels of **unconjugated bilirubin**. If red cell destruction occurs outside the vasculature, for example in the spleen, then the patient's symptoms will be anemia and jaundice. Intrinsic hemolytic anemias are due to **primary disorders of the RBC**. They usually are **hereditary**.

1. **Hereditary Spherocytosis (HS) (*Slide 5.6*)**. HS is characterized by an **autosomal dominant** inherited **defect in the RBC membrane**, which makes it less resilient, resulting in sequestration and destruction of erythrocytes in the spleen. This disease commonly occurs in Northern Europeans. Mutations in genes coding for several different RBC cytoskeletal proteins can cause HS, with defects in **spectrin** or **ankyrin** being the most significant. Consequently, the red cell is unstable and forms a sphere, which permits the least amount of surface area for a given volume. These rigid spherocytes cannot easily "squeeze" through splenic capillary beds and are thus destroyed, resulting in moderate splenomegaly. Normally, HS patients have a clinically stable course unless infection with parvovirus challenges them, causing an aplastic crisis.

Spherocytes can be detected in patients by the osmotic fragility test in which the abnormal cells lyse when incubated in hypotonic saline.

2. **Paroxysmal Nocturnal Hemoglobinuria (PNH)** is a rare form of intrinsic hemolytic anemia that is actually acquired due to a somatic mutation in a gene that results in decreased synthesis of an important membrane protein called GPI. Since some GPI-linked proteins inactivate complement, in the absence of GPI, red cells are susceptible to hemolysis by complement. Although the name would suggest that patients wake up in the middle of the night with bloody urine, this phenomenon only occurs in 25% of the cases. Most patients have symptoms of chronic hemolysis.

3. **Glucose-6-Phosphate Dehydrogenase Deficiency (G6PD Deficiency)**. Oxidation reactions producing hydrogen peroxide are destructive to RBCs if they do not have the means to combat the oxidative stress. Erythrocytes reduce hydrogen peroxide and other oxidants by a biochemical redox cascade that begins with glucose-6-phosphate dehydro-genase (G6PD). G6PD is an enzyme that produces NADPH. NADPH is used to reduce glutathione which, in turn, reduces hydrogen peroxide. Therefore, if an RBC is deficient in G6PD, it is susceptible to damage by oxidants.

Fig. 5-6. The G6PD pathway. A deficiency in this pathway is destructive to RBCs due to the loss of the redox pathway.

G6PD Deficiency is an **X-linked recessive** genetic disorder that is typically seen in African Americans and Mediterraneans. Patients experience hemolytic anemia after exposure to an oxidant stress, most commonly an infection but also certain drugs (antimalarials and sulfonamides) and fava beans. The RBC hemoglobin becomes oxidized and precipitates as **Heinz bodies**. Splenic macrophages then remove the Heinz bodies by "biting" them out of the cell, leaving characteristic **bite cells** (they look like they were bitten) and **spherocytes** (*Slide 5.5*).

G6PD Deficiency might **provide protection from falciparum malaria**. To remember the salient features of this disease, think of the famous Hannibal saying, "**I ate his RBCs** (think of bite cells) **with some fava beans and some nice Heinz ketchup. Phtt, phtt, phttb (disturbing slurping noise)**."

4. **Sickle Cell Anemia** is caused by a **point mutation in the beta globin gene on chromosome 6, which results in the substitution of valine for glutamic acid**. This altered hemoglobin (called **HbS**) will

THE G6PD PATHWAY

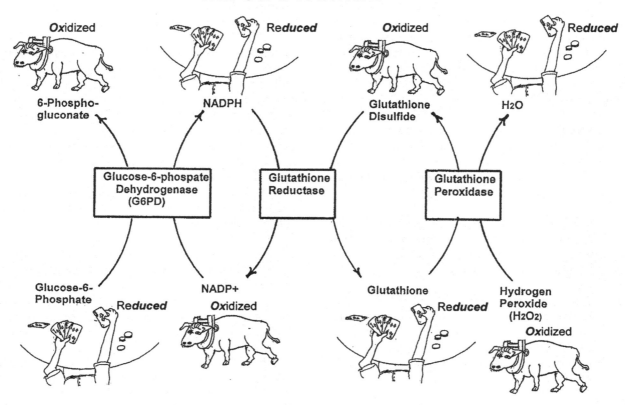

Figure 5-6.

initially form reversible aggregates in conditions of low oxygen tension, which distort the RBC membrane into sickle shapes (the RBCs look like a banana). With repeated episodes of hypoxia and sickling, the HbS polymers will permanently stiffen and distort the RBC shape. (*Slide 5.7*)

As in the case of hereditary spherocytosis, the abnormal RBC morphology in sickle cell anemia doesn't traverse small vessels well, leading to obstruction of the microvasculature and hemolysis. This process causes **young children with sickle cell disease to have congested, enlarged spleens.** Repetitive occlusion of the splenic vessels throughout life will cause ischemia and splenic infarct usually by age 6. The spleen is thus replaced by fibrous tissue—a process called **autosplenectomy.**

The microvasculature of many organs is in jeopardy in sickle cell anemia. Exposure to infection, dehydration, or acidosis can cause a severely painful vaso-occlusive crisis in which the small blood vessels of the bones, lungs, liver, brain, spleen, and penis can become occluded, leading to ischemia. Patients will have a lifelong chronic hemolytic anemia that also makes them susceptible to infection.

Sickle cell trait is carried in 30% of Africans and 8% of African Americans, perhaps due to its ability to protect the patient from falciparum malaria. The heterozygous state results in an asymptomatic carrier, whereas the homozygous state leads to sickle cell disease. Sickle cell trait is also commonly seen in association with other genetic disorders of hemoglobin, such as thalassemia. The other hemoglobinopathy can reduce or worsen the course of sickle cell disease. (Or the sickle cell trait can reduce or worsen the course of the other disease!)

Extrinsic Hemolytic Anemias: Extrinsic hemolytic anemias are due to forces outside of the RBC itself. They are **acquired** disorders.

1. **Immunohemolytic Anemias** are **antibody-mediated,** whether caused by an autoimmune reaction or an adverse drug reaction. They are detected by a **positive direct Coombs' test.**

Fig. 5-7. The direct Coombs' test. Anti-human globulin precipitates RBCs coated with endogenous antibodies.

Warm antibody immunohemolytic anemia is the most common form. It is caused by **IgG** or

IgA class antibodies to the red cell that are active at normal body temperature. These antibodies cause the cell membrane to be destroyed partially by phagocytes, resulting in **spherocytosis** and **splenomegaly**. **Cold Agglutinin Immuno-hemolytic Anemia** is caused by **IgM** class antibodies that are active at cold temperatures. You can actually agglutinate the patient's blood at the bedside by cooling it in ice and then unclotting the blood by warming it in your hand! This phenomenon is characteristic of antibodies produced in response to mycoplasma pneumonia and infectious mononucleosis.

Patients with cold agglutinins are usually asymptomatic but can be particularly susceptible to Raynaud phenomenon (cyanosis in body parts exposed to cold).

Cold Hemolysin Hemolytic Anemia is a more severe hemolytic anemia with hemoglobinuria after exposure to cold temperatures (called paroxysmal cold hemoglobinuria). It is caused by **IgG class antibodies and complement**.

2. **Mechanical.** Obviously, physical trauma can cause hemolysis. The most significant cause of mechanical trauma to the RBC is by **artificial mechanical heart valves**, which cause turbulent flow and essentially "rip" the RBCs as they pass, producing **schistocytes**.
3. **Microangiopathic** hemolytic anemias are another form of trauma to the RBC. They are due to pathologically narrowed vessels through which RBCs are forced to squeeze, and thereby are "sliced" into pieces, producing **schistocytes** (*Slide 5.8*).

Schistocytes are seen in **disseminated intravascular coagulation (DIC)**, **thrombotic thrombocytopenic purpura (TTP)**, and **hemolytic-uremic syndrome (HUS)**, but **not** in ITP. (Refer to Bleeding Disorders.)

BLEEDING DISORDERS

Bleeding disorders, or **hemorrhagic diatheses**, are disorders of excessive bleeding. They can be caused by abnormalities in blood vessels, platelets, or clotting factors. To understand these diseases and how they are clinically diagnosed, it is important to review the coagulation cascade.

Fig. 5-8. The clotting cascade. Although the clotting cascade can be very difficult to learn, it can be simplified into a few facts that are important to remember. The clotting cascade is divided into an intrinsic and extrinsic pathway. Each begins with different clotting factors, but they converge at the same step: the **activation of factor X**.

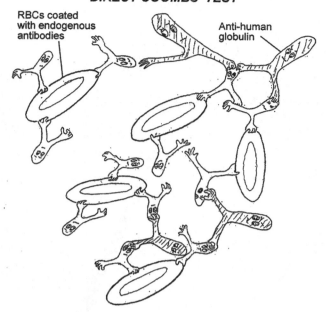

DIRECT COOMBS' TEST

RBCs coated with endogenous antibodies

Anti-human globulin

Figure 5-7.

The **extrinsic pathway** occurs during tissue injury when **tissue factor** is released. Tissue factor activates factor VII, so that it can activate factor X.

On the other hand, the **intrinsic pathway** begins with **factor XII** activation (**XIIa**), which eventually leads to **activated factors XI (XIa) and VIII (VIIIa) together activating factor X**. It is important to remember that **von Willebrand factor is a carrier protein for factor VIII and is essential for its proper activation**. After factor X is activated, the intrinsic and extrinsic pathways are identical as the "common pathway," which concludes with **the formation of fibrin and a clot**.

Laboratory diagnosis of the bleeding disorders depends on an understanding of the difference between the intrinsic and extrinsic coagulation pathways:

• The **prothrombin time (PT)** is an assay that measures the effectiveness of the **extrinsic pathway** and the common pathway. Therefore, problems with factors VII, X, V, II, or I (refer to the right side of Figure 5.8) will prolong the PT.

• The **partial thromboplastin time (PTT)**, in contrast, measures the effectiveness of the **intrinsic pathway** and the common pathway. Therefore, problems with factors XII, XI, IX, VIII, von Willebrand, X, V, II, or I (refer to the left side of Fig. 5.8) will prolong the PTT. **To remember the difference, think of the PTT as being a longer abbreviation, and thus the longer pathway (intrinsic) is measured by the PTT.**

Other important laboratory tests for diagnosis of bleeding disorders include the bleeding time (time it

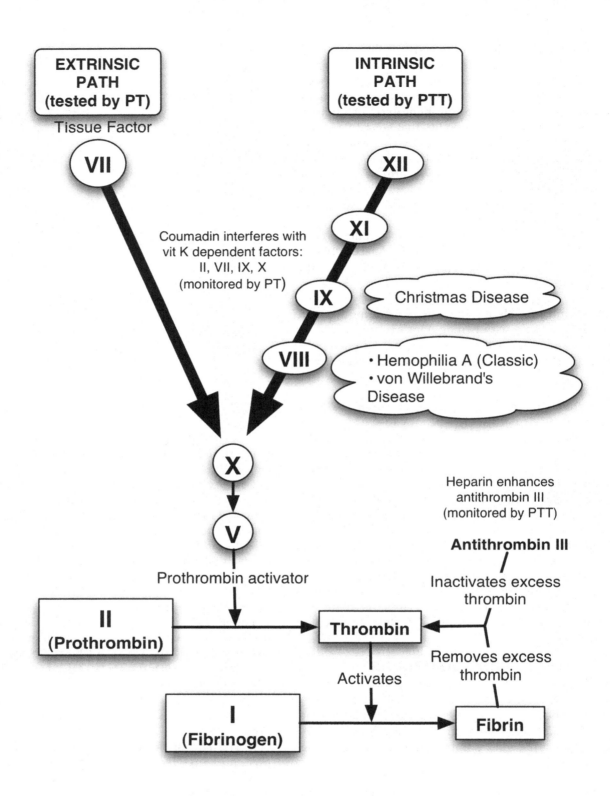

EXTRINSIC PATH (tested by PT)

Tissue Factor

VII

INTRINSIC PATH (tested by PTT)

XII

XI

Coumadin interferes with vit K dependent factors: II, VII, IX, X (monitored by PT)

IX

Christmas Disease

VIII

• Hemophilia A (Classic)
• von Willebrand's Disease

X

V

Prothrombin activator

Heparin enhances antithrombin III (monitored by PTT)

Antithrombin III

Inactivates excess thrombin

II (Prothrombin) → **Thrombin**

Removes excess thrombin

Activates

I (Fibrinogen) → **Fibrin**

Figure 5-8

takes for a cut in the skin to stop bleeding; measures platelet function qualitatively), platelet counts, fibrin split products (d-dimer) level (measurement of how much fibrin has been broken down), and the actual levels of specific clotting factors in the patient.

Vessel Wall Abnormalities

Abnormalities in the vasculature of small blood vessels can cause bleeding disorders. Many diseases can cause blood vessel injury, including drug reactions, infections by organisms such as *Streptococcus pneumoniae*, collagen vascular disorders such as Ehlers-Danlos syndrome or scurvy, and amyloidosis. Laboratory screening tests will usually be normal in the case of vessel wall abnormalities, but the bleeding time might be prolonged.

Platelet Abnormalities

Platelets are necessary for proper blood clotting. Therefore, it is intuitive that platelet abnormalities can cause abnormal bleeding. There are some bleeding disorders in which platelets lack cell surface proteins necessary for adhesion (**Bernard-Soulier Disease**) or for aggregation (**Glanzmann's thrombasthenia**). In these cases, only the **bleeding time will be prolonged** on laboratory diagnosis. Other hemorrhagic diatheses caused by platelets are due to decreased platelet number (**thrombocytopenia**) rather than platelet function abnormalities.

Thrombocytopenia can occur secondary to many causes, including **drugs like heparin, AIDS, SLE, and viral infections**. Four important disease entities exhibit thrombocytopenia. It is worthwhile to learn the differences among the four, because they can be easily confused.

1. **Immune Thrombocytopenic Purpura (ITP)** is an **autoimmune disorder** in which the body makes antibodies to platelets. The antibody-bound platelets are then phagocytosized, leading to thrombocytopenia. Certain risk factors predispose to ITP; it also can occur idiopathically. The **chronic form** of ITP usually involves **women younger than 40 years old** who have an insidious onset of petechiae, ecchymoses, and easy bleeding. If left untreated, ITP can result in intracranial hemorrhage. The **acute form** occurs as a **self-limited childhood disease** that is preceded by **viral illness**. ITP is diagnosed by a prolonged bleeding time, decreased platelet count, and all other normal laboratory values. Also, note that ITP is **NOT a microangiopathic hemolytic anemia** because it does not involve microthrombi occluding blood vessels.

2. **Thrombotic Thrombocytopenic Purpura (TTP)** is a syndrome characterized by **widespread thrombus** formation in the microvasculature. This occlusion of the small vessels will cause a **microangiopathic hemolytic anemia**. TTP is caused by either an inherited or acquired **deficiency in an enzyme that normally degrades multimers of von Willebrand factor**. As a consequence, these multimers accumulate and form thrombi upon which platelets adhere. This widespread thrombotic event will consume platelets, leading to thrombocytopenia and its associated bleeding disorder. The pentad to remember for TTP is: **thrombocytopenia, microangiopathic hemolytic anemia, neurologic deficits, fever,** and **renal failure**. Left untreated, TTP will result in multi-organ system failure and death. Laboratory diagnosis reveals an increased bleeding time, decreased platelet count, and normal PT and PTT.

3. **Hemolytic-Uremic Syndrome (HUS)** is very similar in pathogenesis to TTP. HUS is a syndrome involving **thrombocytopenia and microangiopathic hemolytic anemia**. However, it does not classically cause neurologic problems and fever, and it is associated with **acute renal failure**. Patients typically are **children** who present with thrombocytopenia several days after an episode of **bloody diarrhea** from infection with *E. coli 0157:H7*. This strain of *E. coli* produces **Shiga-like toxin** that is thought to damage endothelial cells, which initiates microthrombus formation. Left untreated, HUS can result in irreversible kidney damage and death. Laboratory diagnosis reveals an increased bleeding time, decreased platelet count, and normal PT and PTT.

4. **Disseminated Intravascular Coagulation (DIC).** On the surface DIC sounds like it has the same pathologic mechanism as TTP and HUS, since it also is a **microangiopathic hemolytic anemia** resulting from microvascular occlusion. However, DIC primarily involves thrombus formation due to **activation of the coagulation cascade**. DIC is a disorder that **occurs secondary** to another disease. For example, **complications of pregnancy, leukemia, or gram-negative sepsis** all can cause DIC. The entire coagulation cascade becomes activated, resulting in widespread microthrombi formation. These thrombi consume not only the patient's clotting factors, but also his platelets and fibrin (plasminogen will be activated to destroy the thrombi). Therefore, patients have symptoms of a **thrombotic disorder** (hypoxia, infarct, and hemolytic anemia) as well as a **hemorrhagic disorder** (purpura, bleeding, etc.). DIC has a laboratory diagnosis distinct from TTP and HUS due to the activated clotting cascade: a prolonged PT, PTT, and bleeding time, as well as an increase in fibrin split products (d-dimers). Management of patients

with DIC can be difficult because the physician must balance between anticoagulants and coagulants.

Abnormal Clotting Factors

There are three important hemorrhagic diatheses that are caused by ineffective levels of clotting factors. (Remember as well that **DIC** could also be placed under this subheading because it involves widespread activation and consumption of the coagulation factors.)

1. **Von Willebrand Disease.** Recall that **von Willebrand factor forms a complex with factor VIII** in order for factor VIII to activate factor X. Von Willebrand factor also **mediates platelet adhesion to the extracellular matrix** when forming a clot. Therefore, a deficiency in von Willebrand factor will affect both the intrinsic coagulation pathway and platelet function. This problem is manifested clinically as a **prolonged PTT and a prolonged bleeding time** with all other laboratory values normal. Von Willebrand Disease is an **autosomal dominant** disorder that causes deficiency in von Willebrand factor. It is the **most common hereditary bleeding disorder**, with a frequency of 1%.

2. **Hemophilia A** is the "classic" form of hemophilia. It is an **X-linked recessive** disorder of **factor VIII deficiency or inactivity**. The severity of the hemophilia depends on the mutation's effect on the level of factor VIII activity. In general, patients bruise easily and hemorrhage at points of trauma, most notably in the joints (**hemarthrosis**). Since factor VIII is deficient and we know factor VIII is part of the intrinsic pathway, the PTT will be prolonged. The PT and bleeding time, however, will be normal (the extrinsic pathway is still intact and the platelets are still functional).

3. **Hemophilia B**, also known as **Christmas disease** (named after a hemophilia B patient, not the holiday), is clinically identical to classic hemophilia. It is caused by an **X-linked recessive** disorder of **factor IX**. Since factor IX activates factor X together with factor VIII in the intrinsic pathway, the PTT also will be prolonged with a normal PT and bleeding time in this form of hemophilia.

LYMPHOID PATHOLOGY

Most clinically relevant pathology of lymphoid cells has to do with neoplasia. Many of us have heard of the terms "leukemia" and "lymphoma" and might have vague understandings of their definitions. But, beware! The classification of these neoplasms is notoriously confusing. **Leukemia** classically refers to neoplasms that present with widespread malignant white blood cell (WBC) involvement of the bone marrow and peripheral blood. **Lymphoma**, on the other hand, usually implies neoplastic WBC proliferations in focal masses, particularly in the lymph nodes. Leukemia and lymphoma were originally believed to be discrete entities, but now their characteristics are not so distinct.

Many untreated lymphomas will progress to a leukemic picture. One particular type of leukemia, chronic lymphocytic leukemia, is identical in every way to small lymphocytic lymphoma, except it has more widespread neoplastic involvement.

To complicate matters even more, there are also malignant proliferations of myeloid cells that fall under the leukemia/lymphoma categories as well as another category, **myeloproliferative diseases**. For ease of discussion, the neoplastic myeloid diseases are included in this section in order to keep all of the neoplastic white blood cell diseases (which share characteristics) together.

Additionally, when considering WBC neoplasia, it is important to remember the cell of origin. All of the precursors to the hematopoietic cells can become cancerous, as well as the terminally differentiated blood cells. Therefore, other classifications of leukocyte neoplasms exist (like **functional B-cell neoplasms** or **cutaneous T-cell lymphomas**), based on the cell of origin. **Also keep in mind that cancerous cells will share characteristics (like cell-surface markers or behavior) with their non-neoplastic counterparts.**

Leukemia

Leukemias can be divided into acute or chronic leukemias. **Acute** leukemias are those in which there is a predominance of immature WBC precursors (**blasts**). They are most often diagnosed in **children** and are, in fact, the **most common cancer in children less than 20 years old**. Untreated acute leukemias have a **short, aggressive course** that will lead to death. **Chronic** leukemias are those in which the neoplastic cells are capable of differentiating into more mature cell types. Typically, chronic leukemias are diagnosed in **middle-aged to older adults** and follow a **less aggressive, longer course**.

Acute Lymphoblastic Leukemia (ALL)

ALL is a group of neoplasms in which the cancer cells are of precursor B- or precursor T-cell origin (**lymphoblasts**); with **precursor B-cells** the most common in the leukemic form. (Precursor T-cells are more common in the lymphoma form. See Acute Lymphoblastic Lymphoma.) The malignant cells infiltrate the bone marrow, causing pancytopenia. As a result, patients have anemia, increased risk for infection, and bleeding disorders. These symptoms are nonspecific and identical to those in acute myeloblastic leukemia (AML). More characteristic features of ALL

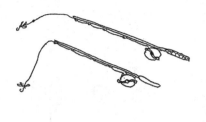
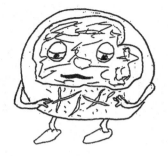

Figure 5-9

include an abrupt onset with bone pain, generalized lymphadenopathy, and hepatosplenomegaly due to tumor infiltration.

Most patients with ALL are **under fifteen years of age** and **white**. There is also an increased incidence of ALL in children with **Down Syndrome**.

Relapses of ALL occur particularly in the **central nervous system** and **testicles**. However, ALL responds favorably to aggressive chemotherapy and greater than ninety percent of children with ALL will achieve complete remission.

Flow cytometry (which looks for cell surface markers on lymphoid cells) and immunostaining for terminal deoxy-nucleotidyltransferase (**TdT**, an enzyme expressed in lymphoblasts) help in the diagnosis of ALL.

Acute Myeloblastic Leukemia (AML)

AML results from the malignant proliferation of **myeloid precursor cells**. It is typically diagnosed in **young adults** of 15-39 years of age. The neoplastic cells infiltrate the patient's bone marrow, causing anemia, thrombocytopenia, and neutropenia, just like in ALL. The malignant cells often contain eosinophilic rod-shaped structures in their cytoplasm, called "**Auer rods**." *(Slide 5.9)*

AML is classified into different categories based on the origin of the myeloid precursor and the level of differentiation of the cells. One distinctive type of AML, named "**acute promyelocytic leukemia**" or "**M3**," contains **multiple Auer rods** in the neoplastic cell.

Fig. 5-9. Auer rods characteristic of AML, "M3" type.

Acute promyelocytic leukemia (M3) is associated with the genetic translocation **t(15:17)**. This translocation produces a protein which halts transcription and the maturation of myeloid cells. Consequently, **all-trans-retinoic acid** can be used to treat M3, because it causes the neoplastic cells to complete their differentiation. Additionally, M3 is a clinically significant AML subtype, as it is associated with a **high incidence of life-threatening DIC**. In general,

AML has a **worse prognosis** and is more difficult to treat than ALL.

Chronic Lymphocytic Leukemia (CLL)

CLL is a neoplastic disease of **B-cells**. CLL is indistinguishable from **small lymphocytic lymphoma (SLL)**, except that it contains a higher level of **lymphocytosis** (increased numbers of lymphocytes in the blood smear). (See Small Lymphocytic Lymphoma.) *(Slide 5.10)*

CLL is the **most common adult leukemia in the Western world**, occurring in adults **over fifty years of age**. CLL/SLL follows a characteristic **indolent course**, in which many patients are either asymptomatic or have nonspecific symptoms. Additionally, the disease interferes with normal immune function. Patients may have **hypogammaglobulinemia** (and increased risk of infection) or develop **warm antibody immunohemolytic anemia**.

CLL/SLL has the capacity to **transform** into prolymphocytic leukemia or diffuse large B-cell lymphoma, both with worse prognosis. The peripheral blood smear will show small, fragile lymphocytes which are commonly destroyed during processing. Thus, these cells are aptly named "**smudge cells**."

Chronic Myelogenous Leukemia (CML)

CML is due to a neoplastic proliferation of a pluripotent stem cell that gives rise to **neoplastic mature myeloid cells**. CML is a **myeloproliferative disease** (see section below). The distinguishing characteristic of this disorder amongst the other myeloproliferative diseases is the presence of the **Philadelphia chromosome**, a reciprocal **t(9:22) translocation** which codes for the *bcr-abl* fusion protein. Bcr-abl results in unregulated excitation of cell division and inhibition of apoptosis. The presence of this fusion protein allows CML to be treated by drugs that inhibit the activity of bcr-abl. (However, this therapy does not elicit full recovery from CML.)

CML has an **insidious onset** and typically occurs in **adults in their fourth and fifth decades**. Extramedullary hematopoiesis is usually stimulated, resulting in **massive splenomegaly**. As the disease progresses,

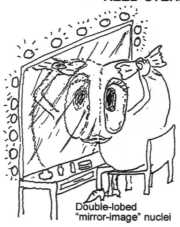

Double-lobed "mirror-image" nuclei

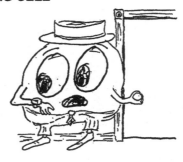

Figure 5-10.

it enters an **"accelerated phase"** in which patients have worsening anemia, thrombocytopenia, and **basophilia** (increased numbers of basophils). Lastly, the disease will terminate as an acute leukemia, with increased levels of blasts (**"blast crisis"**). *(Slide 5.11)*

Lymphoma

Lymphomas are clinically divided into two distinct disease entities: Hodgkin lymphomas and "non-Hodgkin" lymphomas. Regardless of the type, lymphoma typically presents as painless lymph node enlargement.

Hodgkin Lymphoma

Hodgkin lymphoma is characterized by lymphoid neoplasia that **begins in a single lymph node and spreads contiguously to adjacent lymph nodes.** As the disease progresses, it typically will metastasize to the spleen, liver, bone marrow, and lastly other extra-nodal sites. The disease has features of an inflammatory disorder, with high lymphocyte counts, night sweats, and fever.

The diagnostic cell of Hodgkin lymphoma is the **Reed-Sternberg cell**, a multi-nucleated (or a multi-lobulated, single nucleated) neoplastic cell with an inclusion-like nucleolus.

Fig. 5-10. (Slide 5.12) The Reed-Sternberg cell, characterized by large double-lobed "mirror image" nuclei.

The Reed-Sternberg cell is believed to be of **B-cell origin. The more Reed-Sternberg cells there are in the lymph node, the worse the prognosis.** In contrast, **the more reactive inflammatory cells present, the better the prognosis.** Hodgkin lymphoma typically occurs bimodally in young adults and the elderly. It has been associated with infection with Epstein-Barr Virus (EBV).

Non-Hodgkin Lymphomas

In contrast to Hodgkin lymphoma, non-Hodgkin lymphomas usually involve **extranodal sites and multiple lymph nodes in a non-contiguous pattern.** They are associated with **immunosuppression**, particularly in **HIV infected patients**.

1. **Burkitt Lymphoma** is a **B-cell** neoplasm that occurs **endemically in Africa** and **sporadically in developed countries**. The endemic form commonly presents as **jaw and abdominal organ masses**. This form has a **high association with Epstein-Barr Virus (EBV) infection**. The sporadic form of Burkitt lymphoma typically is found in the **abdomen, involving the ileocecum and peritoneum**. This form is sometimes associated with **EBV or HIV** infection.

   Histologically, the forms of Burkitt lymphoma are identical, containing sheets of neoplastic B-cells and diffuse macrophages with ingested apoptotic tumor debris. The presence of the lighter staining macrophages amongst darker-staining lymphocytes yields the classic **"starry-sky"** appearance.

   Burkitt lymphoma is associated with a **translocation of the proto-oncogene c-*myc*** from chromosome 8, most commonly **t(8:14). Children and young adults** are most likely to have Burkitt lymphoma.

2. **Follicular Lymphoma** is the **most common non-Hodgkin lymphoma in the United States**. It is a **B-cell** neoplasm that typically presents as **generalized lymphadenopathy** in **middle-aged adults**. The majority of follicular lymphomas are associated with **t(14:18)**, a translocation that allows the **over-expression of *bcl*-2 protein**. This protein is an inhibitor of normal apoptosis. Therefore, follicular lymphoma follows a more **indolent course** due to

reduced apoptosis (rather than increased cell proliferation).

3. **Acute Lymphoblastic Lymphoma** is a neoplasm of **lymphoblasts** like acute lymphoblastic leukemia. However, this lymphoma form is usually of **precursor T-cell** origin, rather than precursor B-cell. It commonly occurs in **adolescent males** as a **thymic mass**. (The thymus reaches its largest size in adolescence.) Although the precursor T-cell neoplasm presents in a lymphoma pattern, it can evolve to a leukemic pattern and be identical to classic ALL.

4. **Small Lymphocytic Lymphoma (SLL) is identical to CLL.** The only difference between these two diseases is the number of lymphocytes in the peripheral blood smear. SLL is the lymphoma form with lesser amounts of lymphocytosis. (*See Chronic Lymphocytic Leukemia.*)

5. **Diffuse Large B-Cell Lymphoma.** The name for this group of lymphomas is helpful. Diffuse large B-cell lymphoma is comprised of atypical, enlarged neoplastic **B-cells** which grow diffusely. It typically presents as a **rapidly growing lymph node or extranodal mass**. The pathogenesis of diffuse large B-cell lymphoma is varied. In the case of immunodeficiency and HIV infection, EBV and Human Herpes Virus 8 (HHV8) have been associated with the development of this lymphoma. Diffuse large B-cell lymphoma follows an **aggressive, fatal course**. However, **complete remission is possible with chemotherapy**.

Cutaneous T-Cell Lymphomas

Neoplastic proliferations of T-cells are less common than B-cell neoplasms. However, there are some T-cell lymphomas that present in the skin that are worthy of note.

Mycosis Fungoides and Sézary Syndrome: Both mycosis fungoides and Sézary Syndrome are diseases of **neoplastic helper T-cells**. Mycosis fungoides is a lymphoma in which neoplastic cells with **cerebriform nuclei** (folded, like the cerebrum) infiltrate the skin, forming skin lesions. Eventually, the cells also spread to lymph nodes and bone marrow. Sézary Syndrome is a variant of mycosis fungoides with a **leukemic phase**. Instead of discrete skin lesions, patients have diffuse redness and scaling of the skin (**erythroderma**).

Adult T-Cell Leukemia/Lymphoma: This disease is caused by **human T-cell leukemia virus type 1 (HTLV-1)**, a retrovirus endemic to **Japan, West Africa, and the Caribbean**. Patients get skin lesions, hepatosplenomegaly, and hypercalcemia. Involved tissues contain neoplastic T-cells with "**cloverleaf**" **nuclei**.

This disease typically rapidly progresses to death within a year.

MYELOPROLIFERATIVE DISEASES

Myeloproliferative diseases are **neoplasms derived from the myeloid line** of stem cells. Both acute myeloblastic leukemia and chronic myeloid leukemia by this definition can fit into this category. However, "myeloproliferative disease" commonly implies a **chronic disease course**, so that only **CML** is clinically considered to be a myeloproliferative disease. Myeloproliferative diseases commonly occur in patients in their **sixth decade or greater**. The neoplastic cells of a myeloproliferative disease are capable of causing **extramedullary hematopoiesis in the spleen**, resulting in **splenomegaly**. These diseases also can progress to **acute leukemia** or end in **marrow fibrosis**.

Polycythemia Vera

This disease is characterized by neoplasia of a **multipotent myeloid stem cell**. Although the levels of RBCs, granulocytes, and megakaryocytes, thus, are all elevated, the **increase in red blood cell mass is the most significant clinically**. The **high hematocrit** causes blood to be viscous and sluggish, leading to **thrombotic and hemorrhagic phenomena** that can be life threatening. The increase in blood cell mass also acts as a feedback mechanism to **decrease erythropoietin (EPO)** production. A low EPO sets apart this disease from other benign conditions that cause erythrocytosis (like chronic hypoxia or tumors that secrete EPO). Hence, the name polycythemia "vera", or the "true" increase in red cell mass.

Essential Thrombocythemia

Essential thrombocythemia (essential thrombocytosis) is the least common of the myeloproliferative diseases. It is characterized by neoplastic proliferations of megakaryocytes and, thus, platelets. Patients have increased levels of large, dysplastic megakaryocytes in their bone marrow and increased amounts of large platelets in their peripheral blood smear. As a result of the thrombocytosis (increased numbers of platelets), these patients are at risk for **thrombotic and hemorrhagic events**. Essential thrombocythemia typically follows an indolent course.

Primary Myelofibrosis

The hallmark of primary myelofibrosis is the rapid replacement of bone marrow by fibrous tissue, leading to pancytopenia. It is believed that this disease is caused by **fibrogenic factors released by neoplastic megakaryocytes**. As a consequence of bone marrow failure, **extensive extramedullary hematopoiesis** occurs, resulting in an enlarged spleen, liver, and lymph nodes. Red blood cell and granulocyte precursors (**leukoerythroblastosis**) produced by these extramedullary sites will be seen in the peripheral blood smear. Additionally, **teardrop-shaped RBCs** are present from the marrow fibrosis damaging RBC precursors. Primary myelofibrosis resembles the end stage of fibrosis seen in the other myeloproliferative diseases.

FUNCTIONAL B-CELL NEOPLASMS

The neoplasms that fall under this classification are those that originate from the **B-cell/plasma cell line** and, thus, produce copious immunoglobulins. These antibodies will be of one type (since the cancers are monoclonal) and can be detected on electrophoresis as an **M spike**, denoting the **monoclonal protein**. Keep in mind that an M spike does not automatically mean cancer, because 1% of otherwise healthy persons older than 50 will have a benign **mono-clonal gammopathy of undetermined significance (MGUS)**.

Multiple Myeloma

Multiple Myeloma is characterized by **neoplastic plasma cells** that produce **IgG or IgA** class antibodies. The malignant cells also secrete factors that activate osteoclasts to break down bone, resulting in characteristic **bone lytic lesions**. They are detected radiographically as multifocal **"punched out"** lesions, particularly in the skull and axial skeleton. As a result, patients are at risk for **pathologic fractures** as well as neurologic symptoms from **hypercalcemia**. The elevated amounts of monoclonal antibodies will "crowd out" normal production of immunoglobulins, making **infection the number one cause of death**. Additionally, **free immunoglobulin light chains** (called **Bence Jones proteins**) will be excreted in the urine and will contribute to the **second leading cause of death: renal failure** (half of myeloma patients will have renal insufficiency). "Myeloma kidney" is caused by Bence Jones proteinuria, amyloidosis, light chain deposition in the glomerular basement membrane, and hypercalcemia. Another complication of the high levels of monoclonal protein is that they cause RBCs to be "sticky," so that they stack like poker chips (called the **rouleaux formation**). Multiple myeloma occurs most often in **older men of African descent**.

Waldenström's Macroglobulinemia

Waldenström's Macroglobulinemia is caused by **neoplastic lymphoid cells that are in a stage between B-cells and plasma cells, called "plasmacytoid lymphocytes."** In contrast to multiple myeloma, the immunoglobulins produced in Waldenström's are **IgM** class antibodies (*Macro = IgM, the larger antibody*). This disease will also have **Bence Jones proteinuria without renal failure,** because the large IgM molecules cannot be filtered in the kidney. There are **NO** lytic lesions associated with Waldenström's. The major morbidity in this disease is associated with the elevated serum IgM levels, causing the blood to be thick and prone to occlusion of specifically the retinal arteries, leading to blindness (**hyperviscosity syndrome**). Waldenström's macroglobulinemia is typically seen in **men older than fifty**.

LEUKOPENIA

Lymphoid pathology doesn't only include neoplasia. **Leukopenia**, or an abnormally decreased number of WBCs, occurs commonly in clinical practice and is caused by a variety of factors. A decreased amount of neutrophils (**neutropenia; agranulocytosis**) can occur from aplastic anemia, megaloblastic anemia, myelodysplastic syndromes, immunologic disorders, and infections. The most important cause of agranulocytosis is therapeutic drugs, particularly those that suppress bone marrow (i.e., chemotherapeutic alkylating agents and antimetabolites). **Lymphopenia** (decreased amounts of lymphocytes) is less common and is seen typically in AIDS, autoimmune disorders, viral infections, and with certain drugs. As would be expected, a leukopenic patient is at risk for serious infection.

REACTIVE LEUKOCYTOSIS

The leukocyte count can be increased (**leukocytosis**) in cases other than cancer. Typically, it is a "reactive" process, caused by inflammation. Elevation in each specific WBC count is associated with a different type of inflammation. Elevated neutrophil counts are common during pyogenic bacterial infections and tissue necrosis. Eosinophil levels will rise during allergies, asthma, parasitic infections, and collagen vascular disorders. Chronic infections will cause rises in monocyte and lymphocyte levels. Basophils rarely increase in number; therefore, basophilic leukocytosis may be indicative of a myeloproliferative disorder. Reactive leukocytosis can cause palpable, swollen lymph nodes (lymphadenitis).

6

Lung Pathology

NORMAL ANATOMY AND HISTOLOGY OF THE LUNG

The gross and microscopic structure of normal lung allows for efficient exchange of gases between inspired air and the blood.

Anatomy

The right lung has 3 lobes, and the left lung has 2 lobes (the left middle lobe equivalent is referred to as the **lingula**). The upper and middle lobes are anterior, while the lower lobes are posterior.

Fig. 6-1. Gross appearance of the lungs.

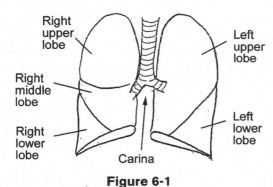

Figure 6-1

Each lobe is divided into 19 bronchopulmonary segments. From the distal trachea, the respiratory tree divides into paired branches of unequal length and diameter (an "arborizing" pattern). The bifurcation of the trachea is called the **carina**, after which the trachea branches into right and left **mainstem bronchi** and enters the lung tissue. The **right mainstem bronchus is more vertical** and thus is more subject to **aspiration**. Progressive branching of the bronchi forms **bronchioles**, which, in contrast to bronchi, **lack cartilage and submucosal glands** within their walls.

The bronchioles continue to divide, giving rise to the **terminal bronchioles**. A cluster of three to five terminal bronchioles and their associated acini (an **acinus**, or **terminal respiratory unit**, is the terminal cluster of alveoli at the end of the airway—"acinus" means "berry" in Latin) form the **pulmonary lobule**. The terminal respiratory unit contains multiple alveolar sacs, which are the site of gas exchange. *(Slide 6.1)*

Fig. 6-2. Terminal bronchioles.

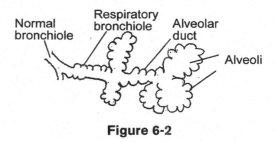

Figure 6-2

Histology

The primary cells of the respiratory tract are **ciliated pseudostratified columnar epithelial cells**. (They are called "pseudostratified" due to the differing heights of the cells, which make the epithelium look like it is multilayered or "stratified".) The epithelial cells are intermixed with mucus-secreting **goblet cells** in the cartilaginous airways. The bronchial mucosa also contains **neuroendocrine cells** that secrete serotonin, calcitonin, and gastrin-releasing peptide. Numerous submucosal mucus-secreting glands are found throughout the walls of the trachea and bronchi—**remember that there are no glands in the bronchioles!** The terminal airway epithelium is composed mostly of **low cuboidal cells** that are **partially ciliated**. Finally, the alveoli themselves are lined by a specialized, gas-permeable epithelium. The blood-gas barrier is described further in the next section.

The only exception to this histology is in the **vocal cords**—they are composed entirely of **stratified squamous epithelium**.

THE BLOOD-GAS BARRIER

Several microscopic structures in the alveolar walls (alveolar septae) constitute the blood-gas barrier:

1. **Capillary endothelium** lines the network of anastomosing capillaries.
2. **Interstitial tissue** is the delicate portion of the alveolar septum, which consists of fused epithelial and endothelial basement membranes.
3. **Alveolar epithelium, which contains:**
   a. **Type I pneumocytes.** These are flattened, continuous cells that cover 95% of the alveolar surface and create a cellular barrier specialized for gas exchange.
   b. **Type II pneumocytes.** These are small, cuboidal cells that secrete **surfactant**, a substance that lubricates the alveoli and decreases surface tension. Surfactant is made by **lamellar bodies** within the cytoplasm of the type II pneumocyte and is necessary for the normal expansion of the alveoli. When surfactant is decreased or completely absent, a condition called **hyaline membrane disease** results (to be discussed later). Type II pneumocytes also help repair damaged alveoli by **regenerating into Type I cells**.
4. **Alveolar macrophages** are loosely attached to the epithelial cells or lie freely within the alveolar spaces. They are derived from blood monocytes and ingest foreign particles in the airway.

Fig. 6-3. Microanatomy of pulmonary gas exchange.

The alveolar walls are not solid but are perforated by **Pores of Kohn**—apertures in the alveolar septum that allow two adjacent alveoli to communicate. These pores equalize the pressure in alveolar sacs and play an important role in the extrusion of bacteria and exudates.

PULMONARY DISEASE

Atelectasis refers to **incomplete expansion of the lungs** (in neonates) or the **collapse of previously inflated lung substance** (in adults). Three basic types of atelectasis exist, all of them reversible:

1. **Obstruction/Resorption atelectasis** results from **complete obstruction of an airway** that eventually causes resorption of the oxygen trapped in the dependent alveoli. This type of atelectasis often is caused by **excessive secretions** (e.g., mucus plugs) or exudates within smaller bronchi, as seen in

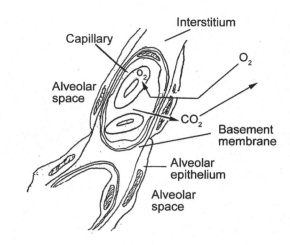

Figure 6-3

asthma, chronic bronchitis, aspiration, and bronchial neoplasms.
2. **Compression atelectasis** generally involves the entire lung and occurs when the **pleural cavity is expanded by fluid, tumor, blood (hemothorax), or air (pneumothorax)**. This type of atelectasis most commonly is found in congestive heart failure and cancer patients with pleural effusions.
3. **Patchy atelectasis** involves small segments of all lobes and usually is due to **loss of surfactant**, as seen in neonatal and adult respiratory distress syndromes.

VASCULAR DISORDERS

Pulmonary edema (accumulation of edema fluid in the alveolar spaces) and **congestion** (excessive accumulation of blood in the lungs) *(Slide 6.2)* can occur either as separate entities, or more commonly, together as a consequence of hemodynamic instability.

Fig. 6-4. Pulmonary edema and its causes.

The main causes of pulmonary edema are:

1. **Increased hydrostatic pressure**, as occurs with left-sided congestive heart failure or stenosis of the mitral valve.
2. **Increased alveolar capillary permeability**, usually seen with infectious agents, inhaled irritant gases, aspiration, drug overdose, or any other substance that causes direct microvascular injury to the alveolar capillaries. Proteins and fluid then leak from the capillaries into the interstitial spaces, leading to alveolar inflammation.
3. **Lymphatic insufficiency**, resulting from lymphangitic carcinomatosis (cancer cells plugging up the lymphatics in the lung), or fibrosing lymphangitis, seen in silicosis.

PULMONARY EDEMA AND ITS CAUSES

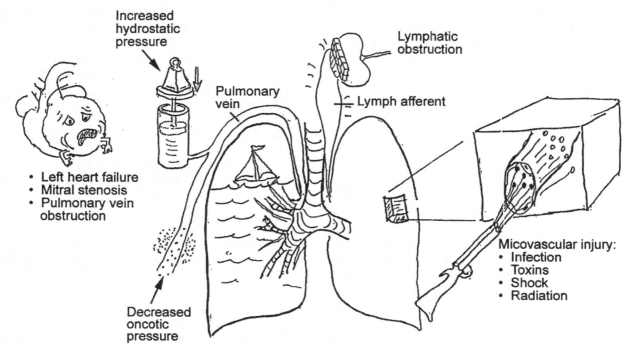

Figure 6-4

Hyaline Membrane Disease

In adults, **hyaline membrane disease** goes by many names, most commonly **Adult Respiratory Distress Syndrome (ARDS)** and **Diffuse Alveolar Damage (DAD)**. The salient clinical features of ARDS include the rapid onset of life-threatening respiratory insufficiency and severe hypoxia, associated with severe pulmonary edema.

An important diagnostic clue to ARDS is microscopic **thickening of the alveolar walls** and **deposition of hyaline membranes**. *(Slide 6.3)*

Alveolar thickening impairs gas exchange and leads to eventual multiorgan system failure. ARDS is fatal in 60% of cases.

The causes of ARDS can be classified into two categories—direct lung injuries and systemic conditions.

1. **Direct injuries:** Inhalation of toxins and irritants, aspiration of gastric contents, oxygen toxicity, and diffuse pulmonary infections (note that these conditions also will cause pulmonary edema).
2. **Systemic causes:** septic shock (usually due to gram negative bacteria), trauma, surgical complications, severe burns, acute pancreatitis, and drug reactions (especially heroin overdose).

The pathogenesis of ARDS is complex. The initial injury, whatever the cause, leads to **infiltration of the** **alveoli by inflammatory cells** (especially neutrophils) and activation of the **coagulation cascade**, as evidenced by microemboli within the vessels. The inflammatory cells release substances that are toxic to the alveolar wall, resulting in further damage to the capillary endothelium and alveolar epithelium. This situation is further complicated by the need for aggressive oxygen therapy, which may result in the formation of oxygen free radicals, leading to oxygen toxicity.

In infants, hyaline membrane disease is known as **neonatal respiratory distress syndrome**. Clinically, the disease is marked by dyspnea, tachypnea, and cyanosis shortly after birth. Most often, neonatal respiratory distress syndrome results from a deficiency of surfactant due to lung immaturity in premature babies.

Pulmonary Embolism (PE)

The pulmonary arteries can become occluded by thrombi, which almost always are embolic in origin. In approximately 95% of cases, pulmonary emboli **originate in the deep veins of the leg**. Common risk factors for thrombotic PE include:

1. **Immobilization:** Clinically, long episodes of bed rest due to severe illness or advanced age, as well as extended periods of sitting during travel may predispose to PE by causing venous stasis.

2. **Congestive Heart Failure (CHF)**: Heart failure causes venous stasis when the heart no longer is capable of pumping blood efficiently.
3. **Postpartum and oral contraceptive use**: In both of these situations, **increased estrogen** in the body leads to hypercoagulability and increased risk for thromboses. Immediately postpartum, women also are at risk for amniotic fluid emboli (see later).
4. **Cancer**: Tumors often release pro-coagulant factors as they grow, leading to multiple thromboses.

When a PE develops, several different outcomes are possible:

Large emboli (approximately 5% of cases) may block one of the major pulmonary arteries or lodge astride the bifurcation of the right and left pulmonary arteries—called a **"saddle embolus."** Sudden death often occurs, owing largely to the blockage of blood flow through the lungs. **A large pulmonary embolus represents one of the few causes of immediate and instantaneous death.** Acute dilation of the right side of the heart (acute cor pulmonale), resulting in hemodynamic collapse, is a major contributing factor in sudden death due to PE.

Fig. 6-5. Saddle embolus, blocking the right and left pulmonary arteries.

Small emboli (approximately 60-80% of cases) may be **clinically silent** in patients with normal cardiac function. On the other hand, in patients with inadequate pulmonary circulation (i.e., patients with heart or lung disease), even a small PE can cause **infarction**. Grossly, **the classic pulmonary infarct is hemorrhagic ("red**

infarct") and wedge-shaped. With time, an infarct may resolve with fibrous replacement and scarring.

Several non-thrombotic events also may cause PE. Important **non-thrombotic emboli** include:

1. **Air emboli**: usually iatrogenic in nature.
2. **Bone marrow emboli**: most often seen in resuscitory efforts (i.e., CPR) and trauma to the ribs.
3. **Fat emboli**: occur in trauma with multiple fractures, especially of the long bones (e.g., femur).
4. **Amniotic fluid emboli**: arise immediately postpartum and are composed of sloughed fetal cells and hair mixed with amniotic fluid.
5. **Foreign body emboli**: as seen in intravenous drug abusers (usually talc emboli).

Pulmonary Hypertension

The pulmonary circulation is a low-resistance system. Consequently, the pulmonary blood pressure is approximately 1/8 of the systemic pressure. Clinically, pulmonary hypertension can be diagnosed when the pulmonary blood pressure increases to 1/4 of the systemic pressure.

Primary (a.k.a. "idiopathic") **pulmonary hypertension** is a rare disorder with a poor prognosis. The etiology remains unknown. Much more frequently, pulmonary hypertension is **secondary** to cardiopulmonary conditions that increase pulmonary vascular resistance. Such conditions include:

1. **Chronic obstructive pulmonary disease (COPD) or interstitial lung diseases**.
2. **Left-sided heart disease**, such as mitral stenosis or a congenital right-to-left shunt.

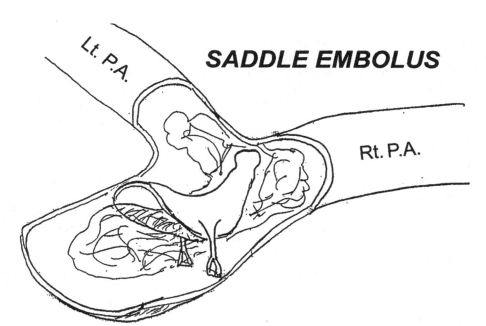

SADDLE EMBOLUS

Lt. P.A.

Rt. P.A.

Figure 6-5

3. **Recurrent thromboemboli** in the lung vasculature.
4. **Autoimmune disorders**, most notably systemic sclerosis, as in **scleroderma**.
5. **Drugs** (especially fenfluramine and phentermine), toxins, and certain herbal remedies.
6. **Increased blood viscosity**, as in polycythemia.

The pathogenesis of secondary pulmonary hypertension involves dysfunction of the pulmonary vascular endothelial cells.

Endothelial cell dysfunction is caused by increased shear, mechanical, and/or biochemical injury to the vessel, which is manifested as vascular lesions.

Vascular lesions can involve the entire arterial tree, from the main pulmonary arteries down to its branches and arterioles. In the most severe cases, **atheromas** ("plaques") form in the pulmonary artery and its major branches. The arterioles and small arteries are most prominently affected, with striking thickening of the medial vessel layer (called **"medial hypertrophy"**) and **intimal fibrosis**.

OBSTRUCTIVE AND RESTRICTIVE PULMONARY DISEASES

Obstructive diseases (airway diseases) are characterized by an **increase in resistance to airflow, owing to partial or complete obstruction** from the trachea and larger bronchi to the terminal and respiratory bronchioles. Pulmonary function tests in patients with this type of disease always show a **decrease in expiratory flow rates**. Major obstructive lung diseases include:

- **Emphysema**
- **Chronic bronchitis**
- **Bronchiectasis**
- **Bronchial asthma**
- **Foreign body inhalation**

Restrictive diseases are characterized by **reduced expansion of lung parenchyma with decreased total lung capacity**. The hallmark of this pattern is a decrease in lung volume, manifested as a **decrease in inspiratory capacity** during pulmonary function testing. Restrictive disease may be caused by chest wall disorders in the presence of normal lungs or in interstitial/infiltrative lung diseases. Common conditions leading to restrictive lung disease include:

- **Neuromuscular diseases**
- **Severe obesity**
- **Pleural diseases**
- **Kyphoscoliosis**
- **ARDS**
- **Pneumoconioses (dust diseases)**

Obstructive Lung Diseases

Chronic Obstructive Pulmonary Disease (COPD) includes a group of conditions that share one major symptom, **dyspnea** (shortness of breath), accompanied by **chronic or recurrent airflow obstruction** within the lungs. The incidence of COPD has increased considerably in recent years, largely due to cigarette smoking and environmental pollutants. The most frequent causes of death in patients with COPD are the development of respiratory acidosis and coma, cor pulmonale with right-sided heart failure, or massive collapse of the lungs secondary to pneumothorax. The different conditions classified as COPD are included in **Table 6.1**.

Emphysema is defined as the abnormal, permanent dilation and destruction of the air spaces distal to the terminal bronchiole. The four main types of emphysema are classified according to anatomic distribution within the lobule:

1. **Centriacinar:** affects the **central or proximal parts of the acini** (the respiratory bronchioles), whereas the distal alveoli are spared. The lesions generally are localized to the **upper lobes** of the lungs, especially the apical segments. The walls of the affected spaces often contain abundant black (**"anthracotic"**) pigment. Centriacinar emphysema often occurs in **heavy smokers** and accounts for more than 95% of emphysema cases.

Table 6.1. Chronic Obstructive Pulmonary Disease (COPD)

Clinical term	Anatomic site	Pathologic changes	Etiology	Signs/Symptoms
Chronic Bronchitis	Bronchus	Mucous gland hyperplasia/hypersecretion	Tobacco smoke, air pollution	Cough, sputum production
Emphysema	Acinus	Airspace enlargement, wall destruction	Tobacco smoke	Dyspnea
Asthma	Bronchus	Smooth muscle hyperplasia, excess mucus, inflammation	Immunologic or undetermined causes	Episodic wheezing, cough, dyspnea
Bronchiectasis	Bronchus	Airway dilation, scarring	Persistent or severe infections	Cough, purulent sputum, fever
Bronchiolitis	Bronchus	Inflammation, scarring, obliteration	Tobacco smoke, air pollutants	Cough, dypnea

2. **Panacinar:** affects the **entire acinus** (alveoli, alveolar ducts, respiratory bronchioles, and terminal bronchioles). It occurs more frequently in the **lower basal zones** of the lung and is strongly associated with **alpha-1-antitrypsin deficiency.**
3. **Paraseptal:** affects mainly the **distal acinus** (alveoli and alveolar ducts). It tends to localize to the **pleura** and **interlobar septae**, causing large bullae ("blebs"). Rupture of these bullae may lead to **spontaneous pneumothorax.**
4. **Irregular:** affects the acinus irregularly and almost always is associated with **scarring**.

The pathogenesis of alveolar wall destruction is a complex process. Basically, **destruction results from an imbalance between proteases, mainly elastases and antielastases, in the lungs**.

Fig. 6-6. The pathogenesis of emphysema. Elastase, an enzyme capable of digesting human lung, is released by neutrophils and macrophages that infiltrate the lung during chronic inflammatory states.

Neutrophil elastase is inhibited by alpha-1-antitrypsin ("antielastase"). On the contrary, alpha-1-antitrypsin does not inhibit macrophage elastase, and over time, chronic lung disease can lead to alveolar destruction and emphysema. **Congenital deficiency of alpha-1-antitrypsin** (due to an aberrant gene in ~10% of the population) leads to symptomatic emphysema at an early age, even more severe if the individual smokes. Oxidants in cigarette smoke inhibit a-1-antytripsin and thus decrease net antielastase activity in smokers.

Grossly, emphysematous lungs appear voluminous and often overlap the heart, diminishing the cardiac tones upon auscultation. Large apical bullae may be seen grossly and are characteristic of irregular emphysema, secondary to scarring.

Microscopically, abnormally large alveoli are separated by thin, fibrotic septae *(Slide 6.4).* With advanced disease, the air spaces enlarge further, with complete destruction of the alveolar walls. Often, the respiratory bronchioles and vasculature are deformed and compressed by the large airways.

Chronic bronchitis is clinically defined as persistent cough with sputum production for at least 3 consecutive months over at least two consecutive years. The earliest feature of chronic bronchitis is **hypersecretion of mucus** in the large airways, associated with **hypertrophy of the submucosal glands** in the trachea and bronchi. With disease progression, the number of goblet cells (mucus secreting cells) in the small airways markedly increases.

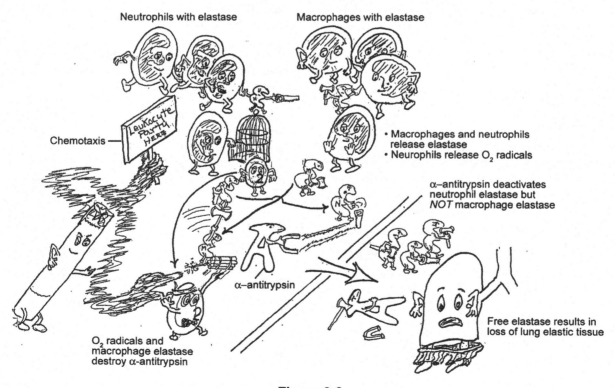

THE PATHOGENESIS OF EMPHYSEMA

Figure 6-6

Excess mucus production, is initially protective against irritants (especially cigarette smoke), but it eventually contributes to airway obstruction.

Fig. 6-7. How smoking leads to chronic bronchitis.

Macroscopically, the main features of chronic bronchitis are edema and congestion of the mucous membranes, accompanied by excessive mucinous or mucopurulent secretions covering the epithelial surfaces. Microscopically, the mucus secreting glands are enlarged. The degree of glandular hypertrophy is assessed via the **Reid Index**.

Fig. 6-8. The Reid Index (B/A). This is the **ratio of the thickness of the mucous gland layer to the thickness of the wall between the basement membrane of the epithelium and the cartilage.** The Reid Index is increased in chronic bronchitis due to hypertrophy and hyperplasia of mucous glands. The normal Reid Index value is 0.4.

Additionally, goblet cell metaplasia causes marked constriction of the bronchioles, as well as mucous plugging, inflammation, and fibrosis. In the most severe cases, obliteration of the bronchiole lumens, called **bronchiolitis obliterans**, further aggravates the clinical course. Finally, with long-standing severe chronic bronchitis, **cor pulmonale** causes right-sided heart failure and eventual death.

Bronchial asthma is a chronic, relapsing inflammatory disorder of the lungs manifested as **tracheobronchial hyperreactivity** to various stimuli. Asthma patients experience unpredictable, disabling attacks of severe dyspnea, coughing, and wheezing, triggered by sudden **bronchospasm**. Between attacks, most patients are asymptomatic. **Status asthmaticus**, the most severe form of asthma, is an acute, sustained attack that may persist for days to weeks and can threaten ventilatory function enough to cause severe cyanosis and death.

Typically, asthma is categorized into two groups:

1. **Extrinsic (atopic or allergic) asthma** is induced by exposure to an extrinsic allergen and elicits a **type I IgE-mediated hypersensitivity reaction**. This reaction has two phases, including:
   - An **acute phase**, caused by antigen binding to presensitized, IgE-coated mast cells on the mucosal surface, which causes release of specific mediators. These mediators induce bronchospasm, edema, mucus secretion, and recruitment of inflammatory cells (particularly **eosinophils**).

HOW SMOKING LEADS TO CHRONIC BRONCHITIS

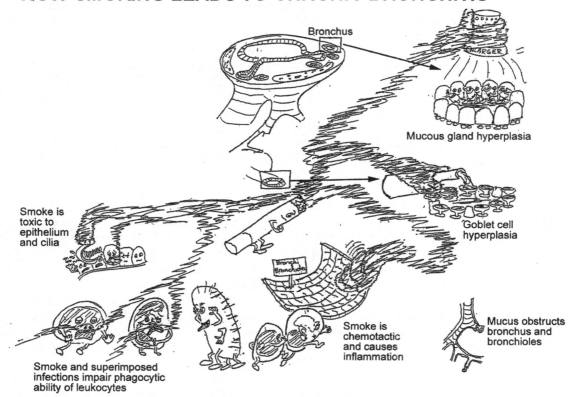

Figure 6-7

THE REID INDEX

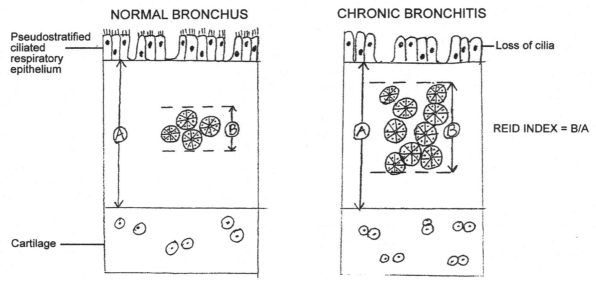

Figure 6-8

• A **late phase**, mediated by inflammatory cells (e.g., neutrophils, monocytes, lymphocytes, basophils, and eosinophils). This late-phase response occurs 4-8 hours after exposure and may be severe, lasting for 12 hours or more.

Extrinsic asthma **begins in childhood**, generally in patients with a **family history** of allergy ("atopy").

2. **Intrinsic (idiopathic) asthma** is initiated by diverse, **non-immune mechanisms**, including drug reactions (e.g., aspirin), respiratory tract infections (especially viral), and inhaled irritants. Intrinsic asthma **begins in adult life**, and patients usually have **no family history** of asthma. **Exercise- and cold-induced asthmas** are variants of intrinsic asthma.

The chemical mediators of the acute phase reactants are seen in **Table 6.2**.

Grossly, asthmatic lungs are over-inflated with small areas of atelectasis. Perhaps the most striking macroscopic finding is bronchial and bronchiolar occlusion by thick, tenacious **mucous plugs**. Histologically, the plugs contain whorls of shed respiratory epithelium, forming characteristic **Curschmann spirals** *(Slide 6.5)*. Numerous eosinophils are present, and their sloughed membrane protein forms **Charcot-Leyden crystals** *(Slide 6.6)*. The basement membrane of the bronchial epithelium is thickened; the bronchial walls are edematous and infiltrated by inflammatory cells. Submucosal glands are increased

in size, while the bronchial wall muscle is hypertrophied due to prolonged bronchoconstriction.

Occasionally, bronchial asthma spontaneously regresses. Complications of prolonged asthma include recurrent **respiratory tract infections**, **chronic bronchitis**, and superimposed **emphysema**. In the most severe cases, **cor pulmonale** and right-sided heart failure may develop.

Bronchiectasis is a permanent abnormal dilation of bronchi and bronchioles, caused by destruction of the muscle and elastic tissue in association with chronic necrotizing infections. Patients present with cough, fever, and expectoration of copious amounts of foul-smelling, purulent sputum.

Bronchiectasis develops in association with a number of conditions:

1. Necrotizing **pneumonia**: caused by *Mycobacterium tuberculosis*, *Staphylococcus aureus*, *Haemophilus influenzae*, among other organisms
2. **Destructive viral diseases**: caused by adenovirus, influenza virus, and HIV
3. **Fungal infections**
4. **Bronchial obstruction**: as seen with tumors, foreign bodies, and obstructive airway diseases
5. **Congenital and hereditary conditions**: such as **cystic fibrosis**, immunodeficiency, and primary ciliary disease (e.g., **Kartagener syndrome**, to be described later)
6. **Systemic diseases**: including rheumatoid arthritis, systemic lupus erythematosus, inflammatory bowel disease, and post-transplantation

Table 6.2. Chemical mediators of the acute phase reactants.

Chemical mediator*	Site of action	Action
Leukotrienes C4, D4, E4	Bronchus, pulmonary vessels, mucous glands	Prolonged bronchoconstriction, increased vascular permeability, increased mucus secretions
Acetylcholine	Airway walls	Smooth muscle constriction
Histamine	Bronchus	Bronchoconstriction
Prostaglandin D2	Bronchus, pulmonary vessels	Bronchoconstriction, vasodilation
Platelet activating factor (PAF)	Platelets	Aggregation, serotonin and histamine release from platelet granules

*Additional mediators implicated in asthma include interleukins (IL-1 and IL-6), tumor necrosis factor (TNF), chemokines, neuropeptides, nitric oxide, bradykinin, and endothelins. However, their precise roles are not well understood.

In order for full-blown bronchiectasis to develop, **obstruction** and **infection** both are necessary. Early bronchial wall inflammation and intraluminal secretions initially result in **reversible** dilation of the patent airways. However, if the obstruction persists, along with recurrent superimposed infection, the changes become **irreversible**. After prolonged bronchial obstruction, air is resorbed from the airways distal to the obstruction, resulting in atelectasis.

The mechanisms of obstruction and infection are most apparent in the severe form of bronchiectasis associated with **cystic fibrosis (CF)**. In CF, **a defect in chloride transport causes impaired chloride secretion into mucus, leading to low sodium and water content, defective mucociliary action, and accumulation of thick, viscous secretions that eventually obstruct the airways**. Repeated infections ensue, causing irreversible damage to the airways, supporting smooth muscle, and elastic tissue. Ultimately, the bronchi dilate further, and fibrosis develops. The genetic aspects of CF are further elaborated in Chapter 3.

Primary ciliary disease (immotile cilia syndrome) is another congenital condition that causes bronchiectasis. Approximately half of patients with primary ciliary dyskinesia have **Kartagener syndrome**, characterized by the triad of **bronchiectasis, sinusitis,** and **situs inversus** (complete mirror-image reversal of the thoracic and abdominal organs). These abnormalities are caused by a primary defect in ciliary motility due to an **absence or shortening of the dynein arms** that are responsible for the coordinated bending of the cilia. When this occurs in the respiratory tract, mucus becomes entrapped with resultant obstruction and eventual bronchiectasis. Kartagener syndrome is inherited as an **autosomal recessive** trait. Males with this condition often are infertile due to ineffective sperm mobility.

Macroscopically, bronchiectasis usually affects the **lower lobes** and is most severe in the **distal bronchi** and **bronchioles**. The disease may be sharply localized when caused by foreign body aspiration or compression by tumor masses.

Microscopic findings in bronchiectasis vary with activity and chronicity of the disease. In active cases, **intense acute and chronic inflammatory exudate** is apparent within the bronchi and bronchiole walls. Areas of **necrotizing ulceration** show desquamation of the epithelium. Extensive necrosis may lead to a **lung abscess**. Finally, **fibrosis** develops, obliterating the bronchiolar lumina.

Restrictive Lung Diseases

Intrinsic restrictive (interstitial, infiltrative) lung diseases are a heterogeneous group of conditions that share **diffuse, chronic changes of the pulmonary connective tissue**, principally in the interstitium of the alveolar walls. Clinically, patients display dyspnea, tachypnea (rapid breathing), and eventual cyanosis without evidence of airway obstruction. **Secondary pulmonary hypertension** and **right-sided heart failure** develop with long-standing disease. In advanced stages, the different types of restrictive lung disease are nearly impossible to differentiate morphologically. For all restrictive lung diseases, the end result is the same— **scarring** and **cystic destruction of the lung**, referred to as end-stage lung disease or **honeycomb lung**.

Regardless of type, the earliest common manifestation of intrinsic restrictive lung disease is **alveolitis**. Alveolitis is an **accumulation of inflammatory cells** (i.e., macrophages, neutrophils, eosinophils, and lymphocytes) **and immune effector cells within the alveoli**. Accumulation of these cells distorts the alveolar structures and causes the release of mediators that injure parenchymal cells and stimulate fibrosis. The consequence is end-stage fibrotic lung disease in which the alveoli are replaced by cystic spaces, with thick bands of connective tissue infiltrated with inflammatory cells *(Slide 6.7)*.

Sarcoidosis *(Slide 6.8)* is a common disease of unknown etiology, distinguished by **noncaseating granulomas** in multiple organ systems. Women are affected more frequently than men, and blacks are affected more frequently than whites. Sarcoidosis usually presents in early adulthood as **bilateral hilar and**

mediastinal lymphadenopathy on routine chest x-ray. Other common pathologic changes include:

- **Interstitial lung disease**
- **Cutaneous lesions (e.g., erythema nodosum)**
- **Ocular lesions (e.g., anterior uveitis)**
- **Peripheral lymphadenopathy**
- **Polyarthritis**

Histologically, all involved tissues show classic non-caseating granulomas, composed of aggregates of tightly clustered epithelioid cells, often with multinucleated **giant cells**. Additionally, two specific histologic hallmarks may be found in up to 60% of the granulomatous lesions. **Schaumann bodies** are laminated concretions composed of calcium and proteins. **Asteroid bodies** are stellate inclusions often found enclosed within giant cells. However, the histologic diagnosis of sarcoidosis is a **diagnosis of exclusion**, since mycobacterial infections, fungal infections, and berylliosis also can produce noncaseating granulomas.

Patients who develop sarcoidosis also have several well-documented immunologic derangements, which include the following:

- **Lymphocytic alveolitis** (intra-alveolar and interstitial accumulation of CD4+ T cells)
- **Activated helper T cells**, leading to macrophage recruitment and additional granuloma formation in tissue
- **Cutaneous anergy** (lack of sensitivity) to skin test antigens (e.g., tuberculin)
- **Polyclonal hypergammaglobulinemia**
- **Absolute lymphopenia** due to reduced levels of circulating T cells (circulating B cells are normal in number)

The clinical course of sarcoidosis is varied. Approximately 65-70% of affected patients recover with minimal or no residual manifestations. Twenty percent exhibit some permanent loss of lung function or permanent visual impairment. The remaining 10% die from severe organ damage, including progressive pulmonary fibrosis and cor pulmonale.

Usual interstitial pneumonia (UIP; idiopathic pulmonary fibrosis; Hamman-Rich syndrome) is a disease of unknown etiology. Clinically, UIP is characterized by severe hypoxemia and cyanosis. Pathologically, the hallmark of UIP is the presence of **chronic inflammation in the interstitial spaces with widespread fibrosis of alveolar septa (honeycomb lung). Exclusion of other diseases causing end-stage lung pathology is mandatory before making this diagnosis.** Average survival is less than five years.

Hypersensitivity pneumonitis refers to a group of immunologically-mediated conditions caused by **intense and prolonged exposure to organic dusts**. It is important to recognize these diseases early, because progression to end-stage lung disease can be prevented by removal of the causative agent.

Salient histologic findings in hypersensitivy pneumonitis include interstitial pneumonitis, fibrosis, obliterative bronchiolitis, and granuloma formation. Specific diseases include:

- **Farmer's lung**: due to actinomycete spores in hay.
- **Pigeon breeder's lung**: due to bird feathers or guano.
- **Humidifier or air-conditioner lung**: due to thermophilic bacteria.
- **Byssinosis (cotton worker's lung)**: due to inhaled cotton fibers.

Pneumoconioses

Up until recently, the pneumoconioses were defined as pulmonary diseases caused by the inhalation of inorganic dusts. Today, use of the term is broadened to include **diseases induced by organic and inorganic particulates, as well as chemical fumes and vapors.** The major types of pneumoconioses, categorized by their causative agents, are:

- **Anthracosis (carbon)**
- **Silicosis (silica)**
- **Asbestosis (asbestos)**
- **Berylliosis (beryllium)**
- **Siderosis (iron)**

The development of a pneumoconiosis depends on several factors. First, the amount of dust accumulated in the airways is key—a larger duration and magnitude of exposure yields a greater chance for disease. Second, and most important, is the size of the inhaled particles. **The most dangerous particles range from 1 to 5 micrometers because they are tiny enough to reach the small terminal airways and airs sacs, settling in their linings.** Solubility and physiochemical reactivity of the particles, as well as additive effects of other irritants (e.g., concomitant tobacco smoking), also are factors. Lastly, the overall condition of the lungs plays a role in the development of pneumoconioses.

Coal worker's pneumoconiosis (CWP) is caused by inhalation of coal dust, which contains silica and carbon. The spectrum of lung findings in coal workers is varied. Black anthracotic pigment may accumulate in the lungs without a perceptible cellular reaction, allowing the patient to remain asymptomatic. **Simple CWP** is characterized by accumulation of coal macules (1-2 mm) with little to no pulmonary dysfunction. **Complicated CWP ("progressive massive fibrosis")** requires many years to develop and is characterized by extensive fibrosis with large black, necrotic nodules

(>2 cm), resulting in severe respiratory insufficiency ("**black lung disease**").

Silicosis, caused by inhalation of crystalline silicon dioxide (silica), is the most prevalent chronic occupational lung disease in the world. **Miners, glassblowers, sandblasters, and stonecutters commonly are affected.** Early on, silicosis is characterized by tiny, discrete **silicotic nodules** in the upper lungs. With disease progression, the nodules coalesce into hard, collagenous scars that may obstruct airways and/or compromise blood flow. Often, thin sheets of calcification occur in the lymph nodes, seen radiographically as **eggshell calcification**.

Histologically, the nodular lesions in silicosis consist of concentric whorls of hyalinized collagen. Polarized light microscopy reveals birefringent silica particles within the nodules.

Silicosis often is asymptomatic and detected incidentally on chest x-ray. Most patients do not develop dyspnea until late in the course, after progressive massive fibrosis is present. Silicosis also is associated with an **increased susceptibility to tuberculosis**.

Asbestosis is caused by exposure to asbestos fibers. Asbestos is a crystalline hydrated silicate that forms two types of fibers: **serpentine** (curly and flexible) and **amphibole** (straight, stiff, and brittle). Amphiboles, while less prevalent, are more pathogenic. Asbestosis is marked by diffuse interstitial fibrosis, which begins in the lower lobes and subpleural areas.

The histologic hallmark of asbestos exposure is the presence of **asbestos bodies**, which appear as golden brown, dumbbell-shaped, beaded rods with translucent centers. Asbestos bodies arise when macrophages attempt to ingest the asbestos fibers, coating them with proteinaceous material and hemosiderin (iron pigment). Other inorganic particulates may become coated with similar iron-protein complexes and are called **ferruginous bodies. Dense fibrocalcific plaques**, found on the pleura and/or diaphragm, are the most common feature of asbestos exposure.

The risk of **bronchogenic carcinoma** is increased about fivefold for asbestos workers, and the risk for developing **malignant mesothelioma** (cancer of the pleura or peritoneum *(Slide 6.9)* is more than a thousand times greater than the general population. Concomitant cigarette smoking greatly increases the risk of bronchogenic carcinoma but not of mesothelioma. When complicated by lung or pleural/peritoneal cancer, the prognosis of asbestosis is particularly grim.

Pulmonary Hemorrhage Syndromes

Important diseases whose main clinical presentation is **hemoptysis** (coughing up blood) include:

Goodpasture's syndrome is characterized by the simultaneous appearance of rapidly progressive, proliferative **glomerulonephritis** and necrotizing **hemorrhagic interstitial pneumonitis**. Both the lung hemorrhage and the glomerulonephritis improve with intensive plasma exchange.

Idiopathic pulmonary hemosiderosis presents as insidious onset of productive cough, hemoptysis, anemia, and weight loss with diffuse pulmonary infiltrations. The disease is episodic and chronic, generally occurring in young adults and children. Affected lung tissue demonstrates areas of red-brown consolidation, prominent hemosiderin deposition, fibrosis, and marked alveolar capillary congestion. The cause of this disease is unknown.

Vasculitis-associated hemorrhage is seen in hypersensitivity angiitis, Wegener granulomatosis, and systemic lupus erythematosus (SLE).

PULMONARY INFECTIONS

The respiratory system, more than any other organ system, is an extremely common site for infection and accounts for the largest number of workdays lost in the general population. While **viruses cause the vast majority of upper respiratory tract infections** (e.g., "the common cold" and pharyngitis), **lower respiratory tract infections** (e.g., pneumonia) **may be bacterial, viral, fungal, or atypical** (e.g., due to mycoplasma) in origin. Salient clinical features of pneumonia include fever, chills, productive cough with rust-colored sputum, and dyspnea.

Pneumonia is classified in many ways, depending on the causative agent, the nature of the host reaction (fibrinous, suppurative, etc.), or the distribution of infection (lobar versus lobular).

Bacterial pneumonia is defined as any bacterial infection of the lung parenchyma and is characterized by exudative solidification (consolidation) of the pulmonary tissue. According to gross anatomic distribution, bacterial pneumonia is classified into the following categories:

1. **Lobular pneumonia (bronchopneumonia)** is marked by **patchy consolidation** of the lung, usually due to extension of a preexisting bronchitis or bronchiolitis. It tends to occur more frequently in age extremes (i.e., infancy and old age). The consolidation tends to be **multilobar** and **bilateral**, usually affecting the basal portions of the lungs.
2. **Lobar pneumonia** is an acute bacterial infection with consolidation of a **large portion of one lobe**. In severe infections, an **entire lobe** may be involved.
   The **stages of lobar pneumonia** follow a classic pattern, but appropriate treatment with antibiotics generally does not allow full progression:
   a. **Congestion**, characterized by heavy, red lungs, is apparent within the first 24 hours. Microscopic characteristics include vascular engorgement

and intra-alveolar fluid, often with the presence of numerous bacteria.

b. **Red hepatization** is marked by a "liver-like" consolidation of the lung. The affected lung tissue is red, firm, and airless. Histologically, the alveolar spaces are filled with red blood cells, neutrophils, and fibrin.

c. **Gray hepatization** manifests as a grayish-brown, dry lung surface. Microscopic examination shows progressive disintegration of red blood cells and the persistence of fibrinosuppurative exudates.

d. **Resolution** is the final stage in which consolidated exudates within the alveolar spaces are enzymatically digested, producing a semi-fluid debris that is cleared. Normal lung structure generally is restored, but fibrous thickening of the pleura or permanent adhesions may remain.

Recall that the respiratory system has excellent defense mechanisms that protect against infection. Pneumonia can result whenever defense mechanisms are impaired or host resistance is decreased. Factors contributing to the development of bacterial pneumonia include:

1. **Loss or suppression of the cough reflex**, often due to alcohol intoxication, drug overdose, coma, anesthesia, and/or debilitation
2. **Damage to the ciliated epithelium** owing to cigarette smoke, inhalation of hot or corrosive gases, or genetic causes (i.e., immotile cilia syndromes)
3. **Interference with the phagocytic ability of alveolar macrophages**, which clear debris from the alveolar spaces
4. **Pulmonary edema and congestion** and/or **accumulation of secretions** as seen in cystic fibrosis and bronchial obstruction
5. **Presence of pathogenic bacterial agents**

Fig. 6-9. Contributory causes of pneumonia.

Streptococcus pneumoniae **(the "pneumococcus") is the most common cause of acute bacterial pneumonia.** A Gram stain of the patient's sputum is needed for diagnosis. The presence of numerous neutrophils containing Gram-positive, lancet-shaped diplococci supports the diagnosis of pneumococcal pneumonia. Isolation of the organism via culture is more specific but less sensitive, especially in the early phase of the illness. Pneumococcal pneumonias generally respond to penicillin, but

Table 6.3. Pneumonia caused by fungal and fungus-like organisms.

Disease	Fungal organism	Morphology in tissue	Notes
Candidiasis	*Candida albicans*	Pseudohyphae	Only in the immunocompromised, disseminated candidiasis can cause pulmonary abscesses and pneumonia
Aspergillosis	*Aspergillus flavus*	Hyphae	In immunocompromised patients, hyphae mat grow into blood vessels, causing invasive pneumonia with hematogenous spread. Fungal balls may grow in pre-existing lung cavitations.
Histoplasmosis	*Histoplasma capsulatum*	Yeast inside macrophages	Primary pneumonia (in immunocompetent) or secondary disseminated disease (in immunocomprimised), similar to TB in symptoms.
Coccidiomycosis	*Coccidioides immitis*	Endospores inside spherules	Primary pneumonia (in immunocompetent) or secondary disseminated disease (in immunocomprimised).
Cryptococcosis	*Cryptococcus neoformans*	Encapsulated yeast, visualized by mucicarmine stain or India ink	In immunocomprimised patients, cryptococcal pneumonia may lead to severe meningitis.
Pneumocystis carinii (PCP)	*Pneumocystis carinii*	Cyst-like protozoan structures	PCP is the most common opportunistic infections in AIDS patients.
Actinomycosis **	*Actinomyces israelii* — a mycelia-forming Gram positive, anaerobic bacterial rod	Beaded, filamentous, Gram-positive rods	Actinomycetes produce "sulfur granules" – clumpy yellow exudates.
Nocardiosis **	*Nocardia asteroids* — a partially acid-fast bacterial rod	Thin, partially acid-fast, branching rods	Often confused with TB.

**These diseases are not caused by fungal organisms, but by fungus-like organisms.

CONTRIBUTORY CAUSES OF PNEUMONIA

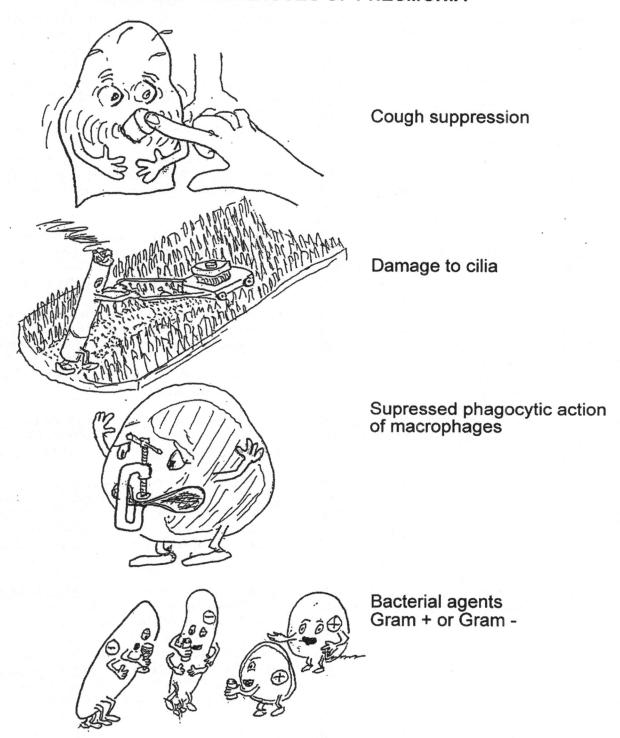

Cough suppression

Damage to cilia

Supressed phagocytic action
of macrophages

Bacterial agents
Gram + or Gram -

Figure 6-9

antibiotic sensitivity always should be determined. Vaccines for high-risk patients are available.

Haemophilus influenzae, another important cause of pneumonia, is a **pleomorphic, Gram-negative rod** that is ubiquitous in the pharynx. *H. influenzae* is a major cause of life-threatening, acute lower respiratory tract infections and meningitis in young children. *H. influenzae* pneumonia, which may follow a viral infection, is a pediatric emergency and has a high mortality rate. Although there are six encapsulated serotypes, **type b is the most frequent cause of invasive disease**. With the advent of conjugate vaccines, the incidence of disease caused by serotype b has declined significantly. In contrast, infections with the non-encapsulated forms are increasing, especially in older patients with pre-existing lung disease. *H. influenzae* is the most common bacterial cause of acute exacerbations of COPD.

Staphylococcus aureus is an important cause of secondary bacterial pneumonia in **children and healthy adults, following a viral respiratory illness**. *S. aureus* pneumonia is associated with a high incidence of complications, such as **abscess** formation and **empyema** (an intrapleural fibrinosuppurative reaction). Intravenous drug abusers have a high risk of developing staphylococcal pneumonia in association with bacterial endocarditis. *S. aureus* also is an important cause of **nosocomial** (hospital-acquired) pneumonia.

Other causes of bacterial pneumonia include *Klebsiella pneumoniae, Moraxella catarrhalis, Pseudomonas aeruginosa,* and *Legionella pneumophilia.* Coliform bacteria also can be causative agents.

Several complications can occur as a consequence of bacterial pneumonia, including abscess formation, empyema, and organization of exudates. In susceptible individuals, bacteremia with hematogenous dissemination can occur, giving rise to metastatic abscesses, endocarditis, meningitis, or suppurative arthritis.

Fungal pneumonia is caused by a variety of pathogenic fungal organisms, by inhaling either spores or fungal hyphae. Most often, fungal pneumonia occurs in **immunocompromised** patients. (*Slides 6.10 through 6.15*)

Table 6.3. Pneumonia caused by fungal and fungus-like organisms.

Atypical pneumonia is an acute febrile respiratory disease characterized by **patchy inflammation** in the lungs, largely **confined to the alveolar septa and pulmonary interstitium**. The term **atypical** emphasizes the **lack of consolidation**. A much more accurate term is **interstitial pneumonitis**. This type of pneumonia is caused by a variety of organisms, the most common being *Mycoplasma pneumoniae*. Other agents include *Chlamydia, Coxiella burnetti* (Q-fever), respiratory syncy-

tial virus (RSV), adenovirus, rhinovirus, rubeola, and varicella. In some cases, the cause cannot be determined.

Grossly, the affected areas are red-blue and congested. Microscopically, the alveolar septae are widened and edematous with a mononuclear inflammatory infiltrate. Frequently, **hyaline membranes**, similar to those seen in ARDS, are present. Superimposed bacterial infections are common and may cause ulcerative bronchitis and bronchiolitis.

Pulmonary abscesses are **local, suppurative, lesions of infectious origin**, characterized by **necrosis of lung tissue**. Commonly isolated organisms include aerobic and anaerobic streptococci, *Staphylococcus aureus*, and gram-negative bacteria. Common causes include:

1. **Aspiration.** This is the **most common cause**, especially when the cough reflex is suppressed
2. **Primary bacterial pneumonia.**
3. **Septic embolism** due to infected thrombi or vegetations of the cardiac valves.
4. **Bronchial obstruction**, especially due to tumors.
5. **Direct traumatic penetration** of the lung tissue.
6. **Direct extension of infection** from a neighboring organ.
7. **Hematogenous seeding** by pyogenic organisms, as in severe bacteremia.

Pulmonary abscesses may affect any part of the lung and may be single or multiple. **Abscesses caused by aspiration are more common in the right lung due to the more vertical main bronchus.**

The cardinal histologic change in all abscesses is suppurative destruction of the tissue within the central area of cavitation.

Tuberculosis (TB), caused by *Mycobacterium tuberculosis*, is a cause of high morbidity and mortality worldwide, especially in underprivileged populations. TB occurs in two stages—primary and secondary:

Primary TB results from inhaling highly infectious aerosols from an infected person. The initial focus of infection, called the **Ghon complex**, consists of a subpleural parenchymal lesion and hilar lymph nodes draining the infection. Granulomatous inflammation with central **caseous ("cheesy") necrosis** is characteristic of primary TB lesions. TB granulomas, called **"tubercles,"** generate a **type IV delayed hypersensitivity reaction**, which is the basis of the purified protein derivative (PPD) test. Most frequently, patients with this initial infection are **asymptomatic**, and the lesions undergo fibrosis and **calcification**, which can be seen on x-ray.

Secondary ("reactivation") TB represents active disease in a previously sensitized person. When TB reactivates, it settles in sites with high oxygen tension, most

Table 6.4. Histologic classification of bronchogenic lung carcinoma.

Type of cancer	Location in the lung	Notes
Non-small cell carcinomas		
Adenocarcinoma (25 – 40% of all lung tumors)	Peripheral	Microscopic gland formations with surrounding desmoplastic tissue response. Bronchioloalveolar-type adenocarcinoma is unrelated to smoking.
Squamous cell carcinoma (25 – 40% of all lung tumors)	Central	Strong correlation to smoking. Tumors arise near the hilum. Microscopic squamoid or anaplastic (poorly differentiated) cells.
Large cell carcinoma (10 – 15% of all lung tumors)	Peripheral	Rare tumors. Undifferentiated large cells.
Small cell carcinomas		
Small cell ("oat cell") carcinoma (20 – 25%) of all lung tumors)	Central	Strong correlation to smoking. Most aggressive type of bronchogenic carcinoma. Metastasizes widely. Surgery is not indicated. Often responds to chemo and radiation. Microscopic small, blue cells in sheets and nests (no gland formation). Electron microscopy reveals neurosecretory granules — often associated with paraneoplastic syndromes (i.e. ectopic hormone production).

Remember that metastatic lung cancer is more common than primary lung cancer!

notably the **lung apices** (since *M. tuberculosis* is an obligate aerobe). These lesions may progress to **cavitary TB, TB pneumonia,** or **miliary TB**. Miliary TB refers to the presence of multiple, small tuberculous granulomas (like millet seeds) in many organs. Favored targets are bone marrow, liver, spleen, kidneys, and retina.

M. tuberculosis can be demonstrated in the early exudative and caseous phases by staining affected tissue for acid-fast bacilli **(AFB stain)** *(Slide 6.16)*.

Histologically, tuberculous sites with active disease are marked by granulomatous inflammation that forms both caseating and non-caseating tubercles. Multinucleate giant cells are present in the granulomas. One exception—immunocompromised people do not form the characteristic granulomas for lack of immune response.

LUNG CANCER

Lung cancer currently is the **most common cause of cancer mortality worldwide**. The vast majority of lung cancers are **bronchogenic** carcinomas *(Slide 6.17)*, comprising about 90-95% of cases. Bronchogenic carcinomas are classified according to their histologic type. *(Slides 6.18 through 6.21)*.

Table 6.4. Histologic classification of bronchogenic lung carcinoma.

Additionally, lung carcinomas can be divided into two main groups, which help determine the therapeutic modality and prognosis: **small cell carcinomas** (often metastatic, usually responsive to chemotherapy, not amenable to surgery) and **non-small cell carcinomas** (less likely to metastasize, less responsive to chemotherapy, often surgically resectable).

Carcinoid tumors represent approximately 1-5% of lung tumors and are **not bronchogenic** in origin. Grossly, carcinoids are finger-like or polypoid masses that grow into the bronchial lumen.

Microscopically, carcinoid tumors show neuroendocrine differentiation and may secrete hormonally active polypeptides that cause **paraneoplastic syndromes** (described later).

Overall, carcinoids follow a fairly benign course with little to no risk of metastasis.

The **most common site for lung cancer metastasis is the pleural surface**, sometimes followed by dissemination to the pleural cavity or into the pericardium. Many patients experience eventual spread to the tracheal, bronchial, and mediastinal lymph nodes. Distant spread of carcinoma results from both lymphatic and hematogenous dissemination. The most common sites of distant metastases are the adrenal glands, liver, brain, and bones. In lymphatic dissemination, subpleural lymphatics may be outlined by the contained tumor, with a characteristic gross appearance referred to as **lymphangitis carcinomatosis.**

Systemic manifestations of lung tumors may include:

1. **Lambert-Eaton myasthenic syndrome**, in which muscle weakness is caused by autoantibodies directed to **neuronal calcium channels.**
2. **Pancoast's tumor**: cancer in the apex of the lung may involve the **cervical sympathetic plexus**, causing **Horner's syndrome** (ptosis, miosis, anhydrosis).
3. **Superior vena cava syndrome**, due to tumor obstruction or compression of the superior vena cava, leading to **dyspnea, cyanosis,** and **facial swelling.**
4. **Dermatologic abnormalities**, including **acanthosis nigricans** (dark, velvety plaques on intertriginous skin due to stimulation of dermal growth factors by tumor secretions).
5. **Paraneoplastic syndromes**: ectopic hormone or hormone-like production.

The most common paraneoplastic syndromes are:

1. **Cushing's syndrome**, caused by excess **ACTH** in association with **small cell carcinoma.**
2. **Hyponatremia.** caused by too much antidiuretic hormone (**ADH, vasopressin**) due to **small cell carcinoma.**
3. **Hypercalcemia**, caused by secretion of **parathyroid hormone**-related peptide in association with **squamous cell carcinoma.**
4. **Carcinoid syndrome** (flushing, diarrhea, cyanosis) associated with excess **serotonin** and **bradykinin** secretion by **carcinoid tumors.**

DISEASES OF THE PLEURA
Pleural Effusions

Normally, no more than 15 mL of clear, serous fluid occupies the pleural space. Increased accumulations occur in several settings:

1. **Increased hydrostatic pressure**, as in congestive heart failure
2. **Increased vascular permeability**, seen with infection
3. **Decreased oncotic pressure**, as in nephrotic syndrome

4. **Increased negative intrapleural pressure**, seen in atelectasis
5. **Decreased lymphatic drainage**, as in mediastinal carcinomatosis

Hydrothorax is a **collection of serous fluid within the pleural cavity** and most commonly arises in the setting of cardiac failure, but also can result from renal and liver failure.

Hemothorax is **blood in the pleural cavity** and may represent a fatal complication of a ruptured aortic aneurysm or severe vascular trauma.

Chylothorax is an **accumulation of milky, lymphatic fluid**, generally caused by thoracic duct trauma or obstruction. Chylothorax also is associated with **rheumatoid arthritis.**

Pneumothorax refers to **accumulation of air or gas in the pleural cavity.** Four types of pneumothorax exist:

1. **Spontaneous ("secondary") pneumothorax** is a common complication of any pulmonary disease that causes **rupture of alveoli** (e.g., emphysema, asthma, and tuberculosis). Spontaneous pneumothorax **may be idiopathic** in young people, caused by the accidental rupture of small, apical blebs.
2. **Traumatic pneumothorax** is caused by a perforating **injury to the chest wall** (e.g., rib fracture) and often is accompanied by hemothorax.
3. **Tension pneumothorax** often occurs in patients who are mechanically ventilated (i.e., intensive care patients), due to **compression of the lungs and mediastinal structures** by positive pressure ventilation.
4. **Iatrogenic pneumothorax** is a possible **surgical complication**, especially in transthoracic needle aspiration and thoracentesis.

Clinically, pneumothorax causes **compression, collapse, and atelectasis** of the lung, leading to marked respiratory distress and **deviation of the trachea to the contralateral side.** Insertion of a chest tube can release the unwanted gas and return the intrathoracic pressures to normal.

Pleural Tumors

Pleural tumors can be primary (e.g., malignant mesothelioma, described earlier), but most commonly are **due to metastatic disease.** Most frequently, the metastatic malignancies arise from primary neoplasms of the **lung** and **breast**.

7

Gastrointestinal Tract Pathology

OVERVIEW

Fig. 7-1. The gastrointestinal (GI) tract, affectionately known as "The Gut."

The GI tract is essentially a long tube that extends all the way from the mouth to the anus. This tube has many different parts, and the different sections have different functions. Nevertheless, anatomically, there are always 3 distinct layers of tissue throughout the entire length of the gastrointestinal tract. In order from the inner surface to the external surface, they are the **mucosa, muscularis,** and **serosa** *(Slides 7.1 and 7.8)*. Different disease processes affect these 3 layers in various manners, and this fact is essential in understanding the nature of gastrointestinal pathology.

The suffix "-itis" literally implies inflammation and is often applied to disease processes. Every organ can become inflamed and can have an associated "-itis," and it is important to focus on the associated causes and complications that arise from inflammation.

A common finding associated with the gastrointestinal system is jaundice, and many diseases, not just those associated with the GI tract, can cause jaundice. Jaundice is caused by an accumulation of bilirubin, which under normal circumstances is conjugated in the liver and excreted in the feces in the form of bile.

Jaundice is divided into two types: **obstructive** and **non-obstructive**. This distinction can help to make a large list of differential diagnoses shorter in order to help close in on the true diagnosis.

Obstructive jaundice is caused by any kind of post-hepatic obstruction, blocking the output of bile, causing conjugated bilirubin to be found in the blood.

Non-obstructive jaundice is due to pre-hepatic causes, in which the bilirubin has not even passed into the liver to be conjugated yet, and often these diseases are not associated with gastrointestinal tract. For example, the lysis of red blood cells in hemolytic anemia causes unconjugated bilirubin to be found in the blood.

Diverticula are also common findings in many parts of the gastrointestinal tract, and occur in two forms: true and false diverticula. A **diverticulum** is simply an outpouching of the wall of the gastrointestinal tract. A true diverticulum is an outpouching of the wall that is covered by all of the 3 main layers of tissue and is usually a congenital malformation. A false diverticulum is an outpouching that is not covered by all 3 layers and develops as weakness in the muscular layer allows the mucosal layer to push through the muscular layer.

THE ESOPHAGUS
Congenital Disorders

Fig. 7-2. Tracheoesophageal fistulas and atresias. These are congenital malformations seen in newborns that involve abnormal formations of the trachea and esophagus, often allowing abnormal communication between the two organs. Each type of formation has a unique presentation, depending on combination of fistula formation (abnormal communication between the esophagus and trachea) and atresia (ending in a blind pouch). Symptoms commonly present when the newborn tries to feed. The common indications are cyanosis, choking, and coughing, which of course vary depending on the type of malformation.

The **most common** variant (90% of cases) involves the upper esophagus ending in a blind pouch (atresia) with communication between the lower esophagus and the trachea (fistula). Another variant involves the upper portion of the esophagus communicating with the trachea, and the lower esophagus is not connected. Finally, the third variant involves fistula between the trachea and the esophagus, but with a patent esophagus throughout its length.

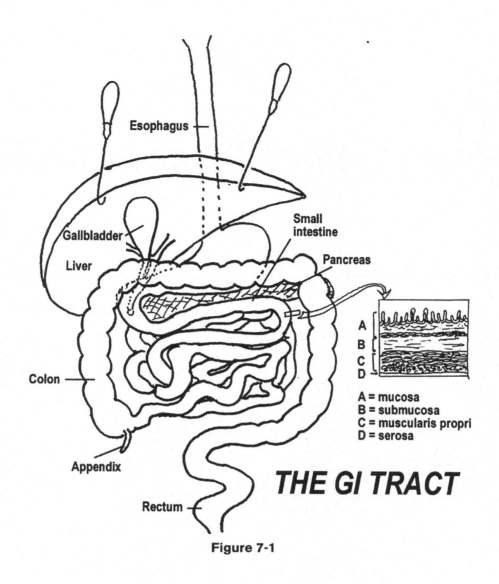

THE GI TRACT

A = mucosa
B = submucosa
C = muscularis propri
D = serosa

Esophagus

Gallbladder

Liver

Small intestine

Pancreas

Colon

Appendix

Rectum

Figure 7-1

TRACHEOESOPHAGEAL ATRESIAS AND FISTULAS

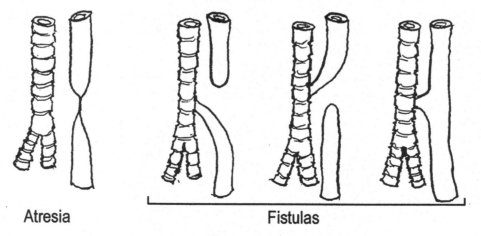

Atresia

Fistulas

Figure 7-2

Structural Disorders

Esophageal Constrictions

An esophageal constriction is a stenosis (narrowing) of the esophageal lumen due to fibrous thickening of the submucosa. This process usually results from inflammation due to injury and can progress to an obstruction in severe cases.

Mucosal webs are protrusions of the esophageal mucosa into the lumen of the esophagus forming "ledges." They are classified based upon their location and are described as "webs" when they occur in the upper esophagus and "Schatzki rings" when they occur in the lower esophagus. Esophageal webs are often associated with **Plummer-Vinson syndrome**, which also includes iron deficiency anemia, glossitis, and cheilosis.

Esophageal Diverticula

Fig. 7-3. Esophageal diverticulae. These are outpouchings of the esophageal wall. They are categorized as **true** (contain full-thickness esophageal wall) or **false** (no muscular wall) **diverticula**. Diverticula of the esophagus are also classified into 3 types based upon their location along the length of the esophagus.

Achalasia

Achalasia is a lack of the ability of the lower esophageal sphincter to relax, as well as lack of motility of the esophagus, due to a loss of the ganglion cells in the myenteric plexus. Therefore, the esophagus remains in the contracted state, making the movement of food into the stomach difficult and resulting in marked dilation of the esophagus. The mechanism of this loss of innervation is poorly understood, and it is often considered to be an idiopathic condition, which is just a fancy way of saying that we do not know what causes it. ("Idiotpathic" is probably a more honest term.) It can also be caused by the organism *Trypanosoma cruzi* (the causative agent of Chagas disease), which destroys the myenteric plexus in the esophagus and other parts of the gastrointestinal tract as well. Achalasia also **predisposes to esophageal carcinoma.**

Esophageal Stricture

Esophageal stricture is caused by severe irritation of the esophageal lining due to long-standing gastroesophageal reflux disease (GERD – see below) or the ingestion of corrosive acids. Ingestion of corrosive acids may be either due to a **suicide attempt** (more common in adults), or accidental (more common in children). The irritation of the esophageal mucosa results in fibrosis, which happens in any sort of healing process, and the end result is narrowing of the esophageal lumen. The severity of an esophageal stric-

ESOPHAGEAL DIVERTICULA

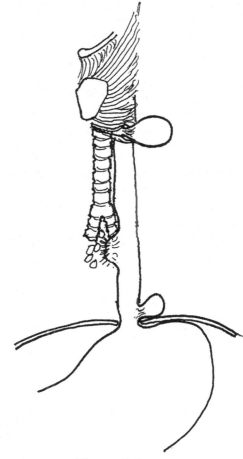

Figure 7-3

ture can vary, depending on the type and extent of injury to the esophageal tissue.

Vascular Disorders

Esophageal Varices

Esophageal varices are dilated veins in the submucosal layer of the esophagus *(Slide 7.2)*. They occur most often in the lower esophagus and proximal stomach. There is a strong association between esophageal varices and portal vein hypertension. These varices appear grossly as dilated submucosal veins that protrude into the lumen of the esophagus, leading to rupture, the most common complication, which may lead to massive bleeding that can be severe enough to result in death.

Mallory-Weiss Syndrome

Mallory-Weiss syndrome is a condition characterized by severe tears or lacerations that occur in the esophagus in a linear fashion and are commonly found near the junction of the stomach and the esophagus. Although the exact mechanism is unknown, Mallory-Weiss syndrome has been linked with alcoholism and most likely results from the mechanical stress of **vomiting**. Like varices, Mallory-Weiss syndrome can lead to severe bleeding and death.

Esophagitis

OK, this is a "no-brainer." The word itself means inflammation of the esophagus. That was easy. The bigger battle is to know the various causes of the inflammation.

Gastro-Esophageal Reflux Disease (GERD)

Fig. 7-4. GERD, with predisposing factors. GERD is caused by reflux of gastric acid into the esophagus resulting in, yes, inflammation! Patients may have complaints of a burning sensation in their thoracic region, otherwise known as heartburn. A common cause of GERD is a **hiatal hernia**. Several other factors predispose a patient to the condition, including **alcohol** and tobacco use. A large increase in gastric volume can also cause this condition, which along with an incompetent lower esophageal sphincter (LES) can allow stomach contents to exit into the esophagus. Microscopically, as with any inflammatory process, inflammatory cells such as neutrophils, eosinophils, and lymphocytes will be present.

Barrett's Esophagus

Long-standing GERD can be dangerous, and it causes changes in the epithelial lining of the esophagus that predisposes the patient to developing **adenocarcinoma**. This change is known as **Barrett's esophagus**, and is a metaplastic process of the esophageal mucosa. Grossly, this metaplastic area appears red and velvety.

GERD: PREDISPOSING FACTORS

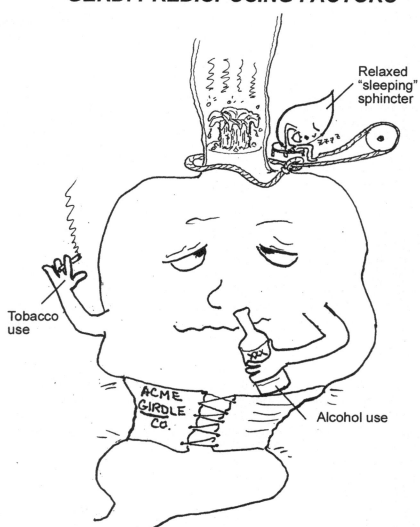

Relaxed "sleeping" sphincter

Tobacco use

Alcohol use

ACME GIRDLE Co.

Figure 7-4

Microscopically, this change is termed columnar metaplasia, which is essentially a change of the normal stratified squamous epithelium of the esophagus to a columnar epithelium normally found in the stomach. There can also be "intestinalization" of the epithelium, characterized by the presence of goblet cells, which are normally found in the intestine.

Candidiasis

Fig. 7-5. Candidiasis. This is a fungal infection caused by the species *Candida*, most commonly *Candida albicans.* It can occur in the oral cavity, vagina, and more rarely in the esophagus. White, painful patches that can be scraped off mucosa surfaces characterize candidiasis. The ability to scrape this lesion off is important because it helps to differentiate candidiasis from other diseases of the oral cavity. Immunosuppression allows oral candidiasis to develop. Cases involving the esophagus usually progress from oral candidiasis and are associated with AIDS, immunosuppression, **diabetes mellitus**, malignancy, and antibiotic treatment.

Other Causes of "-Itis"

Other common causes of esophagitis include infection with viruses such as HSV-1 and CMV as well as radiation treatment and graft-versus-host disease.

Carcinoma of the Esophagus

Carcinomas are the most common type of esophageal malignancy. There are two types: **squamous cell carcinoma** and **adenocarcinoma**. Worldwide, squamous cell carcinoma is the most common, but in the United States there is an **equal incidence** of the two types, which is important to note. The difference is likely related to the declining use of alcohol and tobacco in the United States, a risk factor for squamous cell carcinoma. Both types may become large lesions that can protrude into the lumen of the esophagus, causing

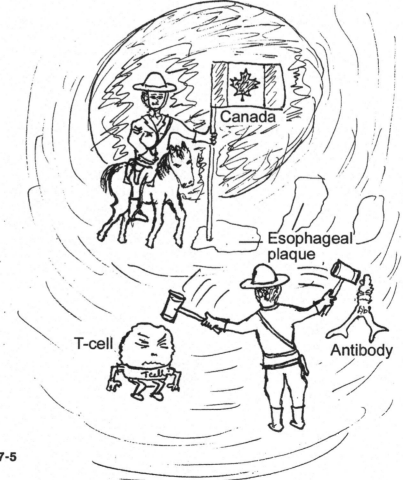

ESOPHAGEAL CANDIDA ("CANADA") IN IMMUNOCOMPROMISED PATIENTS

Canada

Esophageal plaque

T-cell

Antibody

Figure 7-5

obstruction. Spread to adjacent organs occurs by extension through the wall of the esophagus. Predisposing conditions include achalasia, Barrett's esophagus, alcohol and tobacco use, corrosive esophagitis, diverticula, and familial causes.

Squamous Cell Carcinoma of the Esophagus

As discussed, the main risk factors for squamous cell carcinoma of the esophagus *(Slide 7.3)* are **tobacco and alcohol** use. Again, it is the more common of the two types of carcinoma worldwide and usually presents in the **upper two thirds** of the esophagus. It is more common in males and in African-Americans.

Adenocarcinoma of the Esophagus

The main risk factor for adenocarcinoma of the esophagus *(Slide 7.4)* is GERD, which leads to **Barrett's esophagus**. Barrett's esophagus is a premalignant lesion that can develop into adenocarcinoma. It usually arises in the **lower third** of the esophagus, because it is primarily this area that is insulted with stomach acids in patients with GERD, and large lesions can grow in size to involve the cardiac portion of the stomach. It is less common worldwide, but it occurs at the same frequency as squamous cell carcinoma in the United States. It affects men more than women, but different from squamous cell carcinoma, whites more often than blacks.

THE STOMACH
Congenital Disorders

Pyloric Stenosis

This congenital condition, more common in boys, is due to hypertrophy of the circular muscle layer of the pyloric sphincter. It presents within the first few weeks of life as **projectile vomiting** following feeding, and often a mass can be palpated in the epigastric region. It is easily correctable with surgery.

Heterotopic Rests

Normal pancreatic tissue can sometimes be found in the stomach. These rests (nest of normal tissue in an abnormal place), if large, can cause inflammation due to the release of pancreatic enzymes.

Gastritis

This is another "no-brainer," except now it involves the stomach. Again, same story as with any "-itis", there can be many causes of inflammation. Gastritis is divided into two categories: acute and chronic, which is based upon the type of inflammatory cells present.

Acute Gastritis

This is also referred to as "**erosive gastritis**." Grossly, areas of erosion of the mucosa may be present.

Microscopically, all the signs of an acute process are present. Neutrophils (the key cell type seen in acute inflammation) and hemorrhage can be seen, along with areas of necrosis. Common causes include cigarette and alcohol use, long-term **NSAID** (non-steroidal anti-inflammatory drug) use, burn injury (Curling ulcer), brain injury (Cushing ulcer), and many other forms of gastric irritators. Depending on the severity of mucosal injury, the presentation can be variable from mild epigastric pain to bleeding that, in the most extreme cases, can result in death.

Chronic Gastritis

The microscopic picture of chronic gastritis is what one would expect: chronic inflammatory cells such as lymphocytes and sometimes plasma cells in the mucosa. There is atrophy of the mucosal glands, and sometimes metaplasia, changes that can lead to the development of **adenocarcinoma**. Chronic gastritis is divided into two groups based upon their location of occurrence in the stomach. The most common cause is bacteria, specifically *Helicobacter pylori*, comprising **type B** ("antral"). The organism has been linked to both gastric and duodenal ulcers, and is associated with **increased risk** of gastric carcinoma. **Type A** ("fundal") is associated with other conditions, including pernicious anemia, chronic thyroiditis, Addison's disease, achlorhydria, and other autoimmune conditions.

Structural Disorders

Hiatal Hernias

Fig. 7-6. Hiatal and rolling hernias. A hiatal hernia is a protrusion of the stomach through the diaphragm into the thoracic cavity. There are several different types. The **sliding hiatal hernia** is a protrusion of the cardiac portion of the stomach through the diaphragm, causing the stomach to take on a bell shape. This protrusion occurs in the opening of the diaphragm through which the esophagus passes. It is associated with GERD and thought to contribute to the reflux of gastric acid into the esophagus by increasing the pressure of the lower esophageal sphincter.

The **rolling hiatal hernia** is formed when a portion of the stomach protrudes through the diaphragm in a separate location other than at the point where the esophagus passes through to the abdominal cavity. This protruding portion can become **entrapped** and necrotic.

Peptic Ulcer Disease of the Stomach

Peptic ulcers are ulcers of the stomach, small intestine or esophagus. In the stomach they are referred to as gastric ulcers. Ulcers in the stomach occur most

HIATAL HERNIAS

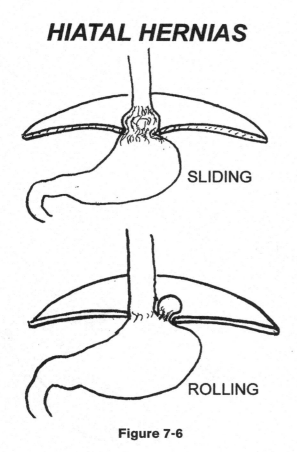

SLIDING

ROLLING

Figure 7-6

avoiding eating decreases pain. Duodenal ulcers, on the other hand, feel better with meals, and there is often associated weight gain, since eating alleviates pain.

Stomach Carcinoma

Adenocarcinoma is the most common tumor of the stomach, and it occurs at ages fifty and older. It is also more common in males than females. The etiology is not well understood, as there appear to be both genetic and environmental components. There is increased frequency in **blood group A**, indicating a genetic predisposition. Environmental components also play a large role in the pathogenesis. *Helicobacter pylori* infection, diets rich in nitrosamines (dietary amines used as food preservatives in smoked fish and other meats), diets high in salt and low in fiber, achlorhydria, and chronic gastritis all increase the risk. Common sites of involvement are the lesser curvature of the antrum and the distal stomach.

Grossly, stomach adenocarcinomas appear as areas with irregular borders, which is a very different appearance from the well-circumscribed appearance of gastric ulcers. They can be exophytic (protrude from the wall), flat, or excavated. The term **linitis plastica** is used to describe stomach cancer that is diffusely infiltrative. They are aggressive tumors that tend to metastasize early to regional lymph nodes. Metastatic involvement of a supraclavicular node is known as a **Virchow node**.

Fig. 7-8. The Krukenberg tumor. This is a type of adenocarcinoma of the stomach that **metastasizes bilaterally to the ovaries**. The tumor cells are called **signet-ring cells**. There is abundant **mucin**, appearing as clearing in the cytoplasm, which pushes the nucleus to one side of the cell, giving the appearance of a ring. **(Think of the nucleus as the diamond, and the mucin in the cytoplasm as the open area that slips around the finger.)**

THE SMALL INTESTINE
Congenital Disorders

Meckel Diverticulum

A Meckel diverticulum is a congenital anomaly that results from a failure of the **vitelline duct** to involute. These are true diverticula because all 3 layers of the wall surround them. Remember, congenital diverticula tend to be of the "true" variety. In half of cases they will contain ectopic tissue from other parts of the gastrointestinal tract such as pancreatic, gastric, duodenal, and colonic tissue. These are usually asymptomatic, and are discovered as an incidental finding, but occasionally they present as bleeding, perforation, and even ulceration when there is ectopic tissue present.

commonly in the lesser curvature, antrum, and prepyloric regions of the stomach, but the most common location overall is the duodenum. They occur more commonly in men and twice as often in smokers. Grossly, they appear as ulcerations with a smooth base and well circumscribed, or "punched-out" appearing, borders. The most common cause is the bacteria *Helicobacter pylori*, which interferes with the normal protection mechanisms of the gastric epithelium, making it more susceptible to the corrosive effects of the normally low pH of the stomach. The treatment is antibiotic therapy.

Fig. 7-7. Peptic ulcers and Helicobacter pylori.

Several other causes of gastric ulcers include gastric hypertrophy, Zollinger-Ellison syndrome (resulting from a benign gastrin-producing tumor), chronic **NSAID** use, and cigarette smoking. Regardless of the mechanism, stomach ulcers can be precursors to **carcinoma**.

Finally, there are several important distinctions between gastric and duodenal ulcers. Duodenal ulcers, unlike gastric ulcers, **do not** have an increased risk of malignancy. Also, gastric ulcers have pain associated with meals, secondarily causing weight loss, since

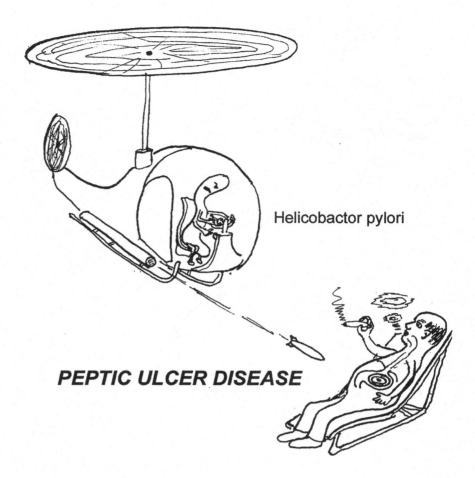

Helicobactor pylori

PEPTIC ULCER DISEASE

Figure 7-7

Malabsorption Syndromes

Celiac Sprue

Celiac sprue is a disease mostly of whites. It is caused by sensitivity to **gluten** (found in wheat products). The disease is immune mediated, and gliadin antibodies can be detected, but there is also a genetic component. HLA types HLA-B8, HLA-DQ2 and HLA-DW3 are all associated with the disease. Patients present with diarrhea and weight loss. The stools are characterized as being **frothy and foul smelling**.

Microscopy of celiac sprue shows plasma cells and lymphocytes, and the mucosal surface is flattened and the **villi are blunted**. These changes are most severe in the proximal duodenum, making this disease a cause of malabsorption.

The treatment of celiac sprue is avoidance of all gluten-containing products in the diet. Progression to malignancy occurs in 10-15% of cases, most commonly T-cell lymphoma.

Tropical Sprue

The microscopic changes in tropical sprue are similar to celiac sprue, and therefore, also cause a malabsorption syndrome. It is thought to have an infectious origin, which is supported by the disease response to antibiotic treatment. However, no specific agent has been linked.

Whipple Disease

Tropheryma whippelii is the bacterium that causes this disease, and it can infect any organ system. The small bowel is a common site, along with the joints and the central nervous system. For this reason, arthralgias and neurologic and cardiac symptoms are common.

Microscopically, macrophages that stain with PAS are seen in the mucosa of the small bowel in Whipple disease. However, electron microscopy is necessary to visualize the organism itself. The treatment is antibiotic therapy.

Peptic Ulcer Disease of the Small Intestine

Peptic ulcers are found in the first part of the duodenum and were discussed with gastric ulcers. Comparing and contrasting these two types of ulcers is very important. Along with the causes already mentioned in the gastric ulcer discussion, duodenal ulcers are also

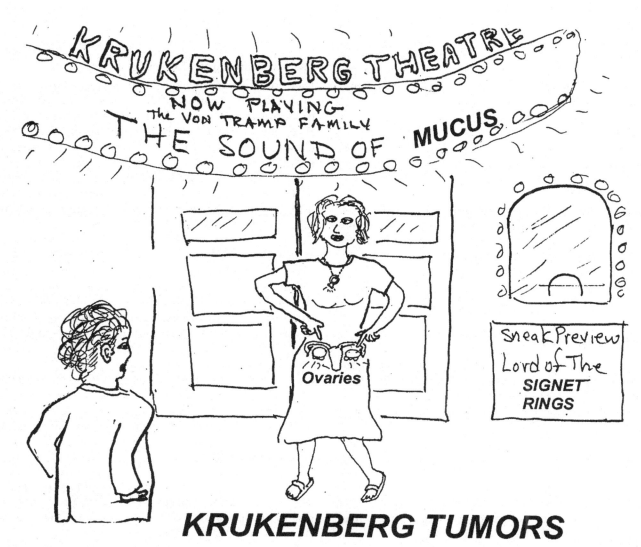

KRUKENBERG TUMORS

Figure 7-8

associated with increased secretion of gastric acid and pepsin, but there is no association in gastric ulcers. Genetic factors may also play a role in the pathogenesis of duodenal ulcer disease, as it is more common in blood group O. Several other medical conditions that are known to be associated with duodenal ulcers specifically include primary hyperparathyroidism, multiple endocrine neoplasia (MEN) type 1, and Zollinger-Ellison syndrome.

Zollinger-Ellison Syndrome

This syndrome presents as recurrent ulcers, most often in the jejunum. They develop as a result of an islet cell tumor of the pancreas that secretes gastrin. It is this secretion that causes the ulcer formation.

Tumors of the Small Intestine

Tumors of the small bowel are relatively uncommon, and compromise only 3-6% of all gastrointestinal tumors.

Carcinoid Tumors

Carcinoid tumors can occur in multiple areas of the body, with 30% occurring in the small bowel (*Slide 7.5*). In general, they produce vasoactive amines (mainly **serotonin**) that cause a **carcinoid syndrome**, which is characterized by cutaneous flushing, diarrhea, abdominal cramping, bronchospasms, and valvular lesions and heart failure on the right side of the heart. This specificity for only the right side of the heart is due to the inactivation of the amines in the lung, thus rendering them harmless by the time they reach the left side of the heart.

Carcinoid tumors of the small bowel, however, do **not** cause valvular lesions of the heart, as the vasoactive amines are also inactivated in the **liver**, and are thus already inactivated by the time they reach the heart. It is carcinoid tumors located in other organs that cause right-sided heart valve damage.

Lymphoma

Lymphoma can arise from the lymphoid tissue that is scattered throughout the small bowel.

Adenocarcinoma

This is the **most common** primary malignancy of the small bowel. It can present early with obstructive symptoms. Usually it presents as fatigue and rectal bleeding and often is very large at the time of discovery, increasing the mortality of this cancer.

THE COLON

Hirschsprung Disease

Hirschsprung Disease, also known as **congenital aganglionic megacolon**, is a congenital condition in which there is a **lack of neural crest migration**, leading to an absence of ganglion cells in both the submucosal and myenteric plexuses. This results in the inability of the colon to accommodate the passage of waste products, causing a dilation of the colon proximal to the region devoid of ganglion cells. The enlargement can become so massive that rupture of the bowel occurs. As this is a congenital disorder, it presents immediately after birth as a failure to pass meconium (the first bowel movement of a newborn).

Other conditions can also lead to a similar picture. **Chagas disease** can cause dilation of the colon as trypanosomes destroy the neural elements in the bowel. **Ulcerative colitis** also has an associated complication known as **toxic megacolon**, in which inflammation from the disease process destroys the neural plexuses. These conditions combined belong to the disease grouping of **acquired megacolon.**

Inflammatory Diseases

More "-itis" diseases! This time it is the colon, with the term "colitis".

Infectious Enterocolitis

Through ingestion, the gastrointestinal tract can easily become infected with all sorts of microorganisms including viruses (rotavirus and Norwalk virus), bacteria (*Staphylococcus aureus, Vibrio cholerae, Clostridium perfringens, E. coli, Shigella*, and *Salmonella*), and parasites (*Entamoeba histolytica*, and *Giardia lamblia*). All of these microorganisms can cause various degrees of diarrhea and inflammation of the gastrointestinal tract through different mechanisms.

Pseudomembranous Colitis

Pseudomembranous colitis *(Slide 7.6)* is a common hospital complication after patients are placed on broad-spectrum antibiotics. It presents as massive diarrhea. It is caused by an overgrowth of the bacteria *Clostridium difficile* due to the loss of normal gastrointestinal flora secondary to antibiotic use. The bacterial colonies form a gray-colored exudate on the mucosal surface of the bowel, appearing as a **pseudomembrane**, and produce an exotoxin, which causes fibrinous necrosis of the mucosa.

Ulcerative Colitis

Ulcerative colitis is an autoimmune disease causing inflammation that is limited to the large bowel. It is the first of two entities encompassed in the category of Inflammatory Bowel Disease, the other being Crohn's disease (see below). The inflammation starts in the rectum, and progresses **continuously** to involve greater areas of the colon. In serious cases it can involved the entire colon. It presents in early adulthood as diarrhea containing large amounts of blood and mucus.

Besides the intestinal symptoms, there are associated extraintestinal manifestations, including polyarthritis, uveitis, episcleritis, pyoderma gangrenosum, and sclerosing cholangitis.

Grossly, the ulcerations of the mucosa in ulcerative colitis give the appearance of **pseudopolyps** *(Slide 7.7)*. These are **not true polyps**, but only appear polypoid due to the appearance of small areas of normal mucosa surrounded by large areas of ulceration.

Microscopically, the inflammatory changes in ulcerative colitis affect **only the mucosa**. "Crypt abscesses" also occur, consisting of neutrophils in the crypts of Lieberkühn.

Common complications that arise in ulcerative colitis include toxic megacolon, perforation, and the development of **adenocarcinoma**. (There is a much greater risk to patients with ulcerative colitis than patients with Crohn's disease.)

Fig. 7-9. Ulcerative colitis. It starts at the rectum and contains pseudopolyps ("soda-pop"). The cooking delicacy is a crepe ("crypt abscesses").

Crohn's Disease

Crohn's disease is the second inflammatory bowel disease. The etiology of Crohn's disease is unknown, but it is believed to be infectious. It is more common in females and in the Jewish population. It is **not limited to the colon**, and in fact, any part of the gastrointestinal tract can be affected, with the small intestine being

ULCERATIVE COLITIS

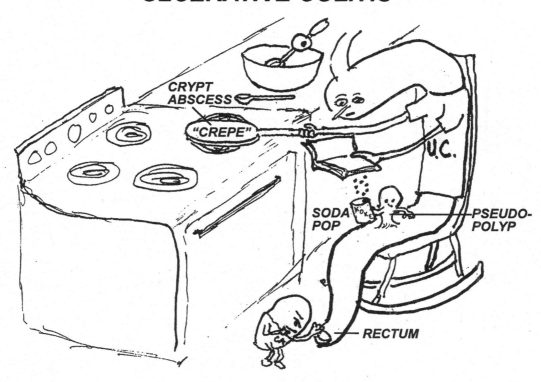

Figure 7-9

most common. Other common sites include the distal ileocecum and the colon, but for the most part the disease spares the rectum. Symptoms include abdominal pain, diarrhea, and malabsorption.

Grossly, there is thickening of the involved segments of bowel, which can result in narrowing of the lumen, called the **"string sign"** on x-ray, and there can even be eventual obstruction. There are also linear ulcerations, creeping fat, and edema of the surviving mucosa, causing elevation of the remaining mucosa, and giving a characteristic **"cobblestone"** appearance to the bowel wall. The lesions are not continuous; there are sections of affected bowel immediately next to a section of normal bowel, and then another area of affected bowel, a pattern known as **"skip lesions."**

Microscopically, there is **transmural** (all 3 layers) involvement of the bowel wall in Crohn's disease, and often noncaseating granulomas.

Fig. 7-10. Crohn 's disease. An old Crohn is **skipping** over **cobblestones**, laying a path of **string** so he does not get lost while going **transmural**.

A common complication of transmural ulceration is the formation of **fistulas** (connections between two organs) and strictures. Fistulas can form with other portions of the small bowel, bladder, vagina, and skin. Other symptoms of the disease that do not involve the gastrointestinal tract are known as **extraintestinal manifestations** and can include migratory polyarthritis, ankylosing spondylitis, erythema nodosa, and sacroiliitis. There is also an increased risk of developing cancer, but this risk is greater with ulcerative colitis.

It is **very important** to distinguish ulcerative colitis from Crohn's disease; while they are both lumped into the category of Inflammatory Bowel Disease they have several very important characteristics that distinguish one from the other.

Vascular Disorders

Ischemic Bowel Disease

The bowel, like any organ, can become ischemic due to lack of blood flow. Infarction of the bowel is characterized by the extent of wall involvement: **mucosal** (limited to the mucosal surface), **mural** (extending into the muscular wall), or **transmural** (extending to the entire thickness of the bowel wall). The most common cause of an ischemic bowel is atherosclerotic disease. Because of the collateral nature of the large blood supply to the bowel (superior mesenteric artery, the inferior mesenteric artery, and the internal iliacs), infarctions usually

CROHN'S DISEASE

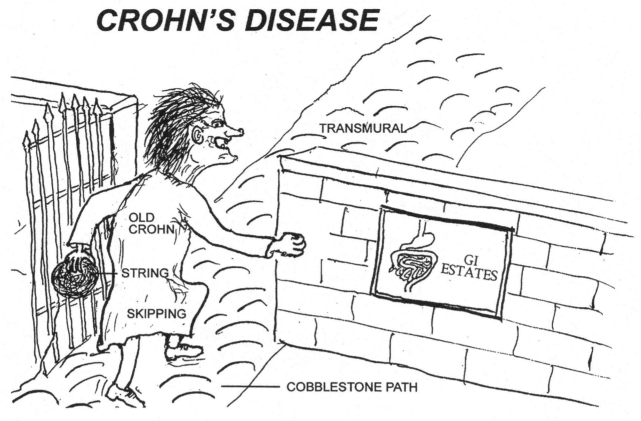

Figure 7-10

occur when two or more of the supplying vessels are occluded. The superior mesenteric artery is the most common vessel to be occluded.

The "watershed" areas (those that are the farthest away from the supplying vessels and have low oxygen tension with normal amounts of perfusion) are affected first when there is any decrease in blood supply. These watershed regions are the splenic flexure and the rectosigmoid junction. They bear the brunt of any ischemia. There is a very high death rate, which nears 50-75%, due to the rapid progression of this disease.

Angiodysplasia

Angiodysplasia presents with unexplained rectal bleeding. It is caused by abnormal dilation of vessels in the mucosa, which rupture easily when subjected to trauma (which can occur easily in the bowel with the passage of stool).

Hemorrhoids

Hemorrhoids are caused by a dilation of the perianal and anal veins as a result of elevated venous pressure within the portal system. Two different venous systems exist in this area, the inferior and superior rectal plexuses. **External hemorrhoids** develop with the dilation of the veins of the

inferior rectal plexus, and there is associated **pain** due to the innervation of the area by the inferior rectal nerves. **Internal hemorrhoids** are dilations of the superior rectal plexus. They usually have no associated pain, as there is autonomic innervation in that area.

Both types have associated rectal bleeding, since they are close to the mucosal surface, and rupture easily with the trauma of bowel movements. Hemorrhoids rarely develop in people under the age of 30, except in pregnancy (in which it is common to have hemorrhoids). They can be an early warning sign of other diseases that have associated portal hypertension.

AV Malformations

Arteriovenous (AV) malformations are large, tortuous, congenital vessel collections that form in the wall of the colon. They are prone to rupture and are one of the leading causes of the bleeding per rectum in the elderly.

Diverticular Disease

Diverticulosis

Diverticulosis is a condition of multiple false diverticula *(Slide 7.9)*. They are most often seen in the sigmoid colon and associated with increased age. In the Western world approximately 50% of people who are over the age of 60 have this condition. The pathogenesis makes sense, since as a person ages, the muscular layer of the bowel wall becomes weaker due to years of intraluminal pressure from fecal material. Eventually the mucosa pushes through these areas of weakness. There is no associated inflammation (if there were, it would then be called **diverticulitis**), and they are usually asymptomatic, but can cause alternating symptoms of diarrhea and constipation.

Diverticulitis

Inflamed diverticula present as abdominal pain, tenderness, fever, bright red rectal bleeding, and leukocytosis, resulting from the entrapment of fecal material within the diverticula. The sigmoid colon is a common site, since this is where diverticulosis is most common, causing pain in the left lower quadrant. Complications include perforation, peritonitis, and abscess formation.

Obstructive Disorders

Hernias

Hernias result from weaknesses in the abdominal wall (common areas are the femoral and inguinal canals, umbilical region, and scarred regions from previous abdominal surgeries), which allow abdominal contents such as loops of bowel to move through these points, making a pouch. Hernias are important to treat because the blood supply to the herniated abdominal contents can become compromised (**"strangulation"**), leading to infarction, perforation, and obstruction of the gastrointestinal tract.

Adhesions

Adhesions have many causes, **such as abdominal surgery**, peritonitis, Crohn's disease, and endometriosis. Any process that causes intra-abdominal injury can cause adhesions. Adhesions form as a result of the fibrous scarring that occurs in the healing process. They can sometimes choke off portions of the bowel and its blood supply, causing infarction and obstruction.

Intussusception

A portion of bowel that invaginates into a more distal segment causes intussusception. This can cause bowel obstruction and infarction by pinching off the mesenteric blood supply. It is most common in **children** and infants with no apparent gastrointestinal abnormalities, but when it occurs in adults it is associated with **tumor masses** and conditions that increase gastrointestinal tract motility.

Volvulus

Volvulus is an uncommon twisting of the gastrointestinal tract around its mesenteric attachment, causing obstruction and infarction. The sigmoid colon is most often involved, so rigid sigmoidoscopy is the treatment of choice to relieve the volvulus.

Benign Tumors and Polyps

Polyps are outgrowths of rapidly dividing mucosal cells into the lumen of the colon (and rarely the small intestine). There are a large variety of polyps, which are listed below.

Hyperplastic Polyps

Hyperplastic polyps occur anywhere along the length of the bowel and have no significance clinically.

Inflammatory Polyps

Inflammatory polyps consist of granulation tissue and are most commonly caused by the inflammation that occurs with the inflammatory bowel diseases (Ulcerative colitis and Crohn's disease).

Hamartomatous Polyps

Juvenile Polyps: These occur most often in children (no surprise according to the name). They can affect both the large and small bowel, but the most frequent site of occurrence is the rectum. There is no increased potential to develop malignancy.

Peutz-Jeghers Polyps (Peutz-Jegher syndrome): In this **autosomal dominant** syndrome hamartomatous polyps can be found in the small and large bowel. They have no increased malignant potential. Along with polyps in the gastrointestinal tract, melanotic accumulations are seen on the hands, mouth, lips, and on the genitals. There is also an association with malignancy in other organs.

Adenomatous Polyps

There are 3 different configurations of adenomatous polyps. The polyps themselves are not malignant, but depending upon the configuration, there is an increased potential to develop into a malignancy. They are considered true neoplasms. Presentation ranges from being asymptomatic to rectal bleeding.

Tubular Adenoma (*Slide 7.10*): This is the most common configuration and appears small and pedunculated. There is a slightly increased risk of developing malignancy, but the malignant potential is **low**.

Tubulovillous Adenoma: This configuration comprises 5-10% of adenomatous polyps and appears similar to tubular adenomas; however, their surface is covered by finger-like projections. They are of **intermediate** malignant potential.

Villous Adenoma (*Slides 7.11 and 7.12*): This configuration comprises 1% of adenomatous polyps and appears somewhat flattened and sessile with a velvety surface. They have the **highest** associated malignant potential of the 3, with approximately 30% transforming into malignancy.

Fig. 7-11. The three forms of adenomatous polyps of the colon, each associated with a different cancer risk.

Malignant Tumors

Familial Polyposis Syndrome

Familial polyposis syndrome is an **autosomal dominant** syndrome *(Slide 7.13)*. It involves countless adenomatous polyps that have a greatly increased risk of malignant transformation, such that as the patient ages the risk approaches **100%**! For this reason **colectomy** is recommended for these patients as the only means to prevent malignancy.

Adenocarcinoma

Adenocarcinoma is the **most common** malignancy found in the colon *(Slides 7.14 and 7.15)*. Peak incidence is in the 6th and 7th decades of life. There are many predisposing factors including **ulcerative colitis**, inherited multiple polyposis syndromes (such as familial polyposis syndrome), adenomatous polyps (most especially the villous configuration), genetic factors (there is an increased risk in relatives), and low fiber/high fat diet. Diet is thought to play a role since a low fiber/high fat diet leads to a decreased transit time through the gastrointestinal tract, which increases the time that carcinogens are in contact with the bowel wall.

THE APPENDIX

Acute Appendicitis

Episodes of acute appendicitis occur most often in the 2nd and 3rd decades of life and initially present with vague periumbilical pain progressing to severe, focal right lower quadrant pain. Fever and an acute increase in immature inflammatory cells (the so-call "**left shift**") are often accompanying signs. Bacterial proliferation in the appendix and invasion of the appendiceal wall give rise to these symptoms.

Grossly the appendix is swollen and contains a purulent exudate (pus). An impacted fecalith (inspissated fecal material) is occasionally present. Microscopically, neutrophils can be seen within the appendix wall. Without surgical intervention, this condition can rapidly progress to perforation or abscess formation.

Carcinoid Tumors

These tumors, discussed in greater detail in the tumors of the small bowel, favor, in part, the appendix.

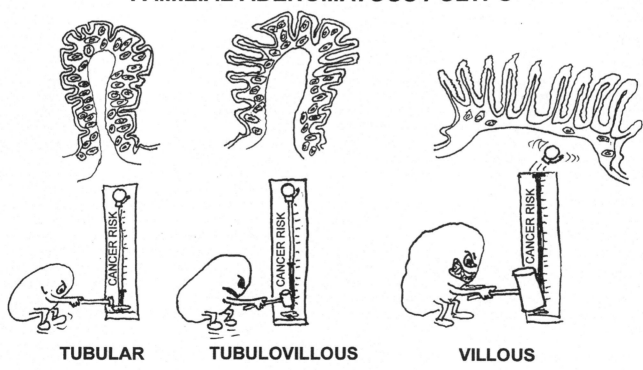

FAMILIAL ADENOMATOUS POLYPS

TUBULAR   **TUBULOVILLOUS**   **VILLOUS**

Figure 7-11

THE LIVER (Slide 7.16)
Hepatitis

There are many different etiologies of liver inflammation. The best-known causes are infectious, but many other conditions can cause hepatitis as well.

Hepatitis A

Hepatitis A is caused by an **RNA virus** of the same name that is transmitted by the **fecal-oral route**. A common cause is eating raw seafood, such as oysters. There is no carrier/chronic state, and the patient merely becomes ill with an acute bout of hepatitis, almost always **recovers**, with only the rare case leading to death. There is no increased risk of developing hepatocellular carcinoma, since there is no long-term chronic inflammation. After the bout, the patient becomes immune to future infections by the same virus.

Hepatitis B

Hepatitis B differs from hepatitis A in almost every way. The virus that causes this form of hepatitis is a **DNA virus** (notice that this one is the only hepatitis DNA virus). It is transmitted **parenterally, sexually, and by vertical routes** (from mother to offspring). There are several disease states, as a patient can have complete remission, become a chronic carrier, or have chronic active disease. There are several portions of the virus that become active during infection, and antibodies to many of these portions are detectable in the patient's serum at different points during the infection. It is the development of the antibody to the surface antigen (anti-HBsAg) specifically that is necessary to completely clear the infection from the body. Without the development of this specific antibody (antibodies to other parts of the virus will develop), the infection will not be cleared, and the patient will have chronic infection.

Therefore, close monitoring of a patient's antibodies is very important for following the disease. (Remember that we immunize with the surface antigen in order to evoke an antibody response to the surface antigen. If a person is immunized, they will have made antibodies to the surface antigen, too, but will not have made antibodies to other viral parts because they were not exposed to the entire virus during the immunization process.) Once a patient has either been infected and developed the anti-HBs antibodies on their own or developed it through immunization, they will then have protective immunity for life. Not all people infected with the virus will develop the anti-HBs antibodies, in which case they will be chronic carriers for life, susceptible to reactivation and a continually active disease.

Microscopically, hepatocytes affected by an ongoing infection will have a "**ground glass**" appearance of the cytoplasm. With chronic infection there is a strong association with the development of **hepatocellular carcinoma** due to the continuous insult from inflammation.

Hepatitis C

This **RNA virus** is transmitted **parenterally** and is a common contaminant of blood in our blood bank system. Other frequent methods of transmission include **IV drug use**, unclean tattoo equipment, and unclean needles used for body piercing. Once infected there is no way for the body to rid itself of the infection. It develops into a carrier state and eventually chronic hepatitis. It is because of the chronic course of the disease that this type of hepatitis is associated with **hepatocellular carcinoma**.

Hepatitis D (Delta Agent)

Hepatitis D is a small piece of RNA (nicknamed the delta agent) that **cannot replicate** on its own, and is therefore not infective on its own. It requires the presence of the **hepatitis B** virus to replicate, so for this reason immunization against hepatitis B is the means of controlling the risk of contracting hepatitis D. A combined infection of hepatitis B with the delta agent is a much more serious disease than hepatitis B alone. For unknown reasons the delta agent is more common in the IV drug-using population.

Hepatitis E

This virus is transmitted **enterically** and is often the cause of water-borne epidemics in underdeveloped countries. For the most part it is not dangerous, and has a disease course similar to hepatitis A, but for unknown reasons has an increased mortality rate in **pregnant women**.

Remember A and E you get **A**fter **E**ating and B and C you get from **B**lood **C**ontamination.

There are many other infectious causes of hepatitis including the Epstein-Barr virus, cytomegalovirus, herpes simplex virus type 1, yellow fever, and schistosomiasis.

Fatty Liver Diseases

Many things can cause the development of fat vesicles in the liver, and these diseases are categorized by the size of the fat vacuoles that accumulate in the liver (**microvesicular** and **macrovesicular liver diseases**). The focus will be on the microvesicular causes, as they are more commonly encountered.

Microvesicular Liver Disease

Reye's Syndrome

This rare, but often fatal syndrome is seen in young children who are given aspirin (salicylates) or aspirin-containing products during an acute viral infection, most commonly varicella-zoster virus (VZV) and influenza B infections. For unknown reasons, this combination can result in microvesicular fatty liver, encephalopathy, coma, and death. For this reason, parents are encouraged not to give their children aspirin or aspirin-containing products if there is a possible ongoing viral infection.

Fatty Liver of Pregnancy

Microvesicular fatty liver disease during pregnancy most often occurs in the 3rd trimester and has a **high mortality** rate.

Alcoholic Liver Disease

Excessive alcohol consumption is the most common cause of liver disease in the United States. Three histologic changes can come about from alcoholic insult: **fatty change**, **hepatitis**, and **cirrhosis**. A liver that has been undergoing alcohol insult for many years can progress either to fatty change or hepatitis, from which the liver can recover if the alcoholic insult is stopped; either of these conditions can progress to cirrhosis if the alcohol insult continues.

Fatty change is the most common change seen with chronic alcohol consumption. The normal liver parenchyma becomes replaced by fat and grossly appears a bright yellow color, but it is completely reversible if alcohol ingestion is stopped. It can progress to cirrhosis if it is not stopped (which is not a reversible condition and predisposes to cancer).

Alcoholic hepatitis is characterized microscopically by focal areas of necrosis, neutrophils, **Mallory bodies** (eosinophilic intracytoplasmic inclusions), and sclerosis around the central vein. An important laboratory feature is that the liver function enzyme **AST will be elevated**, but very often its close cousin **ALT will be normal**.

Cirrhosis

Cirrhosis is a scarring of the liver and the death of hepatocytes *(Slides 7.17 and 7.18)*. It is the end stage of many different types of liver disease, not just alcohol insult! As already mentioned, with chronic alcohol consumption the liver can progress to cirrhosis from both fatty change and hepatitis if alcohol consumption is continued. Cirrhosis will develop from many other types of insults to the liver besides alcohol, such as certain drugs/chemicals, viral hepatitis, biliary obstruction, and hemochromatosis, just to give a few examples.

Fig. 7-12. Causes of cirrhosis.

The clinical signs that result include jaundice, hypoalbuminemia (albumin is made in the liver), coagulation factor deficiencies (all coagulation factors except von Willebrand's factor are made in the liver), gynecomastia, loss of sexual hair, **asterixis** (tremor of the hand), anemia, coma, and hypertension of the portal system. **Portal hypertension** itself causes a specific constellation of symptoms including esophageal varices, rectal hemorrhoids, **caput medusae** (engorgement of the periumbilical veins visible on the abdomen in the umbilical region), ascites, testicular atrophy, and splenomegaly. When any of these symptoms are seen, cirrhosis as a cause must be in the differential diagnosis, and then the cause of the cirrhosis must be investigated.

Grossly, a cirrhotic liver is shrunken and nodular. Microscopically, fibrous bands surrounding nodules of distorted liver cells are seen. Lymphocytes and plasma cells are also characteristic. Remember that cirrhosis results from some sort of injury, so cirrhosis is a product of the liver's attempt at a **repair process** that is ultimately counterproductive. If the injury is large (such as chronic insults that are chemical or viral), then the response will be large and, in the end, destructive to the liver itself. This is why a cirrhotic liver becomes smaller and shrinks down. Think back to a cut on your skin, and how the scar tissue (fibrosis) contracts. The liver is exactly the same way. As bands of scar tissue form, they contract, making the liver small and nodular. With cirrhosis also comes an increased incidence of **hepatocellular carcinoma**.

Biliary Cirrhosis

Primary biliary cirrhosis is an autoimmune phenomenon associated with destruction of the small bile ducts within the liver. As with many other autoimmune diseases, it is more common in **women**. It occurs in middle age. Patients commonly present with severe obstructive jaundice (often causing itching) and hypercholesterolemia (remember that the liver plays a role in cholesterol transport as well), often causing cutaneous xanthoma formation. A helpful laboratory diagnostic tool is the detection of **anti-mitochondrial antibodies** in the serum.

Secondary biliary cirrhosis is due to extrahepatic biliary obstruction arising from many different situations. Tumors in the head of the pancreas and gallstones lodged in the duct system can obstruct the bile flow, causing dilation of the duct and increased pressure in the intrahepatic bile ducts. Fibrosis occurs as a result. Microscopically, bile stasis can be seen as visible bile accumulation in the hepatic parenchyma from the backed-up flow of bile.

Primary Sclerosing Cholangitis

Primary sclerosing cholangitis is a very rare condition that, when it does occur, is usually found associated with inflammatory bowel disease, most specifically ulcerative colitis. The inflammation and fibrosis of the biliary tubules eventually lead to biliary cirrhosis (this

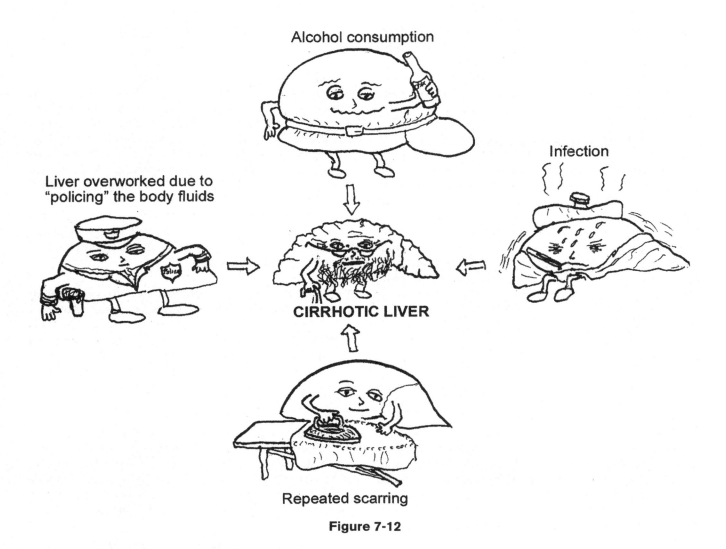

Alcohol consumption

Infection

Liver overworked due to "policing" the body fluids

CIRRHOTIC LIVER

Repeated scarring

Figure 7-12

would be a cause of secondary biliary cirrhosis). Patients with this condition are at increased risk for developing cholangiocarcinoma.

Hemochromatosis

Hemochromatosis is a condition in which the body becomes overloaded with iron. **Primary hemochromatosis** is an **autosomal recessive** condition that results in a defect in iron absorption. **Secondary hemochromatosis** is most often due to ineffective erythropoiesis that requires multiple excess blood transfusions, which in turn result in the hemochromatosis. Thalassemia major is a hematologic disease associated with the secondary form because it commonly requires blood transfusions. Regardless of the cause of the iron overload, the symptoms are the same, since iron accumulates in certain organs such as the liver, skin, heart, and pancreatic islet cells. These accumulations lead to cirrhosis, skin pigmentation (looks like a dark "bronze" tan), and "diabetes" (due to the destruc-

tion of the pancreatic islet cells) leading to the nickname "**bronze diabetes**."

The serum iron levels will be increased, but the total iron binding capacity (TIBC) will be decreased, an important pattern to remember. (Recall that the TIBC increases when the body is low in iron stores because there is a need to build them up, but in this case the body has too much, so the body has no need to bind all the iron for keeping). Ferritin and transferrin levels will both be increased since these proteins are needed to transfer and store the increased iron present in the body.

Microscopically, tissue in hemochromatosis that is stained with Prussian blue (a special stain for iron) will show hemosiderin in the parenchyma of many organs, not just the liver.

Wilson's Disease

Wilson's disease is an **autosomal recessive** condition that results from impaired **copper** excretion in the bile, causing accumulations of copper in the liver, kidney, basal ganglia (causing Parkinsonian symptoms), and cornea (**Kayser-Fleischer rings**). There is also a reduction of serum ceruloplasmin, the protein that carries copper in the blood. Accumulation of copper in the liver causes chronic hepatitis and cirrhosis.

Budd-Chiari Syndrome

Budd-Chiari syndrome results from occlusion or compression of major hepatic veins, such as the inferior vena cava. Liver congestion results and causes centrilobular congestion and necrosis. This causes abdominal pain, jaundice, hepatomegaly, liver failure, and ascites. Many conditions can cause this syndrome, including pregnancy and abdominal neoplasms, which can both cause compression. Polycythemia vera, a hematologic disease, causes this syndrome due to increased blood stasis.

Benign Tumors of the Liver

Hemangioma

Hemangioma is the **most common benign** tumor of the liver and consists of neoplastic growth of vasculature.

Adenoma

Adenoma is a common benign tumor of the liver that is most often found in women, because it has a strong association with the use of **oral contraceptives**. It tends to be **subcapsular** and can cause severe intraperitoneal hemorrhage if rupture occurs. It will resolve on its own if oral contraceptive use is discontinued.

Malignant Tumors of the Liver

Metastatic Tumors

The majority of malignant tumors in the liver are metastatic tumors that originate primarily in the GI tract (anything that drains into the portal vein).

Hepatocellular Carcinoma

Hepatocellular carcinoma *(Slides 7.19 and 7.20)* is the **most common** primary malignant tumor of the liver in adults. It most often develops in the face of preexisting cirrhosis. There are many causes of cirrhosis, so any condition that can lead to cirrhosis also brings with it an increased risk of developing hepatocellular carcinoma. The hepatitis B virus and aflatoxin B_1 have especially close associations with this cancer. This tumor is especially dangerous because it tends to invade vascular channels early in its course.

A serum increase in **alpha-fetoprotein (AFP)** is associated with hepatocellular carcinoma and is often used to monitor recurrence or metastasis since the AFP levels correlate with the tumor burden.

THE GALLBLADDER
Cholelithiasis

Cholelithiasis is the fancy term for gallstones and is simply the condition of having stones. If there is any inflammation the term **cholecystitis** must also be applied. There are several types of stones. **Cholesterol stones** usually are solitary stones that are large enough so that they cannot enter the ducts and therefore tend to remain in the body of the gallbladder. **Pigmented stones** are caused by an excess of unconjugated bilirubin, which is insoluble. They are found associated with hemolytic anemia because destroyed red blood cells are the source of the unconjugated bilirubin. **Mixed stones** make up the majority of the cases (75-80%); they are comprised of cholesterol and calcium salts.

Fig. 7-13. Factors associated with the development of gallstones. Females are affected more commonly than males, tend to be overweight (Fat), and are in their Forties. They are still usually in their childbearing years (Fertile) and have Fair complexions. So, it is easy to remember the "Five F's": female, fat, forty, fertile, fair.

Cholecystitis

Again, this is an "-itis," so immediately start thinking of "inflammation"! There are two types of cholecystitis: **acute** and **chronic**. The acute form is usually pyogenic (an accumulation of pus) and presents as right upper quadrant pain. Chronic cholecystitis is usually caused by gallstones (**cholelithiasis**); the gallbladder wall is

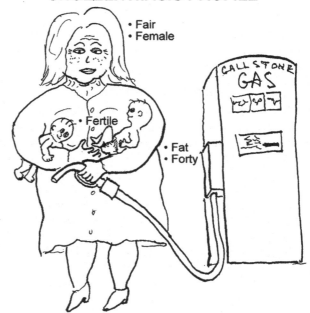

CHOLELITHIASIS PROFILE

Figure 7-13

thickened due to the fibrosis from the chronic inflammatory response caused by the gallstone irritation.

If pain is only intermittent and correlated with ingestion of fatty foods, the disease process is less serious, although very painful. **Biliary colic** arises secondary to the transient obstruction of the cystic duct by a stone. True cholecystitis is characterized by the common triad of symptoms known as **Charcot's triad**, which consists of **fever, jaundice, and right upper quadrant pain**. A worsening of cholecystitis is **ascending cholangitis**, which is a bacterial infection superimposed on the obstruction to bile flow, progressing to **Reynolds' pentad**, the addition of altered mental status and septic shock to Charcot's triad.

Fig. 7-14. Charcot's triad and Reynolds' pentad.

Of course, cholelithiasis can obstruct bile flow when the stones become lodged in the ducts, but **acute pancreatitis, acute cholecystitis,** and **mucoceles** (a distended, mucus-filled gallbladder) can all cause obstruction and lead to ascending cholangitis as well.

Gallbladder Adenocarcinoma

Adenocarcinoma of the gallbladder is associated with gallstones and develops from chronic irritation of the gallbladder wall. It frequently invades the liver before discovery.

Cholangiocarcinoma

Cholangiocarcinoma is a carcinoma of the **bile duct**, as opposed to the above gallbladder carcinoma. It is similar to hepatocellular carcinoma in the fact that it tends to invade vascular channels early in its course, but in contrast, it is not associated with cirrhosis or the hepatitis B virus. It is more common in the Far East, and is associated with *Clonorchis sinensis* infection (a liver fluke found in that part of the world), so think about this tumor if a patient is from that part of the world. Prognosis is dismal.

THE EXOCRINE PANCREAS *(Slide 7.21)*
Acute Pancreatitis

OK, another "-it is," and again the question is "What causes the inflammation?" Excessive **alcohol** intake and gallstones are the main causes of acute pancreatitis. The presentation is severe abdominal pain **radiating to the back**, and an increased serum **amylase** level. Inflammation of the pancreas causes an activation of pancreatic digestive enzymes, which essentially begin to autodigest the pancreas. This results in hemorrhagic

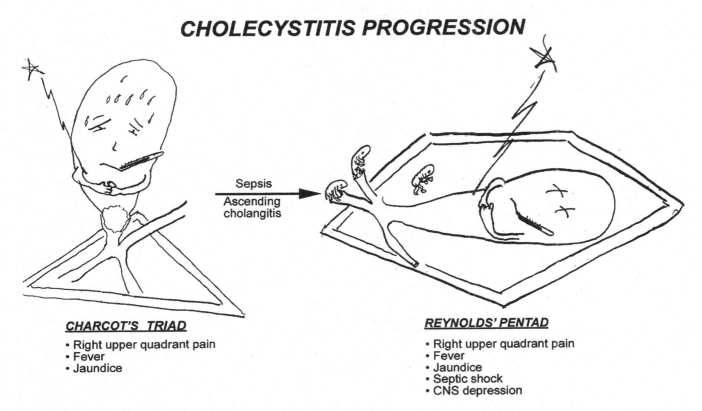

CHOLECYSTITIS PROGRESSION

Sepsis
Ascending
cholangitis

CHARCOT'S TRIAD
• Right upper quadrant pain
• Fever
• Jaundice

REYNOLDS' PENTAD
• Right upper quadrant pain
• Fever
• Jaundice
• Septic shock
• CNS depression

Figure 7-14

fat necrosis and the deposition of calcium soaps, known as **saponification**. The deposition, if severe, can cause hypocalcemia as circulating calcium is pulled out of the circulation and deposited into these soaps.

Another common result is the formation of a pseudocyst (a parenchymal cyst of the pancreas that is not considered a true cyst because it is not lined with ductal epithelium). Two final and possibly life-threatening complications are development of ARDS (acute/adult respiratory distress syndrome) and DIC (disseminated intravascular coagulation). Acute pancreatitis can be superimposed upon an underlying chronic pancreatitis.

Chronic Pancreatitis

Chronic pancreatitis is almost always associated with excessive **alcohol** intake. It presents as complaints of abdominal and back pain, steatorrhea (the loss of the ability to absorb fat due to a lipase deficiency), night blindness, and osteomalacia (due to the inability to absorb the fat soluble vitamins A and D).

The major histologic finding in chronic pancreatitis is progressive parenchymal fibrosis, which is what causes the pancreas to lose its ability to produce lipase. Essentially, the pancreas "burns out" and enzyme pro-duction is dramatically reduced. Calcifications and pseudocysts similar to those found in acute pancreatitis can also be found.

Carcinoma of the Pancreas

The most common kind of carcinoma found in the pancreas is adenocarcinoma. It is more common in smokers. It presents as abdominal pain radiating to the back, migratory thrombophlebitis (**Trousseau sign**), and obstructive jaundice (depending upon the location of the tumor).

Fig. 7-15. Adenocarcinoma of the pancreas (Slide 7-22).

It is most commonly located at the head of the pancreas, where it obstructs bile flow, being near the common bile duct. For this reason, pancreatic cancer is often first recognized by symptoms similar to cholelithiasis. It can also localize in the tail of the pancreas (a less common site), causing islet destruction and secondary diabetes mellitus. Carcinoma in the tail of the pancreas is a particularly aggressive tumor; the prognosis is very poor, average survival being 6 months or less. It is often very advanced by the time it is discovered and has often already metastasized.

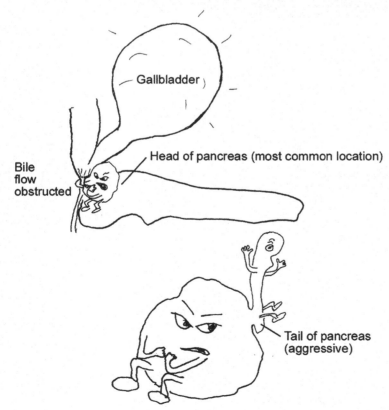

PANCREATIC ADENOCARCINOMA

Gallbladder

Head of pancreas (most common location)

Bile flow obstructed

Tail of pancreas (aggressive)

Figure 7-15

8

Renal and Urinary Tract Pathology

OVERVIEW
Anatomy of the Kidney

The ureter exits the hilum of the kidney at the renal pelvis, which is the confluence of the major calyces. These calyces are in turn formed by the confluence of 12 minor calyces. The kidney proper is divided into an outer cortex and an inner medulla. The medulla contains the renal pyramids. The apices of these pyramids are called papillae and are each associated with a minor calyx. The cortical tissue extends between the pyramids and is termed the *renal columns of Bertini*.

Anatomy of the Nephron

Fig. 8-1A, 8-1B. (Slide 8.1). Kidney, ureter, and nephron. The Nephron is the functional unit of the kidney. It is found in both the medulla and cortex.

Fig. 8-2. The glomerulus. The first part of the nephron, the glomerulus, consists of a capillary network enclosed in an invaginated epithelial structure composed of 2 layers: a fenestrated visceral layer and a parietal layer. The visceral layer and capillary wall are separated by the glomerular basement membrane (GBM). The parietal layer forms the lining of Bowman's space (urinary space).

The epithelium of the glomerulus then extends to form a complex network of tubules, namely the proximal convoluted tubule, the Loop of Henle – which descends toward and sometimes through, and then returns from, the corticomedullary junction – and the distal convoluted tubule. This empties into the collecting ducts, which drain into the papillae and ultimately the renal calyces. The nephron is suspended in a background stroma known as the interstitium.

Basic Renal Physiology

Fig. 8-3. Glomerular filtration and tubular resorption. Blood flow to the kidneys is routed though the afferent arterioles to the glomerular capillaries. The kidney regulates homeostatic balance by filtering small ionic particles and molecules. This process occurs at the interface between the visceral epithelium, at the level of the foot processes, and the intervening basement membrane (slit membrane). Larger molecules (e.g., proteins) are not filtered from the blood, but small molecules may be passed into the filtrate into Bowman's space.

Bowman's space is continuous with the renal tubular lumina. Passing through the tubule, physiologically needed components are reabsorbed and waste materials are retained in the ever-concentrating filtrate, which becomes the urine. Again, the urine flows through the tubules and collecting system to be excreted into the ureter, then collected in the bladder to be released when convenient.

Fig. 8-4. The origins of renal failure. These may be **pre-renal**, **post-renal**, or **intrinsic**.

- **Pre-renal causes** occur in conditions where blood flow is reduced (hypovolemia, sepsis, renal artery stenosis, and low cardiac output) and manifests with a BUN:creatinine ratio greater than 20 due to reduction in the glomerular filtration rate (GFR).
- **Post-renal causes** result from mechanical blockage of urine.
- **Intrinsic causes** may be due to glomerular, tubular, interstitial, or vascular etiologies. If the etiology is glomerular, determine if the disease is nephrotic, nephritic, or both (terms defined later in this chapter). Then determine complement levels. **Low complement**

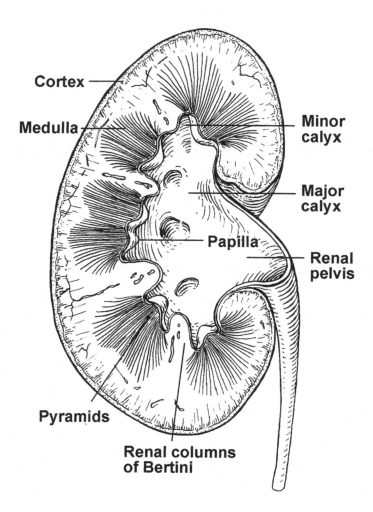

Figure 8-1A

KIDNEY, URETER, AND NEPHRON

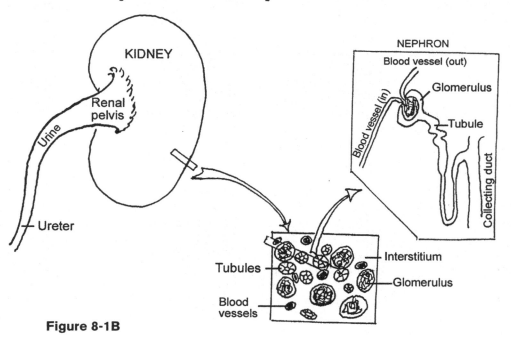

Figure 8-1B

GLOMERULUS

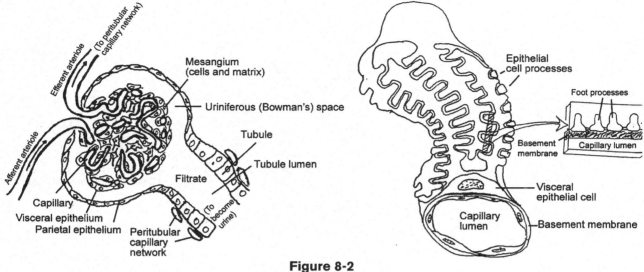

Figure 8-2

GLOMERULAR CAPILLARY

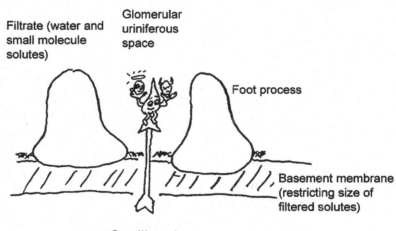

Figure 8-3

Capillary lumen

levels are usually associated with acute proliferative poststreptococcal glomerulonephritis, membrano-proliferative glomerulonephritis (MPGN), and systemic lupus erythematosus (SLE), because these are all autoimmune disorders where the body attacks itself, thus consuming complement.

1. **Acute Renal Failure (ARF):** ARF manifests with either oliguria (scant urine flow) or anuria (no urine flow) and acute onset of azotemia, which is elevation of blood urea nitrogen (BUN), and creatinine levels. These elevations relate to decreased GFR. ARF can result from glomerular, interstitial, or vascular injury, as well as acute tubular necrosis.

2. **Chronic Renal Failure:** Chronic renal failure is the final result of long-standing renal disease.

3. **Diminished Renal Reserve:** This stage is applied when the GFR is close to 50% of normal. BUN and creatinine levels are normal, and the patient is asymptomatic.

4. **Renal Insufficiency:** This stage is applied when the GFR is 20-50% of normal and azotemia appears. Polyuria (excess urine formation) and nocturia (urination at night) may also occur.

5. **Renal Failure:** This stage is associated with edema, metabolic acidosis, and hypocalcemia. The GFR is less than 20% of normal. **Uremia** (azotemia that is associated with clinical signs and symptoms, e.g., uremic fibrinous pericarditis, and biochemical abnormalities, e.g., metabolic and endocrine alterations) is common and may be associated with neurologic, gastrointestinal, and cardiovascular complications.

ORIGINS OF RENAL FAILURE

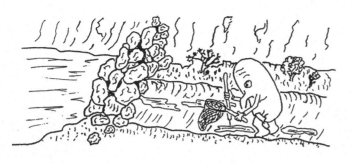
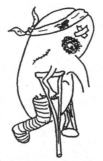
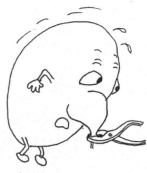

PRE-RENAL IMPAIRMENT	INTRINSIC RENAL IMPAIRMENT	POST-RENAL IIMPAIRMENT
(Blood flow to kidney impeded)	(Injured, compromised renal organ)	(Obstructed or impeded exit of urine)

Figure 8-4

6. **End-Stage Renal Disease**: This entity is the terminal stage of uremia. The GFR is less than 5% of normal. This stage is a major cause of death.
7. **Renal Tubular Defects**: These defects manifest with polyuria, nocturia, and electrolyte disturbances, e.g., metabolic acidosis.
8. **Urinary Tract Infection (UTI)**: UTIs are diagnosed by the presence of **leukocytes and bacteria in the urine.** UTIs may extend to the kidney and cause **pyelonephritis** with **bacteria and white cell casts** seen on urinalysis.

CONGENITAL ANOMALIES
Agenesis of the Kidney

Bilateral agenesis is incompatible with life and is associated with other congenital disorders, e.g., **Potter's Syndrome** (oligohydramnios, limb defects, hypoplastic lungs, and facial deformities). Unilateral agenesis is compatible with life.

Hypoplasia

Renal hypoplasia is failure of the kidney to mature to normal size (150 grams). It is accompanied by a reduced number of lobes and pyramids. This disorder is more commonly seen as a unilateral defect. Scarring is not a characteristic feature (versus acquired atrophic kidney).

Ectopic Kidneys

Ectopic kidneys are most commonly found in the **pelvis** (not to be confused with the renal pelvis). Obstruction and bacterial infections are common because the ureters are more likely to kink and twist due to their abnormal location.

Horseshoe Kidney

A horseshoe-shaped kidney results from fusion of the two kidneys in the midline at the upper or lower poles. This is a common anomaly.

CYSTIC DISEASES OF THE KIDNEY

Cystic diseases of the kidney are important because they are relatively common, create a diagnostic challenge, and cause renal failure.

Cystic Renal Dysplasia

This is a sporadic disorder that presents as a flank mass that usually leads to surgical exploration and nephrectomy, especially when unilateral. The pathogenesis involves abnormal metanephric differentiation and is characterized histologically by undifferentiated islands of mesenchyme, often with cartilage formation, and immature collecting ductules. In unilateral disease, the outcome after nephrectomy is excellent; however, chronic renal failure is common in bilateral disease.

Adult Polycystic Disease

Adult polycystic disease is an **autosomal dominant** systemic disease that involves the **kidneys** and is associated with other extrarenal anomalies, e.g., polycystic liver disease, **intracranial Berry aneurysms**, and mitral valve prolapse. It presents most commonly in the **4th to 5th decades** of life. Three separate genes are involved: PKD1 (polycystic kidney disease), PKD2, and PKD3 genes. Both kidneys are enlarged and may present as a mass on abdominal examination. Other symptoms include pain and hematuria. Progression to chronic renal failure is accelerated in blacks, males (versus females), and in the presence of hypertension. Both kidneys are enlarged, and the external surface is carpeted with **cysts**. The cysts expand and eventually destroy the renal parenchyma; renal failure ensues. Most patients die from coronary or hypertensive heart disease. Other causes of death include infection, ruptured Berry aneurysm, and hypertensive intracerebral hemorrhage.

Childhood Polycystic Disease

Childhood polycystic kidney disease is an **autosomal recessive congenital cystic** disease of **childhood** that usually presents at birth. There are 4 subtypes: **perinatal, neonatal, infantile,** and **juvenile**. In surviving children, many develop **congenital hepatic fibrosis** that leads to portal hypertension and splenomegaly. Hepatic fibrosis may develop even in the absence of polycystic kidney disease.

Histologically, the kidneys in childhood polycystic disease are spongy with small cysts throughout the cortex and medulla. Most infants succumb to renal failure in infancy.

Cystic Diseases of The Renal Medulla

There are 2 major subtypes:
- Medullary Sponge Kidney
- Nephronophthisis – Uremic Medullary Cystic Disease Complex, also known as Hereditary Tubulointerstitial Nephritis . . . whew! (just remember that both terms have medullary in their names)

Medullary Sponge Kidney is defined by innocuous cystic dilations of the collecting ducts and medulla. Usually, medullary sponge kidney is an incidental radiographic finding in adults or sometimes is diagnosed due to secondary complications like hematuria, infection, or calculi. These complications are caused by calcifications within dilated ducts. This disease is relatively common; however, the pathogenesis is unknown.

Nephronophthisis – Uremic Medullary Cystic Disease Complex (Hereditary Tubulointerstitial Nephritis) describes a group of progressive childhood renal disorders that are characterized by cysts in the medulla and cortical interstitial fibrosis. The cause of renal insufficiency is due to the cortical interstitial fibrosis. Children present initially with polyuria and polydipsia (inability of the tubules to concentrate urine), and then with salt wasting and tubular acidosis. Terminal renal failure occurs within 5-10 years. This group of diseases accounts for 20% of chronic renal failure cases in children and adolescents.

Acquired Cystic Disease

Acquired cystic kidney disease manifests in those who have received long-term hemodialysis for end-stage kidney disease. The cysts are thought to be due to tubule obstruction either from interstitial fibrosis or oxalate crystals. These cysts are small (0.5 to 2.0 cm), contain clear fluid, and they are found in the cortical and medullary regions. Renal cell adenocarcinoma is an ominous complication that develops in the cyst walls.

Simple Cysts

Simple cysts are common incidental post-mortem findings. They range from 5-10 cm and are usually found in the renal cortex. These cysts are usually asymptomatic, but occasionally, they can cause distention, pain, or hemorrhage. Radiographically, simple cysts have a smooth contour and are avascular, in contrast to tumors.

GLOMERULAR DISEASE

Glomerular disease is divided into 3 categories: **primary glomerulopathies** (where the predominant organ affected is the kidney), **systemic diseases** (those that involve the kidneys and other organs), and **hereditary diseases**. Glomerular disease is also separated into 5 major syndromes: **acute nephritic syndrome, rapidly progressive glomerulonephritis, nephrotic syndrome, chronic renal failure,** and **asymptomatic hematuria or proteinuria**. These categories are based on the clinical manifestation of each glomerular disease.

Fig. 8-5. Nephritic Syndromes. These include hematuria, azotemia, variable proteinuria, oliguria, edema, and hypertension. (**The Casted NOAH's arc "p" (pee) floats in the red sea** – Casted = red casts, N = nephritic, O = oliguria A= azotemia, H = hypertension, p= proteinuria, red sea = hematuria and edema).

Rapidly Progressive Glomerulonephritis includes acute nephritis, proteinuria, and acute renal failure. (The "R" in Rapidly represents renal failure, the "P" in progressive represents proteinuria, and "itis" in glomerulonephritis represents inflammation).

Nephrotic Syndromes are marked by >3.5 g/day proteinuria, hypoalbuminemia, hyperlipidemia, lipiduria.

Fig. 8-6. Nephrotic syndromes. This may be remembered by the mnemonic: "**A neurotic (nephrotic) plastic surgeon may keep an album (hypoalbuminemia) of lips (lipiduria and hyperlipidemia) that have been injected with collagen (a protein), Oh those thick and edematous (edema) lips!**"

Chronic Renal Failure leads to **azotemia** (excess nitrogenous wastes in the blood) that progresses to **uremia** (the clinical condition), **hematuria**, and **proteinuria**.

NEPHRITIC SYNDROME

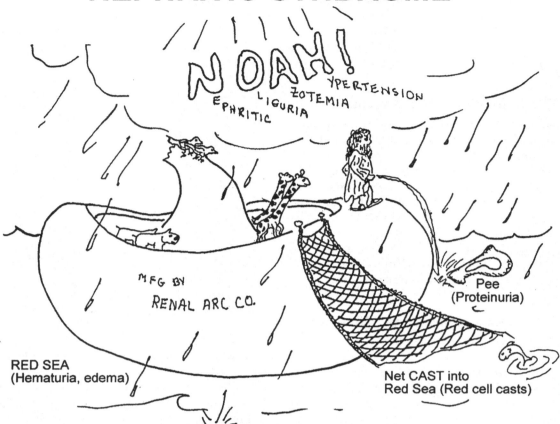

*"The **Cast**ed **Noah**'s Arc **"p"** floats in the **Red** Sea"*

Figure 8-5

NEPHROTIC SYNDROME

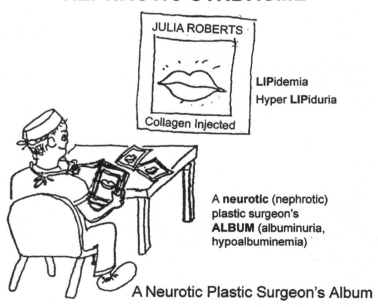

JULIA ROBERTS

Collagen Injected

LIPidemia
Hyper **LIP**iduria

A **neurotic** (nephrotic)
plastic surgeon's
ALBUM (albuminuria,
hypoalbuminemia)

A Neurotic Plastic Surgeon's Album

Figure 8-6

The Nephritic Syndromes

Primary Glomerulonephritis

The pathogenesis of glomerular injury in glomerulonephritis is **immune-related**. In general, there are 3 mechanisms of immune-mediated glomerular injury: **antibody-mediated**, **cell-mediated**, and **activation of alternative complement pathway**. The most important type of immune-mediated injury is antibody-mediated injury, and there are 2 major forms.

The first majors form involves antibodies that react to fixed glomerular antigens or to molecules planted within the glomerulus. Planted antigens include both endogenous (DNA, immunoglobulins, immune complexes, or IgA) and exogenous (drugs and infectious agents) forms. Fixed antigens demonstrate a **linear pattern** on immunofluorescence, while planted antigens will show a **granular pattern**.

The second form involves soluble circulating **antigen-antibody complexes** that become trapped within the glomerulus and cause injury. There are **endogenous** and **exogenous** antigens, which also demonstrate a granular appearance when visualized by immunofluorescence. These circulating immune complexes are seen on electron microscopy as **deposits**, which can settle anywhere within the glomerulus. For example, when they are found in the mesangium, they are seen as **deposits** in the mesangium. When they settle between endothelial cells and the GBM, they are **subendothelial deposits**, and when they occur outside of the GBM between podocytes, they are **subepithelial deposits**. When circulating complexes settle along the GBM, they appear as **granular deposits** on immunofluorescence.

Fig. 8-7. Antibody-mediated glomerulonephritis.

Acute Proliferative (Poststreptococcal, Postinfectious) Glomerulonephritis

Acute proliferative glomerulonephritis is an immune complex-mediated disease caused by **endostreptosin** of streptococcal origin. **Children** (6-10 years old) are most frequently affected. This disease manifests 1-4 weeks following a **group A b-hemolytic streptococcus** infection of the pharynx or skin. The child usually presents with malaise, fever, nausea, oliguria, hematuria that is **"smoky brown,"** and recent recovery from a sore throat.

Histologically, the glomeruli are enlarged due to swelling and hypercellularity *(Slide 8.2)* caused by inflammation and mesangial and endothelial cell proliferation. Immunofluorescence microscopy shows granular deposits of IgG, IgM, and C3 in the mesangium and GBM.

Electron microscopy shows electron-dense deposits (**subepithelial humps or "lumpy bumpy" pattern**) *(Slide 8.3).*

Important laboratory findings include elevated anti-streptococcal antibody titers, decreased serum C3 (because it is consumed), cryoglobulinemia, and microscopic hematuria with mild proteinuria (less than 1 gram). Most children (95%) recover with conservative therapy.

IgA Nephropathy (Berger Disease)

IgA nephropathy is the **most common type of glomerulonephritis worldwide**. It is characterized by IgA (and C3) mesangial deposits seen on immunofluorescence. IgA nephropathy primarily affects children and young adults, who present with gross hematuria following an infection (usually respiratory). Hematuria lasts for several days and then may recur months later. Secondary forms of IgA nephropathy occur and are associated with systemic disorders like Henoch-Schönlein purpura and liver and intestinal disease, e.g., celiac disease.

The pathogenesis of IgA nephropathy relates to **abnormal IgA synthesis** in response to respiratory or gastrointestinal exposure to antigens like viruses, food proteins, and bacteria. The IgA complexes become trapped in the mesangium, and the alternate complement pathway results in glomerular injury. Secondary IgA nephropathy may be genetically acquired because there is an increased association with celiac and liver disease.

When IgA nephropathy occurs as an isolated renal disorder, most patients maintain normal renal function; however, there are some patients where the disease follows an indolent course that progresses to chronic renal failure.

Rapidly Progressive (Crescentic) Glomerulonephritis (RPGN)

RPGN is characterized by a **rapid and progressive loss of renal function and death within weeks to months**, if untreated. The etiology is immune related; however, a specific etiology has not been described, and most cases are idiopathic. This disease is divided into 3 categories: **type I, type II**, and **type III** RPGN on the basis of immunologic features.

Regardless of the cause, the disease is characterized by **crescents in glomeruli**, which are composed of parietal epithelial cells and inflammatory components, e.g., monocytes and macrophages.

Patients with type I and type III RPGN usually respond well to plasmapheresis, steroids, and/or cytotoxic agents. The underlying disease must be treated in Type II RPGN. Some patients, however, progress to renal failure and require either dialysis or transplantation.

The prototype of **Type I RPGN** is **Goodpasture's Syndrome**. The syndrome has a peak incidence in **young men** (mid twenties) and manifests as **pulmonary**

ANTIBODY-MEDIATED GLOMERULONEPHRITIS

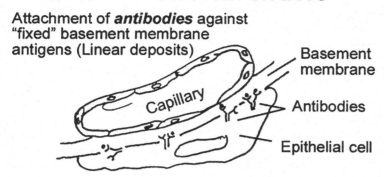

Attachment of *antibodies* against "fixed" basement membrane antigens (Linear deposits)

Basement membrane

Antibodies

Epithelial cell

Capillary

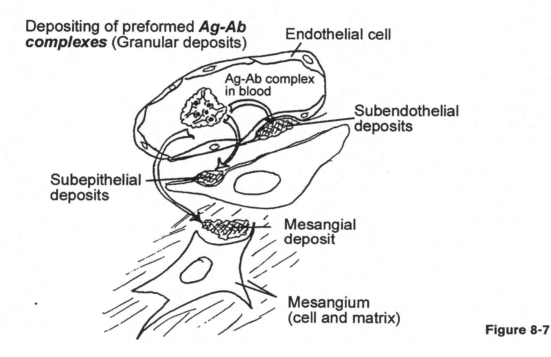

Depositing of preformed *Ag-Ab complexes* (Granular deposits)

Endothelial cell

Ag-Ab complex in blood

Subendothelial deposits

Subepithelial deposits

Mesangial deposit

Mesangium (cell and matrix)

Figure 8-7

hemorrhage or hemoptysis and renal failure. The Goodpasture antigen is directed against the GBM in the kidney and also cross-reacts with the pulmonary alveolar basement membrane to produce pulmonary hemorrhages. Immunofluorescent microscopy shows a **linear deposition of IgG and C3 along the GBM**. Although the etiologic agent that triggers anti-GBM formation is unknown, factors like cigarette smoking, hydrocarbon solvents, and HLA subtypes and haplotypes (HLA-DRB1) are associated with this syndrome.

Type II RPGN is an immune-complex mediated disease that may result from any immune-complex nephritides, like poststreptococcal glomerulonephritis, SLE, or Henoch-Schönlein purpura. Regardless of the underlying cause, immunofluorescence shows a granular pattern of staining.

Type III RPGN is considered "pauci-immune" because antibodies to GBM and immune complexes are **absent,** making immune deposits scarce on immunofluorescence. However, most patients have antineutrophil cytoplasmic antibody (ANCA) in their serum, hence "pauci-immune" ("sort of immune").

Positive ANCA serology is associated with vasculitides like **Wegener's granulomatosis and polyarteritis nodosa**, which may progress to this type of RPGN.

Alport Syndrome

Alport syndrome is defined by the presence of **nephritis and nerve deafness** that occurs most commonly in males (5-20 years old). Eye disorders, including lens dislocation, cataracts, and corneal dystrophy are also associated with this syndrome, but nerve deafness is the most important association. Renal symptoms include hematuria and erythrocyte casts. Renal failure is a complication that occurs between 20-50 years of age. There may be a family history of renal failure.

Fig. 8-8. Alport syndrome. Mnemonic: **Alvin, a member of the chipmunks was so startled by his father that when he screamed at him, Alvin urinated and eventually went deaf. Alvin = Alport; male, urinated = renal, deaf = associated characteristic.**

The mode of inheritance of Alport syndrome is most commonly **X-linked dominant.** The pathogenesis is due to a mutation in the gene encoding the alpha chain of collagen type IV. The result of this mutation is defective GBM synthesis. Histologically, glomerular and epithelial cells appear foamy (from accumulation of neutral fats and mucopolysaccharides). Ultrastructural findings of pronounced **splitting and lamination of the lamina densa** with foci of GBM thickening and thinning are characteristic features of this syndrome.

Thin Membrane Disease (Benign Familial Hematuria)

Thin membrane disease is a hereditary disease that is often discovered incidentally on routine urinalysis in a patient with asymptomatic hematuria with normal renal function. The pathogenesis is related to genes encoding the alpha chains of type IV collagen (as with Alport's Syndrome). Ultrastructurally, there is diffuse thinning of the GBM.

Asymptomatic patients are heterozygotes and have an excellent prognosis; however, homozygotes may progress to renal failure.

The Nephrotic Syndromes

The pathogenesis of nephrotic syndrome (massive proteinuria, hypoalbuminemia, edema, hyperlipidemia,

and lipiduria) is due to **increased capillary permeability to plasma proteins.** Thus, there is massive proteinuria with subsequent depletion of albumin. Because blood protein levels are low, oncotic pressures are altered. Water, in addition to sodium accumulates in the interstitial tissues and causes generalized edema. The genesis of hyperlipidemia is part of the compensatory mechanism by the liver to the loss of protein. Because there are high amounts of circulating lipids, lipiduria occurs secondarily to leaky glomerular capillaries. The lipid may appear as free fat or as **oval fat bodies,** which are complexes of degenerated tubular epithelial cells and lipid.

Fig. 8-9. Causes of nephrotic syndrome. Causes can be remembered using the mnemonic "**My memorable prof's brain (membranoproliferative) can only handle minimal (minimal change disease) segments (focal segmental glomerulosclerosis) of information.**"

Membranous Glomerulonephritis

Membranous glomerulonephritis is the **most common cause of the nephrotic syndrome in adults.** In 15% of cases, the disease is associated with drugs (penicillamine, captopril, gold, NSAIDS), malignancy (melanoma, lung, and colon carcinoma), SLE, infections (Hepatitis B and C, and syphilis), and metabolic disorders (diabetes); however, 85% of cases are idiopathic.

Membranous nephropathy is mediated by antigen-antibody complexes that are related to either exogenous antigens, e.g., hepatitis B, or endogenous antigens, e.g., SLE. The **immune complex is composed of IgG and C3 and is granular on immunofluorescence** *(Slide 8.4).* These complexes cause indirect capillary wall injury by inducing complement (C5b-C9) in glomerular epithelial and mesangial cells, which release enzymes and oxidants that injure the capillary wall.

On light microscopy, the capillary wall is diffusely thickened *(Slide 8.5).*

ALPORT SYNDROME

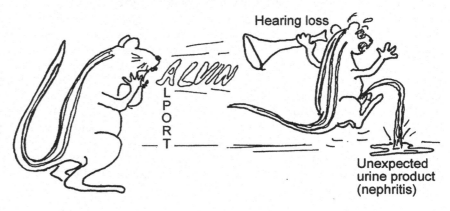

Figure 8-8

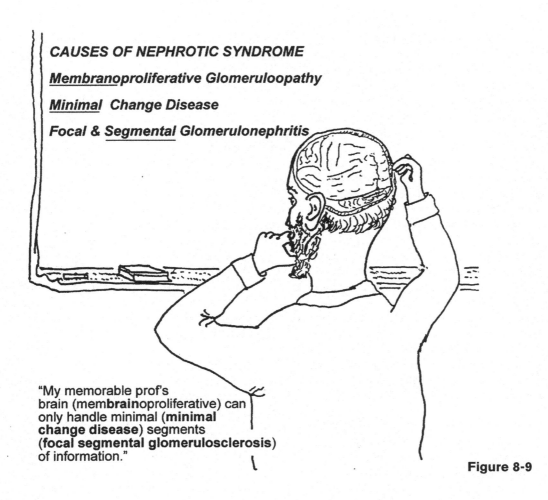

CAUSES OF NEPHROTIC SYNDROME

Membranoproliferative Glomeruloopathy

Minimal Change Disease

Focal & *Segmental* Glomerulonephritis

"My memorable prof's
brain (mem**brain**oproliferative) can
only handle minimal (**minimal
change disease**) segments
(**focal segmental glomerulosclerosis**)
of information."

Figure 8-9

Ultrastructurally, there are deposits within the basement membrane and overlying epithelial cells (**subepithelial**). New basement material is laid down between deposits, and a subendothelial **spiked and dome configuration** results *(Slide 8-6)*.

Membranous nephropathy is an indolent disease that typically is unresponsive to steroid treatment. Disease progression is evidenced by glomerular sclerosis, which is fibrous obliteration of the glomerulus.

Minimal Change Disease (Lipoid Nephrosis)

This disease is the **most common cause of the nephrotic syndrome in children** (2-6 years of age). Minimal change disease or lipoid nephrosis may occur following a respiratory infection or routine immunization. The etiology is based on immune dysfunction, where cytokine-like substances attack the kidney visceral epithelial cells. These cells, in turn, lose their structural integrity, with the disruption of the foot processes, and proteinuria ensues.

On light microscopy, the glomeruli in lipoid nephrosis are normal *(Slide 8.7)*. The proximal tubular cells are lipid laden (hence the term lipoid nephrosis). Immuno-

fluorescence is negative for immunoglobulin or complement deposits. Electron microscopy shows the characteristic **loss of foot processes (due to fusion) of the epithelial cells** *(Slide 8.8)*.

This disease responds very well to corticosteroid treatment; prognosis is excellent. This disease is best remembered by its name, "Minimal Change": normal glomeruli + fusion of the foot processes.

Focal Segmental Glomerulosclerosis

This disease presents similarly to Minimal Change Disease (Lipoid Nephrosis); however, patients are usually **adults**. This disease is often associated with HIV infection. The characteristic features of this disease are described in its name. Within the involved glomeruli, segments of capillary tufts show focal detachment of the visceral epithelial cells with loss of their foot processes.

Light microscopy will show sclerosis of focal glomerular segments. Electron microscopy demonstrates **loss of the foot processes and denudation of the visceral epithelial cells.** Immunofluorescence shows IgM and C3 deposits within the sclerotic areas.

Unlike Minimal Change Disease, Focal Segmental Glomerulosclerosis has a variable course and corticosteroid therapy does not result in disease remission.

Membranoproliferative Glomerulonephritis (MPGN)

Membranoproliferative glomerulonephritis comprises a group of disorders that usually presents as a nephrotic syndrome (occasionally, MPGN may manifest as nephritic or both) in older children or young adults. MPGN is divided into **primary MPGN** and **secondary MPGN** types. Both types are characterized histologically by alterations in the GBM, proliferation of glomerular cells, mainly mesangial cells, and leukocyte infiltration (the name of the disease describes its features).

Primary MPGN is further divided into **type I MPGN** and **type II MPGN**. Type I MPGN is an immune-complex nephritis; however, the antigens involved are unknown. Type II MGPN is caused by an IgG autoantibody that has specificity for the C3 convertase of the alternate complement pathway, which explains why patients have decreased serum C3.

On light microscopy, both types of MPGN have large and hypercellular glomeruli. The hypercellularity is due to mesangial proliferation that gives the glomeruli a lobular appearance. Furthermore, the GBM is thickened and is most prominent in the capillary loops. The thickening is caused by membrane duplication, and by cell processes migrating up into the capillary loop, which gives a double-contour or **tram-track appearance**.

The ultrastructural and immunofluorescent features in types I and II of MPGN are very different. In type I MPGN, **subendothelial electron dense deposits** are present. Immunofluorescence shows **IgG and C3 granular deposits**. In type II MPGN (also known as **dense-deposit disease**), the GBM is ribbon-like and is extremely dense; hence, the term dense-deposit disease. Immunofluorescence shows **C3 distributed in an irregular, granular-linear fashion**. IgG is absent.

Secondary MPGN occurs in chronic immune complex disorders like SLE, hepatitis B and C, HIV, and malignancy. MPGN is a slowly progressive and unremitting disease. Moreover, it tends to recur after kidney transplantation.

Chronic Glomerulonephritis

Chronic glomerulonephritis is the **end-stage of primary glomerular disease**. There are cases, albeit few, where chronic glomerulonephritis occurs in patients who have no previous renal disease.

Morphologically, the kidneys are symmetrically small and contracted. The cortex is thin and has a granular surface. Hypertensive changes like arterial and arteriolar sclerosis are evident. Patients with chronic glomerulonephritis are usually hypertensive and manifest with systemic uremia (uremic pericarditis, uremic gastroenteritis, or uremic pneumonitis). Moreover, secondary hyperparathyroidism and left ventricular hypertrophy also occur. Death is from complications of uremia, or cerebral and cardiovascular problems associated with hypertension. Survival can be prolonged with dialysis or renal transplant in some cases.

Glomerular Manifestations of Systemic Disease

Although there are a myriad of systemic diseases associated with glomerular injury, the focus here will be limited to SLE, diabetic glomerulosclerosis, and amyloidosis.

Systemic Lupus Erythematosus (SLE)

SLE is a systemic autoimmune disease that predominately occurs in women. African-American women of childbearing age are most commonly affected. SLE causes injury to the skin, joints, kidney, and serosal membranes. SLE commonly presents as a nephrotic syndrome.

There are five morphologic classifications of lupus nephritis according to the World Health Organization (WHO): normal (Class I), mesangial lupus glomerulonephritis (Class II), focal proliferative glomerulonephritis (Class III), diffuse proliferative glomerulonephritis (Class IV), and membranous glomerulonephritis (Class V). The pathogenesis of types II-V is the same and is due to **DNA-anti-DNA complex deposition within the glomeruli.**

1. **Class I (Normal):** No changes are seen on light, electron, or immunofluorescent microscopy
2. **Class II (mesangial lupus glomerulonephritis):** This is the mildest lesion. It is characterized by increased mesangial cells and matrix *(Slide 8.9)*. Granular deposits of immunoglobulin and complement are present within the mesangium.
3. **Class III (focal proliferative glomerulonephritis):** This is a focal lesion that affects less than 50% of glomeruli. Typically one or two tufts of the affected glomeruli are swollen due to proliferation of endothelial and mesangial cells, infiltration of neutrophils, fibrinoid deposits, and intracapillary thrombi.
4. **Class IV (diffuse proliferative glomerulonephritis):** This is the **most serious type and is common**. Unlike Class III, the entire glomerulus is affected. There is mesangial, endothelial, and epithelial cell proliferation. Epithelial cell proliferation may fill Bowman's space and cause cast formation. Fibrinoid necrosis and hyaline thrombi are also present. Wire loops, which represent **extensive subendothelial immune complex deposits** *(Slide 8.10)*, are a common light microscopy finding, especially in the

diffuse form. These loops reflect active disease and a poor prognosis.

5. **Class V (membranous glomerulonephritis):** This lesion is morphologically identical to primary membranous glomerulonephritis.

Diabetic Glomerulosclerosis

Diabetes loves to trash kidneys. Grossly, a diabetic kidney has a finely granular cortical surface. There are 3 morphologic lesions encountered in diabetes: glomerular lesions, renal vascular lesions, and pyelonephritis. These features are present in Types I and Type II diabetes, although in Type II diabetes the changes are more heterogenous and less predictable. Patients with diabetes with end-stage diabetic nephropathy are either maintained on dialysis or undergo renal transplantation; however, diabetic lesions do reoccur after transplantation.

Glomerular Lesions: The changes that occur in the glomeruli are capillary basement thickening, diffuse diabetic glomerulosclerosis, and nodular glomerulosclerosis.

1. **Capillary GBM thickening** occurs in all diabetics as early as two years after disease onset regardless of the presence or absence of proteinuria. There is also thickening of the tubular basement membranes.
2. **Diffuse Glomerulosclerosis** is defined as mesangial cell proliferation and mesangial matrix expansion. This process occurs 10-20 years after disease onset.
3. **Nodular Glomerulosclerosis** is also known as **Kimmelstiel-Wilson Disease.** The presence of hyalinized nodules *(Slide 8.11)* within the glomerulus defines this entity. These nodules (**Kimmelstiel-Wilson nodules**) are pathognomonic of diabetes. The acellular nodules contain lipids and fibrin and appear very pink (they look like pink balls). Eventually, the nodules enlarge, compress capillaries and cause renal ischemia. Tubular atrophy and interstitial fibrosis results from the obliterated blood supply.

Renal Vascular Lesions: Arterial vessels show atherosclerosis and arteriosclerosis (amorphous hyaline thickening). These changes are associated with hypertension. The severity of vessel disease is related to the duration of the diabetes and the mean blood pressure.

Pyelonephritis: Acute and chronic inflammation is present in the interstitium and may spread to the tubules and cause papillary necrosis (commonly seen in diabetics) where tubules undergo coagulative necrosis.

Amyloidosis

In disseminated amyloidosis, amorphous pink deposits are also present in the kidney and are best visualized with **Congo-red staining.** Patients with amyloidosis present with the nephrotic syndrome and may have slightly enlarged kidneys (due to the amyloid deposition).

DISEASES OF THE TUBULES AND INTERSTITIUM
Acute Tubular Necrosis (ATN)

Acute tubular necrosis is the major cause of tubular epithelial cellular destruction. It presents as acute renal failure (defined as less than 400 ml of urine output in 24 hours).

There are 2 patterns of ATN: **ischemic ATN** and **nephrotoxic ATN.** Ischemic ATN is usually associated with shock and hypotension; however, hemoglobinuria and myoglobinuria can resemble this type of pattern. Nephrotoxic ATN is caused by drugs, contrast dye, heavy metals, and organic solvents.

The pathogenesis for both types relates to tubule cell injury and persistent alterations in blood flow (intrarenal vasoconstriction). Microscopically, ischemic ATN is characterized by **tubular epithelial necrosis** accompanied by basement membrane rupture (**tubulorrhexis**). Eosinophilic or granular casts are commonly found in the tubular lumen as well as **Tamm-Horsfall protein** (a specific protein secreted by tubular cells).

Microscopically, nephrotoxic ATN is characterized by tubule injury, most commonly in the proximal convoluted tubules. The findings tend to be specific to the toxic agent, e.g., ethylene glycol produces ballooning and hydropic degeneration of the proximal convoluted tubules with calcium oxalate crystals in the tubular lumens.

Pyelonephritis

Pyelonephritis is a renal disorder that affects the renal pelvis, tubules, and interstitium. There are 2 forms: **acute pyelonephritis** and **chronic pyelonephritis.**

Acute pyelonephritis is caused by an ascending bacterial urinary tract infection that may be associated with vesicoureteral reflux (retrograde urine flow into the ureters and kidneys), which results from loss of valvular integrity at the junction of the ureter and bladder. The etiologic agent is most commonly *Escherichia coli* (from endogenous fecal flora), followed by *Proteus, Klebsiella,* and *Enterobacter.*

Microscopically, acute pyelonephritis shows an acute neutrophilic exudate within the tubules and renal parenchyma. Urinalysis will show bacteria and white cell casts. Once the acute phase resolves, the inflammatory cells are replaced with scar formation in the background of tubular atrophy with interstitial fibrosis.

Chronic pyelonephritis is characterized by chronic inflammation of the tubules and interstitium, with renal scarring that extends to the calyces and renal pelvis. Microscopically, there are dilated tubules filled with colloid (protein) casts (**thyroidization-** *Slide 8.12*), chronic interstitial inflammation, and fibrosis.

Acute Drug-Induced Interstitial Nephritis

Acute drug-induced interstitial nephritis is commonly associated with synthetic **penicillins** (methicillin), rifampin, diuretics (thiazides), NSAIDs (phenylbutazone), and cimetidine. The etiology is believed to be immune related. This type of nephritis manifests after **two weeks** of drug exposure and is characterized by hematuria, proteinuria, and leukocyturia (with eosinophils). Creatinine levels are increased and acute renal failure with oliguria may develop.

Histologically, the interstitium is edematous and infiltrated with monocytes and eosinophils. Granulomas may be present. Systemic symptoms include fever, eosinophilia, and rash. Reversal of disease typically occurs when the offending drug is discontinued.

Analgesic Abuse Nephropathy

Analgesic abuse nephropathy disease manifests as chronic renal failure due to excessive intake of phenacetin in combination with other analgesics. The characteristic morphologic features of this disease are **papillary necrosis** followed by chronic tubulointerstitial nephritis.

The pathogenesis is due to oxidative damage caused by the phenacetin metabolite acetaminophen covalently binding to the cells. Moreover, aspirin potentiates papillary damage by blocking prostaglandins' vasodilatory effects, resulting in papillary ischemia. Continued analgesic abuse may progress to chronic renal failure. However, if analgesics are withdrawn, renal function may stabilize or improve. Even if the offending agent is stopped, some patients develop transitional papillary carcinoma of the renal pelvis. **Don't forget that diabetes mellitus also causes papillary necrosis!**

RENAL VASCULAR DISEASE
Benign Nephrosclerosis

Benign nephrosclerosis is defined by sclerosis of the renal arterioles and small arteries. The pathogenesis is due to medial and intimal thickening as well as hyaline arteriolar deposition. On gross exam, the kidneys are normal size, and the cortical surface is finely granular. This disease is asymptomatic, and the GFR is normal; however, it may progress to renal insufficiency in African-Americans and in those patients with diabetes.

Malignant Hypertension

Malignant hypertension is a **medical emergency**, characterized by diastolic pressures greater than 130 mm Hg, papilledema, retinopathy, encephalopathy, cardiovascular abnormalities, and renal failure. The patient may have headaches, vomiting, visual impairment (scotomas), proteinuria, and hematuria. Initially, there is no alteration in renal function; however, renal failure will ensue if prompt antihypertensive therapy is not initiated. This syndrome usually develops in the background of benign hypertension, secondary forms of hypertension, or underlying chronic disease.

The pathogenesis is unclear, but it is likely related to renal vascular damage that results in fibrinoid necrosis and intravascular thrombosis of arterioles (especially the afferents) and small vessels. The kidneys become ischemic, which triggers the renin-angiotensin system and causes further vasoconstriction. Consequently, patients have very high renin levels. Grossly, the cortical surface has pinpoint hemorrhages. Histologically, the arterioles appear eosinophilic and granular (**fibrinoid necrosis**). Furthermore, there is intimal thickening of the arterioles that may be referred to as **"onion-skinning" or hyperplastic arteriolitis.** If an inflammatory infiltrate is present, then the term **"necrotizing arteriolitis"** is applied.

Renal Artery Stenosis

Renal artery stenosis is uncommon, but is important because it is **surgically** curable. The clinical presentation is nonspecific and resembles essential hypertension. The most common cause of stenosis (70% of all cases) is occlusion by an **atheromatous plaque**. A second important cause is **fibromuscular dysplasia** where there is fibrous thickening of the intima, media, or adventitia. Fibromuscular dysplasia is more common in young women.

UROLITHIASIS

Kidney stones (renal calculi) are common and affect men (peak onset is 20-30 years) more than women. Many metabolic diseases, e.g., gout, cystinuria, and primary hyperoxaluria, are associated with stone formation. Sequelae include hydronephrosis (dilation of the renal pelvis and calyces) *(Slide 8.13)* from obstruction of urine outflow by a stone.

There are 4 main types of stones: **calcium oxalate** (or mixed with calcium phosphate), **struvite** stones (magnesium ammonium phosphate), **uric acid** stones, and **cystine** stones.

1. **Calcium stones are the most common** and are associated with hypercalcemia (due to malignancy, hyperparathyroidism, dehydration, sarcoidosis, diffuse bone disease, or milk-alkali syndrome) or hypercalciuria (increased intestinal absorption or impairment of tubular reabsorption of calcium).
2. **Struvite stones** are associated with urea-splitting bacteria like *Proteus*. These stones are the largest. They may form **staghorn calculi** *(Slide 8.14),* which are casts of the renal pelvis or calyces.

3. **Uric acid stones** are common in patients with gout or in diseases with rapid cellular turnover, e.g., leukemias and myeloproliferative disorders.
4. **Cystine stones** are due to genetic defects in amino acid tubular reabsorption that result in cystinuria.

INFLAMMATION OF THE URINARY BLADDER

Cystitis is inflammation of the urinary bladder. There are many types of cystitis but all forms present with **increased frequency of urination, lower abdominal pain** or **suprapubic tenderness**, and **dysuria**. This triad may also accompany other symptoms like fever, chills, and malaise. Bladder infections are **more common in females** because their urethra is shorter and is more susceptible to bacterial colonization from the skin surface. Other predisposing conditions for bladder infections include: diabetes mellitus, bladder calculi, urinary obstruction, instrumentation (e.g., catheterization) and immune deficiency.

Acute Cystitis

Acute cystitis is commonly caused by bacteria, including *Escherichia coli* (most common), *Proteus, Klebsiella*, and *Enterobacter*. Other organisms that cause cystitis include: *Mycobacterium tuburculi, Candida albicans* from long-term antibiotic use, viruses, and *Schistosoma haematobium* infection, which is common in Egypt and Middle Eastern countries. Radiation treatment is also a cause of cystitis when it is directed near the bladder. Finally, **cyclophosphamide** is an important cause of hemorrhagic cystitis.

Grossly, an inflamed bladder appears hyperemic. Microscopically, the inflammatory component consists mostly of neutrophils. When there is a hemorrhagic component, the term *hemorrhagic cystitis* is used, and when there is a suppurative exudate present, *suppurative cystitis* is denoted.

Chronic cystitis

Chronic cystitis is characterized by a predominance of lymphocytes. The bladder grossly shows a friable and granular heaped up epithelial surface. Furthermore, there is fibrous thickening of the muscularis propia.

Malacoplakia

Malacoplakia is a specialized form of inflammatory reaction that occurs in the urinary bladder as well as other sites, including bone, colon, and lungs. It is more common in **immunosuppressed transplant recipients**. *E. coli* and *Proteus* are common etiologic agents.

Grossly, malacoplakia is characterized by soft, yellow, raised plaques. These plaques correspond microscopically to areas containing large foamy, granular, and occasionally multinucleated macrophages, lymphocytes, and **Michaelis-Gutmann bodies** *(Slide 8.15)*.

Michaelis-Gutmann bodies are dense round bodies, which represent laminated mineralized calcium concretions within lysosomes. They are found within macrophages and outside of them as well. These bodies in addition to the foamy and granular character of the macrophages are thought to be due to abnormal degradation of bacterial products.

NEOPLASTIC DISEASE
Benign Tumors of the Kidney

Benign tumors of the kidney are generally incidental findings discovered on radioimaging or at autopsy.

Renal Papillary Adenoma

These are small (less than 5 cm), well-circumscribed and encapsulated nodules that are grossly yellow-gray. Microscopically, they are composed of cuboidal to polygonal cells that grow in a branching pattern with fronds that project into cystic spaces, hence papillomatous (papillary). When these are detected on x-ray as an incidental finding, they are treated as early cancer until their benignity is established.

Renal Fibroma or Hamartoma (Renomedullary Interstitial Cell Tumor)

Renal fibroma is a grossly gray-white tumor found in the renal pyramids. Microscopically, the tumor consists of fibroblast-like cells and collagenous tissue.

Angiomyolipoma

Angiomyolipoma is a tumor consisting of vessels, smooth muscle, and adipose tissue. It is important to remember that angiomyolipomas are common in tuberous sclerosis (cerebral cortex and skin lesions, epilepsy, and mental retardation). This tumor can be symptomatic since is has a tendency to hemorrhage internally, causing pain.

Oncocytoma

Oncocytoma is a common tumor that is usually resected due to its **growth potential**. Grossly, these tumors are encapsulated, tan-brown, and homogeneous (surface is evenly consistent in color and texture). This tumor is believed to arise from the intercalated cells of collecting ducts.

Microscopically, the oncocytoma tumor is comprised of large eosinophilic cells with small round nuclei. EM reveals a tremendous number of **mitochondria**.

Benign Tumors of the Urinary Bladder

Papilloma

There are two types of papillomas, **inverted** *(Slide 8.16)* and **exophytic**. Both types are morphologically identical and consist of papillary finger-like projections that are composed of transitional epithelium. The center of the projections contains a fibrovascular core. Unlike the exophytic type, which manifests as a single discrete red elevated papillary outgrowth, the inverted type extends down into the lamina propria.

Malignant Tumors of the Kidney

Renal Cell Carcinoma (RCC) (Adenocarcinoma of the Kidney)

RCC occurs more commonly in **males in the 6th to 7th decade**. Patients present with costovertebral pain, a palpable mass, and hematuria. **Tobacco** is a prominent risk factor. RCC usually occurs sporadically, but it may occur in genetic diseases that have chromosome 3 alterations (e.g., **Von Hippel-Lindau Syndrome**).

RCC is classified into 3 major types: **clear cell** (the most common) *(Slide 8.17)*, **papillary carcinoma**, and **chromophobe renal carcinoma**.

Grossly, renal cell carcinoma is commonly located in the poles of the kidney, especially the upper pole. The tumor is bright yellow-orange and is spherical. In clear cell carcinoma, the cells are polygonal and have a clear cytoplasm that contains glycogen and lipids.

RCC is a nasty tumor and has a propensity to invade the renal vein *(Slide 8.18)*; metastasis is common even before patients become symptomatic. Moreover, RCC may produce a paraneoplastic syndrome, e.g., hypertension (due to renin production), and secondary polycythemia (due to erythropoietin production). Nephrectomy is the major treatment for RCC. Survival rates are determined by renal vein involvement, extension of tumor into the perinephric fat, and distant metastasis.

Malignant Tumors of the Urinary Bladder

Urothelial (Transitional Cell) Tumors (Slides 8.19, 8.20, and 8.21)

Most tumors of the bladder arise from the urothelial cell layer, which is composed of transitional cells. These tumors range from small benign papillomas (exophytic) to malignant neoplasms (Grades I-III). Grades II and III tend to be multicentric. Carcinoma of the bladder is more common in men (50-80 years old) and in industrialized nations. The most common presentation is **painless hematuria**.

Many factors are strongly associated with bladder carcinoma. These include cigarette **smoking**, arylamines (especially 2-naphthylamine), long-term use of analgesics, and cyclophosphamide (immunosuppressive agent that also induces hemorrhagic cystitis). **Schistosoma haematobium infections** (prevalent in Egypt and Sudan) are associated with **squamous cell carcinoma of the bladder** (70% of cases; the remainder are transitional cell type). The etiology is based on the ova eliciting a chronic inflammatory response that progresses to metaplasia, dyplasia, and possible malignancy.

Urothelial carcinomas tend to recur after resection, regardless of grade. Prognosis relates to grade. Papillomas and Grade I tumors have a 98% 10-year survival whereas 40% of individuals with Grade III disease survive 10 years. Patients with squamous cell have a very poor prognosis with 70% of cases resulting in death within one year.

Finally, transitional cell carcinomas can also arise in the ureteral epithelium.

9

Male Reproductive System

THE PENIS
Congenital Malformations

Most congenital penile malformations are very rare, ranging from a congenital absence to duplication of the penis. Some of the more common anomalies include **hypospadia** (opening of the urethra on the ventral surface of the penis, which occurs in 1/300 live male births) or **epispadia** (urethral opening on the dorsal surface of the penis). Either of these anomalies may also be accompanied by undescended testicles (**cryptorchidism**) or abnormalities of the urinary tract.

Infections

Fig. 9-1. Infection of the glans and foreskin of the penis. This is known as **balanoposthitis** (not to be confused with blepharitis, which is infection of the eyelid). There are a lot of critters that can cause infection down there, including *Candida albicans,* anaerobic bacteria, *Gardnerella,* and pyogenic bacteria. These mostly occur in uncircumcised males, as a result of poor hygiene resulting in the accumulation of **smegma**, which is a collection of desquamated epithelial cells, sweat, and debris.

Repeated infections can lead to scarring of the opening of the foreskin, making it too small to permit normal retraction (known as **phimosis**). This process can lead to the development of secondary infections, and even penile carcinoma.

Chancroid
Chancroid, is condition caused by *Haemophilus ducreyi,* presents as a soft, painful ulcer. This ulceration makes the site more prone to infection with other organisms or fungi, with the tendency to spread along the penis and groin areas.

Fourier's Gangrene
Fourier's gangrene is necrotizing fasciitis of the genitals and perineal area. In adults, the cause is usually gram negative rods or anaerobic bacteria. In children Staph or Strep infections are most likely. The infections are introduced to the area via trauma or burns, or with conditions such as diabetes, leukemia, and alcoholic cirrhosis.

Granuloma Inguinale
Granuloma inguinale is a sexually transmitted disease that is caused by the gram negative rod, *Calymmatobacterium granulomatis.* It starts as a small painful nodule that then ulcerates and may have satellite lesions. You could remember it as a gra-nodule-oma inguinale.

Herpes Simplex
Herpes simplex is a sexually transmitted disease that is usually caused by Herpes simplex virus type 2. It

PROPER HYGIENE

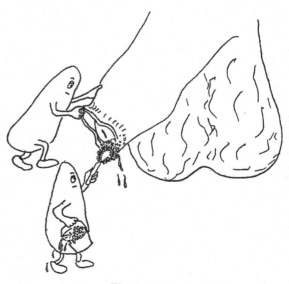

Figure 9-1

causes multiple small vesicles that eventually rupture and ulcerate.

Lymphogranuloma Venereum

Lymphogranuloma venereum is another sexually transmitted disease, caused by *Chlamydia trachomatis*. It causes a painless papule or ulcer, followed by suppurative inflammation of the inguinal lymph nodes and lymphadenopathy. The name will help you remember the clinical course – lympho, and although this condition is not related to lymphomas, you can think a lymphoma is painless, and so is lymphogranuloma venereum.

Syphilis

Syphilis, a sexually transmitted disease, is caused by *Treponema pallidum*, and humans are its only natural host. The clinical disease occurs in stages:

1. **Primary syphilis** is a painless, hard chancre (an indurated ulcer) often at the glans, or site of infection. Because this first stage is painless, the patient may not know he has the disease, and could proceed to infect other people.
2. The **secondary stage** is when there are the largest number of organisms in the body, manifesting in a diffuse rash of small red macules, included on the palms, soles and mucous membranes.
3. In the **tertiary stage**, **gummas** form (which are basically granulomas with giant cells, inflammation of the vessels and necrosis). If this stage is left untreated, the infection may progress to involve the heart and nervous system.

Tumors

Condyloma Acuminatum

Condyloma acuminatum is a benign tumor related to the common wart (**verruca vulgaris**), since both are caused by human papillomavirus (HPV). Condyloma acuminatum tends to be caused by HPV 6 or 11. This is a sexually transmitted disease of males and females that can occur and recur, but will not evolve into a cancerous lesion. Penile lesions range in size and shape, and usually occur on the inner surface of the foreskin or on the coronal sulcus.

Histologically, condyloma acuminatum demonstrates a central fibrovascular core and hyperplastic epithelium with preservation of the normal maturation. **Koilocytes** are also seen (epidermal cells with clear vacuolization of the cytoplasm), which are features of HPV infection.

Carcinoma in Situ

Carcinoma in situ is also known as **high-grade squamous intraepithelial neoplasia**. It is a lesion where malignant cytologic changes do not extend past the epithelium. That, however does not mean that it will never become an invasive cancer – it is still considered precancerous, and is presumably the origination of invasive squamous cell carcinoma of the penis. The DNA of **HPV 16** is found in about 80% of cases of carcinoma in situ.

Bowen's Disease

Bowen's disease (squamous cell carcinoma in situ of the genital region) occurs in males over the age of 35. It presents as a thick whitish plaque on the shaft of the penis. The lesion is HPV positive and transforms into invasive squamous cell carcinoma in about 10-20% of cases.

Bowenoid Papulosis

Bowenoid papulosis, a condition of sexually active young men, around the age of 30, is associated with HPV 16 or 18. These multiple small, pigmented papules (as in, papulosis) occur on the skin of the shaft, glans or scrotum. They may spontaneously regress, and almost never become invasive. The condition grossly resembles condyloma acunimatum and microscopically resembles Bowen's disease, only with greater pigmentation within the lesion.

Penile Squamous Cell Carcinoma

Carcinoma of the penis makes up less than 1% of all cancers in American males; however in other parts of the world (Asian, Africa, and South America) it can compose 10-20% of male cancers. It is a slow-growing, locally invasive lesion that is often present for a year or more before its discovery. Cigarette smoking is a risk factor for the development of invasive penile cancer; most penile carcinomas occur in patients from 40 to 70 years old.

Circumcision is relatively protective against squamous cell carcinoma of the penis, so these cancers are less frequent in cultures where circumcision is widely practiced. This is thought to be due to better hygiene, since circumcision reduces exposure of the penile epithelium to infections and possible carcinogens like HPV. HPV DNA is found in about 50% of patients with invasive carcinoma, mostly **HPV 16** and to a lesser extent **HPV 18**.

Grossly, squamous cell carcinoma of the penis usually begins on the glans or inner surface of the prepuce, near the coronal sulcus. Papillary lesions may produce a cauliflower-like fungating mass, resembling condyloma acuminata. Areas of epithelial thickening are flat and may exhibit ulceration of the mucosa, with possible pain and infection.

Metastasis occurs to inguinal and pelvic lymph nodes in the early stages. More advanced lesions involve the liver, lungs, heart, and bone. About 15% of patients have metastatic disease at the time of diagnosis. Two-thirds of patients survive at least 5 years if the lesions do not involve the inguinal lymph nodes, whereas the survival of patients with lymphatic metastasis is only about one quarter at 5 years.

THE TESTIS AND EPIDIDYMIS

Even though the testis and epididymis are anatomically very close to each other, their pathology can be quite distinct. Pathologic involvement of the epididymis usually is inflammatory, whereas in the testis it is usually neoplastic.

Congenital Malformations

Most congenital malformations of the testis are extremely rare. The exception is the incomplete descent of the testicles, or **cryptorchidism**, found in about 1% of one year-old boys. Testicular descent occurs in 2 phases: transabdominal and inguinoscrotal. Most disorders of descent occur in the inguinoscrotal phase, and the undescended testis can be felt in the inguinal canal. In most cases, the condition is unilateral, and is discovered by physical exam. Histological changes in the undescended testis can occur by 2 years of age. The predominant change is fibrosis of the testicle, including increased thickening and hyalinization of the basement membrane of the spermatic tubules. Most undescended testicles will spontaneously descend into the scrotum during the first year of life. Those that do not spontaneously descend require surgical repositioning. Despite surgical correction, these patients will have an increased risk of cancer in both the undescended and descended testicle.

Inflammation

Inflammatory processes are more common in the epididymis than the testis. Of the major inflammatory diseases, gonorrhea and tuberculosis usually arise in the epididymis, whereas syphilis affects the testis first. Just think of it this way: GET STD... **G**onorrhea, **E**pididymis, **T**uberculosis and **S**yphilis, **T**estis, **D**isease. There are 2 other inflammatory conditions of the testicles (a.k.a. orchitis) to note. **Granulomatous (autoimmune) orchitis** can mimic a testicular tumor, since it is a rare cause of unilateral testicular enlargement. It is characterized by granulomas that are present throughout the testis but confined to the seminiferous tubules. Mumps can also cause orchitis; testicular involvement is most likely to occur in post-pubertal males, most often developing 1 week after the onset of parotid gland swelling.

Nonspecific infections of the epididymis and subsequently of the testis are usually related to infections of the urinary tract that travel via the vas deferens or the lymphatics of the spermatic cord. Epididymitis is uncommon in children, but when it does happen, it is usually associated with a congenital abnormality of the urinary tract, and infection with gram negative rods. This makes sense because congenital anomalies of the urinary tract predispose boys to urinary tract infections, so this is just an extension of that process.

In sexually active men and men under the age of 35, the most common causes of epididymitis come from those STDs *Chlamydia trachomatis* and *Neisseria gonorrhoeae*. In men over the age of 35, urinary tract pathogens, namely *Escherichia coli* and *Pseudomonas*, are most likely to blame.

Microscopically, inflammation of the epididymis can lead to scarring and subsequent infertility.

Vascular Disturbances

The most common vascular disturbance of the testicles and epididymis is **torsion**. This is one of the few urologic emergencies, and occurs when twisting of the spermatic cord cuts off the venous drainage, but the thick-walled arteries remain open.

Fig. 9-2. Testicular torsion.

Testicular torsion can result in vascular engorgement, hemorrhagic infarction, and necrosis of the entire testis. The clinical presentation is that of an abrupt onset of testicular pain which may be associated with trauma or congenital abnormality. The treatment for testicular torsion is surgical, and this should happen within 6 hours of the event, for maximum viability of the testicle.

Testicular Tumors

Testicular tumors have a peak incidence in the 15 to 34 year-old age group, where they are the most com-

TESTICULAR TORSION

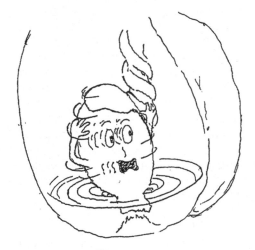

Figure 9-2

mon tumor of men. Overall, they account for about 10% of male cancer deaths. Testicular neoplasms are divided into germ cell tumors and non-germinal tumors. Germ cell tumors compose about 95% of testicular tumors, Most of them are highly aggressive cancers, whereas non-germinal tumors are generally benign. Think of it this way: germ cells are multipotential and can be fairly uninhibited when they become cancerous, and therefore act aggressively.

A common presentation for germ cell tumors is painless enlargement of the testicles. Because biopsy of a possible testicular neoplasm carries the risk of tumor spillage, the standard treatment of a testicular mass (i.e., cancer until proven otherwise) is excision.

Tumors of the testis have a predictable route of spread. Lymphatic spread is common and occurs first to the retroperitoneal para-aortic nodes, then the mediastinal and supraclavicular nodes (in order from the abdomen up to the chest and neck areas). Blood-borne spread is mostly to the lungs, then liver, brain and bones. Sometimes the foci of metastasis are histologically different from the primary tumor, which makes sense, since many of these cells are derived from totipotential germ cells, which progress through different stages of differentiation.

Testicular germ cell tumors are almost always linked to an isochromosome of the short arm of chromosome 12, i(12p).

Germ cell tumors are divided into groups based on whether they are composed of a single histologic pattern, or a combination of histologic patterns. Most (about 60% of testicular tumors) are composed of more than one histologic subtype, which gives rise to the term "mixed tumors."

Most germ cell tumors arise from **intratubular germ cell neoplasias,** or **ITGCN.** ITGCN is basically the in situ stage of germ cell neoplasias, but it can't be called carcinoma in situ, because it's not an epithelial lesion (sigh, semantics!). It's seen adjacent to germ cell tumors in 90-100% of cases. If ITGCN is seen in a testicle without evidence of tumor, there is a 50% chance that area will develop into a germ cell tumor within 5 years. Low dose radiation is used to stop the progression of ITGCN to cancer.

Let's briefly review the stages of testicular cancer:

1. Stage I means the tumor is confined to the testis, epididymis, or spermatic cord.
2. Stage II cancer means distant spread is limited to retroperitoneal lymph nodes below the diaphragm.
3. Stage III cancer means there is metastasis outside the retroperitoneal nodes or above the diaphragm.

A variety of serum markers can be used to detect and follow testicular neoplasms. Serum markers are useful in evaluating testicular masses, staging testicular germ cell tumors, assessing tumor burden, and following a patient's response to therapy:

- **LDH (lactate dehydrogenase)** is useful in following the tumor burden, since its level is proportional to the mass of tumor cells. However, it is produced in a number of tissues, so increased levels are not specific for testicular tumors.
- **Alpha-fetoprotein (AFP)** is the major serum protein of the early fetus and is synthesized by the fetal gut, liver cells, and yolk sac. It is usually undetectable after the first year of life.
- **Human chorionic gonadotropin,** or **HCG,** is usually synthesized and secreted by the placental syncytiotrophoblast.

Increased levels of these markers are most often associated with nonseminomatous tumors (defined as any tumor not classified as a seminoma — see below). Marked elevation of serum AFP is produced by yolk sac tumors, while choriocarcinomas present with a marked increase in HCG. Both of these markers are increased in over 80% of patients with nonseminomatous tumors at the time of diagnosis.

Seminoma vs Nonseminomatous Germ Cell Tumor

Germ cell tumors are further divided into gonadally differentiated **seminomas** and totipotential **nonseminomatous** tumors. Nonseminomatous tumors can remain largely undifferentiated to form **embryonal carcinoma.** If an embryonal carcinoma differentiates along all 3 germ cell layers, the result is a teratoma. Nonseminomatous tumors may also differentiate among extraembryonal lines to form yolk sac tumors or choriocarcinomas. Clinically, the most important distinction is between seminomatous and nonseminomatous germ cell tumors (NSGCT). **The main idea is that seminomas generally have a better prognosis than NSGCTs,** which are more aggressive with a poorer prognosis. Seminomas tend to be slow to metastasize, with about 70% of patients presenting in an early clinical stage. Metastases are usually via the lymphatics, and these tumors are very sensitive to radiation treatment, resulting a cure rate of over 95%. In the case of NSGCT, about 60% of patients present with advanced clinical disease (stages II and III), metastasis is via the blood-borne route, and these tumors are fairly resistant to radiation therapy. Despite the more aggressive behavior of NSGCTs, with aggressive chemotherapy about 90% of patients are still able to achieve complete remission.

Histologic Subtypes of Germ Cell Tumors

Seminomas: These are the most common type of germ cell tumor. The occurrence peaks in men in their 30s, and account for about half of the germ cell tumors.

They are also the most likely to produce one population of cells.

Grossly, seminomas are large tumors which can grow to ten times the size of a normal testicle. Histologically, the classic seminoma has sheets of uniform cells divided into lobules by septa of fibrous tissue *(Slides 9.1, 9.2, 9.3)*. The cells are large and round with a distinct cell membrane, clear cytoplasm, and large central nucleus with one or two prominent nucleoli.

Keep in mind: None of the following are seminomas, so they fall into the category of **nonseminomatous** germ cell tumor (NSGCT).

Spermatocytic Seminoma: This is a distinct entity, although its name closely resembles the classic seminoma. It is one of the two testicular tumors that do not arise from an ITGCN (childhood teratomas are the other exception). This is a rare tumor that generally affects those over 65 years old. In contrast to the classic seminoma, it is a slow-growing tumor that rarely metastasizes.

Grossly, spermatic seminoma is a larger tumor than a classic seminoma and has 3 cell populations (medium-sized, smaller, and giant cells) that are intermixed.

Embryonal carcinomas: These are more aggressive than seminomas and generally occur in 20-30 year olds.

Grossly, embryonal carcinoma is a smaller tumor than the classic seminoma and is poorly demarcated on cut section. The cells may appear in alveolar or tubular patterns, with papillary convolutions, or as sheets of cell *(Slides 9.4, 9.5)*. Immunoperoxidase techniques may detect syncytial cells containing HCG or cells containing AFP.

Yolk Sac Tumor (Infantile Embryonal Carcinoma or Endodermal Sinus Tumor): This is the most common testicular tumor in infants and children up to 3 years old, and carries a good prognosis. The tumor microscopically shows a lace-like network of medium-sized cuboidal or elongated cells. The presence of AFP in the tumor cells is highly characteristic, and it underscores their differentiation into yolk sac cells.

Choriocarcinoma: Choriocarcinomas are a highly malignant form of testicular tumor that is composed of both cytotrophoblastic and syncytiotrophoblastic cells. In its pure form, it is rare (about 1% of all germ cell tumors), but is the most aggressive of the nonseminomatous germ cell tumors. It is more likely to be found as a component of a mixed germ cell tumor. These tumors are usually small and are found by palpation of a small testicular nodule. Testicular enlargement is rare, but hemorrhage and necrosis are common, as these tumors easily outgrow their blood supply. HCG can be readily demonstrated in the cytoplasm of the syncytiotrophoblastic cells.

Teratoma : Teratomas are tumors that consist of tissue from different germ cell lines. Mature teratomas (which contain adult-like tissues, rather than the fetal-type tissues contained in immature teratomas) are more common in infants and children.

Fig. 9-3. Teratoma. The tumor consists of a random arrangement of mesodermal (muscle, cartilage, adipose tissue), ectodermal (neural tissue, skin), and endodermal (gut, bronchial epithelium) tissue.

Miscellaneous Lesions

Leydig (Interstitial) Cell Tumors: These may secrete androgens, mixtures of androgens and estrogens, or even corticosteroids. Remember: Leydig cells are located in the interstitial spaces between tubules, and are the source of testosterone and related androgens. Most tumors occur between the ages of 20 and 60, and may present like most testicular tumors with testicular swelling.

Fig. 9-4. Leydig cell tumor. Due to the hormonal effects, patients can present with gynecomastia or sexual precocity.

Testicular lymphoma: (Slides 9.6, 9.7) A lymphoma is not a primary tumor of the testicle, but is important to know because it may present with a testicular mass. Lymphomas account for about 5% of testicular neoplasms and constitute the most common form of testicular neoplasm in men over the age of 60. The disease (usually diffuse large cell lymphoma) carries a poor prognosis, since disseminated disease is usually present at the time of diagnosis.

The tunica vaginalis is a serosa-lined sac that lies just proximal to the testis and epididymis. Fluids can accu-

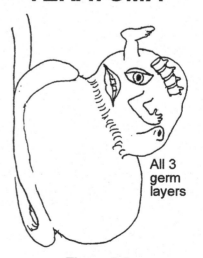

TERATOMA

All 3 germ layers

Figure 9-3

LEYDIG CELL TUMOR

Precocious masculinization

Figure 9-4

mulate in this sac, giving rise to hydroceles, hematoceles, or chyloceles:

- A **hydrocele** occurs when clear fluid accumulates in the sac, due to infection, tumor, or for unknown reasons.
- **Hematocele** is blood within the tunica vaginalis, and usually occurs in cases of direct trauma.
- **Chylocele** refers to the presence of lymph in the sac, and is usually found in patients with elephantiasis who have widespread, severe lymphatic obstruction.

The most common benign paratesticular tumor is an **adenomatoid** tumor. It is usually a small nodule that occurs near the upper pole of the epididymis. Surgical excision of the tumor is curative.

THE PROSTATE

The major conditions of the prostate are: **inflammation, hyperplasia**, and **carcinoma**.

Inflammation

Acute Bacterial Prostatitis

Acute prostatitis is caused by the same bacteria that cause urinary tract infections (*E. coli*, other gram negative rods, enterococci and staphylococci). The organisms usually get to the prostate by reflux of urine, but may also enter by surgical manipulation or sexual contact. Symptoms include fever, chills and painful urination, and the prostate is tender and swollen on physical exam. Pathologic examination may show small diffuse abscesses, areas of necrosis, or edema. However, specimens for prostatic inflammation are rarely examined microscopically. This is because biopsy of an inflamed

prostate may lead to sepsis, and bacterial prostatitis is treated treated medically.

Chronic Bacterial Prostatitis

Chronic prostatitis can commonly be diagnosed by the presence of recurrent urinary tract infections caused by the same organism. Many antibiotics do not penetrate the prostate well, so some bacteria set up camp in the prostate and constantly infect the urinary tract. The patient may present with low back pain, painful urination, and perineal and suprapubic discomfort. Sometimes, the patient is asymptomatic; in most cases the condition appears insidiously without a history of an acute attack. The same organisms that cause acute bacterial prostatitis are responsible for chronic bacterial prostatitis. Diagnosis is based on the presence of white blood cells and bacteria in the prostatic secretions.

The most common form of prostatitis seen today is **chronic abacterial prostatitis**. It presents identically to the clinical picture of chronic bacterial prostatitis, only there is no evidence of recurrent urinary tract infections. This condition may be caused by sexually transmitted disease organisms such as *Ureaplasma urealyticum*, *Chlamydia trachomatis*, and *Mycoplasma hominis*.

Granulomatous Prostatitis

Granulomatous prostatitis is a rare immune-mediated reaction to prostatic secretions from obstructed ducts, which is usually associated with nodular hyperplasia of the prostate. (Makes sense, right? – Nodular hyperplasia predisposes to obstruction of the ducts, which can lead to this condition in susceptible individuals.) About one-fifth of patients present with a high fever, symptoms of prostatic infection, and a hard prostate on digital rectal examination. In the United States, the most common cause is the instillation of Bacillus Calmette-Guerin (BCG) into the bladder for the treatment of superficial bladder cancer. BCG is an attenuated tuberculosis strain that produces a microscopic picture within the prostate that is identical to that seen in systemic tuberculosis. This finding is not clinically significant, and no treatment is indicated.

The prostate is the most common site for tuberculosis of the male genitourinary tract, caused by blood-borne spread from the lungs. Granulomatous prostatitis can also be caused by fungus (usually in immunocompromised hosts) or it can commonly be nonspecific.

Precancerous Lesions

Prostatic Hyperplasia

Nodular hyperplasia, commonly known as **benign prostatic hypertrophy (BPH)** is an extremely common condition in men over the age of 50 *(Slides 9.8, 9.9)*. By age 70, there is microscopic evidence of hyperplasia in about 90% of men, however there is no relationship between microscopic changes and the presence of clinical symptom.

Fig. 9-5. Prostatic hyperplasia. An aging prostate tends to increase in mass.

As many as 50% of men who exhibit microscopic changes will not have symptoms. The prostate increases in size due to hyperplasia of prostatic stromal and epithelial cells, resulting in large, discrete nodules in the inner (periurethral) part of the gland. An increase in periurethral prostate tissue causes symptoms related to a urinary tract obstruction (since the urethra gets squeezed). These can include urinary frequency, nocturia, difficulty starting and stopping the stream, acute urinary retention, and chronic urinary stasis, which could lead to bacterial proliferation and a urinary tract infection. It is important to note that nodular hyperplasia is not a precancerous condition.

The causes of prostatic hyperplasia are thought to be strongly related to hormonal influences. The mediator of prostate growth is a testosterone metabolite called **dihydrotestosterone (DHT)**. The absence of androgenic hormones (in the form of prepubertal castration) has been shown to prevent the development of nodular hyperplasia. Nodular hyperplasia of the prostate occurs almost exclusively in the transition zone, the inner aspect of the prostate gland. The first nodules are composed almost entirely of stromal cells; later, predominantly epithelial nodules arise. The nodules that are mostly glandular will appear yellow-pink and soft, and will exude milky prostatic fluid (because glands secrete stuff). The nodules that are predominantly fibromuscular will appear firm and gray.

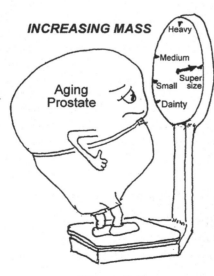

INCREASING MASS

Aging Prostate

Heavy
Medium
Super size
Small
Dainty

Figure 9-5

Microscopically, prostatic hyperplasia shows glandular proliferation with aggregations of cystically dilated glands lined by an inner columnar and outer cuboidal or flattened epithelium, riding on an intact basement membrane. Histologic changes may also include foci of squamous metaplasia or areas of infarction.

Mild cases of nodular hyperplasia can be treated with slight alterations of a person's daily routine. The most commonly used and effective medical treatment for symptoms of benign hyperplasia is alpha-blockers, which decrease prostatic smooth muscle tone. Surgically, transurethral resection of the prostate, or TURP, can be useful in reducing symptoms, and is used as first-line therapy in recurrent urinary tract infections. Currently a number of additional treatments are available.

Carcinoma of the Prostate

"Prostate cancer" – these words strike fear into the hearts of many older men. This is the most common form of cancer in males, and currently the second leading killer of men from cancer. The exact cause of prostate cancer remains unknown, but many factors are thought to play a part, including hormonal influences. The growth of some prostatic carcinomas has been slowed by the administration of estrogen, or by castration. Also, both androgen and estrogen receptors have been shown to exist on normal and neoplastic prostatic tissue.

Most cases of prostate cancer begin in the periphery of the prostate gland (as opposed to prostatic hyperplasia, which begins in the center), particularly the posterior portion. This is why digital rectal exams are a good method of screening for prostate carcinoma.

Fig. 9-6. Prostatic cancer. It is most frequently found posteriorly and can be palpated on rectal exam.

The great majority of these cancers are adenocarcinomas, since the prostate is a glandular structure. Well-differentiated cancers (cancers that still look like their original organ) may be difficult to distinguish from nodular hyperplasia. In prostate cancer, there will be acini that are smaller and more closely spaced (in a "back to back" configuration, important diagnostic criteria for most adenocarcinomas), and a single layer of epithelial cells lines the glands *(Slides 9.10, 9.11)*.

Metastasis of prostatic cancer by blood-borne routes is most likely to go to bone. The grading of prostate cancer defines its histologic properties, such as the growth pattern, nuclear atypia, and the degree of differentiation. Staging is different than grading, and describes the extent of the cancer in relation to the entire body:

1. **Stage A cancer** means it is only a microscopically detectable cancer, so you wouldn't be able to tell

there is cancer by looking at it, you can't feel it, and the patient is probably without symptoms.

2. **Stage B cancer** means there is a palpable nodule of the prostate. Many of these will invade the seminal vesicles and urinary bladder (local invasion), and will spread to distant sites if left untreated. Treatment of localized (stage A and B) cancer is with surgery and/or radiotherapy, and patients generally survive for at least 15 years.

3. **Stage C cancer** means the tumor has spread beyond the capsule of the prostate, but is still contained in the region of the pelvis.

4. **Stage D cancer** means there is tumor metastasis. At the time of diagnosis, about 75% of patients have locally advanced or disseminated disease. These cases will tend to present with urinary obstruction, local pain, or bone pain. Osteoblastic metastasis in an elderly man means metastatic prostate cancer until proven otherwise. Treatment of advanced prostate cancer can include hormonal treatments like orchiectomy or estrogen administration. The 10-year survival rate is between 10-40%.

Serum **prostatic acid phosphatase levels** are useful in the diagnosis and staging of patients with prostatic carcinoma. An increase can show that the cancer has metastasized or extended beyond the capsule. Also helpful is a serum **prostate-specific antigen (PSA)** level, which can be increased in patients with both localized and advanced carcinoma. The PSA level is particularly helpful in monitoring a patient's response to therapy or the progression of cancer.

PALPATION OF PROSTATIC CARCINOMA

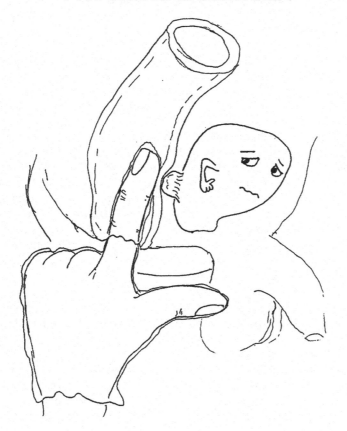

Figure 9-6

10

Female Reproductive System

EMBRYOLOGY

The embryology of the female reproductive system is important for explaining the anomalies and the histogenesis of tumors that occur. For this purpose, embryogenesis of the female genital tract can be divided into two components. The first occurs around the fifth week of gestation and is marked by the arrival of the primordial germ cells into the urogenital ridge. These cells are of endoderm origin because they arise from the yolk sac. The surrounding mesoderm in the urogenital ridge proliferates around the dividing germ cells to form the ovary. At birth, the female's germ cells have already entered meiosis but will remain arrested in meiosis stage I until she enters puberty and begins ovulating. Failure of the germ cells to develop may result in absent ovaries or premature ovarian failure.

The second component occurs around the sixth week of gestation and consists of the development of the **müllerian duct**. This duct is formed from coelomic epithelium (mesothelium). The müllerian ducts grow caudally until they enter the pelvis. The most caudal portions of the duct fuse with one another and connect to the urogenital sinus. The unfused portions of the müllerian ducts become the fallopian tubes, the fused portion becomes the uterus and upper vagina, and the urogenital sinus becomes the lower vagina and vestibule. Thus, the entire lining of the uterus and tubes as well as the ovarian surface is derived from coelomic epithelium. For this reason, one can appreciate why benign lesions like **endometriosis**, and benign and malignant lesions of endometrioid and serous nature arise on the surfaces of these structures and on peritoneal surfaces.

BASIC TERMS

Colposcopic examination is visualization of the patient's cervix using acetic acid and a magnifiying instrument called a colposcope. Acetic acid is applied to the cervix for visualization. When light is applied, the suspicious areas appear white and do not reflect light (due to the large nuclear size). The white areas may indicate dysplasia and are biopsied. This exam is sometimes performed following a pap test that indicates a malignant or premalignant condition.

Cone biopsy is one method used to remove a circular portion of cervix that extends up into the canal especially when dysplasia involves the endocervical canal. The specimen is shaped like a cone.

LEEP (Loop Electrosurgical Excision Procedure) uses an electrified wire loop to remove portions of the cervix. This procedure is a more modern method (compared to the Cone biopsy) used to remove portions of the cervix and can be done in the office.

Proliferative phase *(Slide 10.1)* denotes the time prior to ovulation that is characterized by rapid growth of endometrial glands and stroma. Histologically, the glands consist of tubular structures lined by mitotically active pseudostratified columnar cells. The stroma is composed of mitotically active compacted spindle cells.

Fig. 10-1. Ovulation. Ovulation occurs when the luteal spike (LH) from the pituitary gland stimulates the release of an ovarian follicle.

Fig. 10-2. Secretory phase. The secretory phase follows ovulation. During this time, the endometrial glands become tortuous and serrated (saw-toothed). Progesterone induces compression of the endometrial glands ("spiral" glands), signifying the secretory phase of the menstrual cycle. *(Slide 10.2)*

Histologically, the tubular cells in the secretory phase become vacuolated with glycogen, which is discharged into the glandular lumen. The stroma is

THE LUTEAL SPIKE AND OVULATION

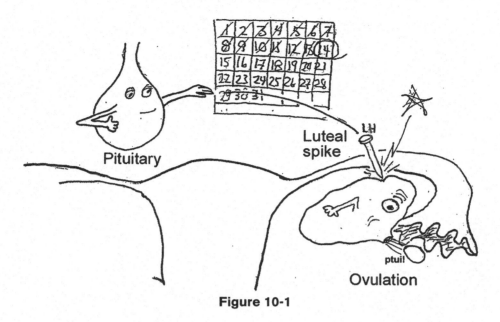

Figure 10-1

SECRETORY PHASE OF MENSTRUAL CYCLE

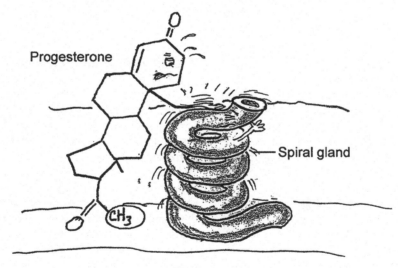

Figure 10-2

marked by edema and an increase in the ground substance, which gives it a "watery" appearance. Within the stroma, tortuous spiral glands develop. These changes do not manifest all at once, and in fact, correspond to a predictable time sequence.

Fig. 10-3. Dating of the menstrual cycle. This can be done by studying the endometrial architecture. Dating is useful to assess endocrine abnormalities (e.g., evaluation of infertility), document ovulation, or determine causes of endometrial bleeding. Based on the endometrial biopsy, the pathologist can discern which one of the 3 phases of the menstrual cycle (**menses, proliferative,** and **early** and **late secretory**) is present. If the secretory phase is encountered, the pathologist can be more specific and predict the post-ovulation day based on the histological appearance of the glands, stroma, and arterioles.

HISTOLOGICAL DATING OF THE MENSTRUAL CYCLE

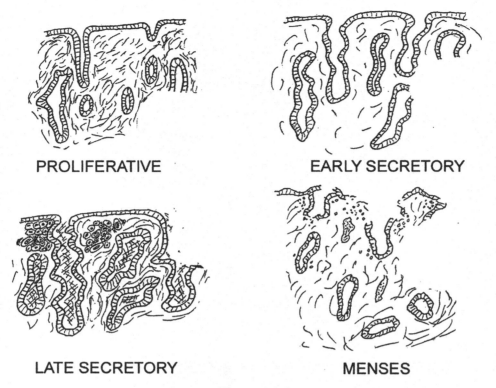

PROLIFERATIVE

EARLY SECRETORY

LATE SECRETORY

MENSES

Figure 10-3

INFECTIONS

There are many organisms that can infect the female genital tract. Some organisms cause major discomfort without serious sequelae, while others can cause infertility, spontaneous abortions, fetal demise, and even be implicated in the pathogenesis of vulvar and cervical malignancies. Below is a list of the most common organisms seen in clinical practice:

Herpesvirus (HSV) *(Slides 10.3, 10.4)* is a sexually transmitted disease (STD) that causes herpes simplex infection. The most common type is HSV type 2, although type 1 may also be a cause. The initial manifestation occurs 3 to 7 days following sexual relations and consists of painful red papules in the vulvar region. The patient may present with fever, malaise, and tender inguinal lymph nodes. There is also heavy white vaginal discharge (leukorrhea). The papules progress to vesicles, which then coalesce and become ulcers. Active infection is marked by the presence of ulcers, and this is when transmission is most likely to occur. Within 1 to 3 weeks the ulcers heal; however, the virus persists in the regional nerve ganglia, which explains why this STD recurs. The most feared complication is neonatal transmission. Diagnosis is made by recovery of the virus by tissue culture.

Chlamydia trachomatis is a small gram-negative bacterium that is an obligate intracellular parasite. There are many different serotypes of *Chlamydia*, which cause different diseases. For example, the venereal form is associated with serotypes D through K, whereas the L serotype causes **lymphogranuloma venereum** (a chronic ulcerative disease endemic in Asia, Africa, and the Caribbean). Patients may present with urethritis, mucopurulent cervicitis, and acute salpingitis (inflammation of the fallopian tubes); however, most times they will have subclinical or asymptomatic infection. Polymerase chain reaction (PCR) or deoxyribonucleic acid (DNA) probe assay is superior to culture for diagnosis. Pelvic inflammatory disorder (PID) can be a sequela.

Neisseria gonorrhoeae is an STD that is limited to the lower genital tract (cervix, urethra, periurethral and vestibular glands). Infection with *N. gonorrhoeae* (gram negative diplococci) presents similarly to chlamydial infection, i.e., mucopurulent discharge and may be asymptomatic. Definitive diagnosis is made by culture although gram staining. can be useful. As with *chlamydia*, PID can be a sequela.

Haemophilis ducreyi is an STD limited to the tropics and causes chancroid. This infection is characterized by soft and painful ulcerated lesions and is unlike syphilis, which produces firm and painless ulcers (see below).

Calymmatobacterium (Donovania) granulomatosis is a gram-negative rod that causes **granuloma inguinale** and is characterized histologically by **Donovan bodies** (histiocytes containing multiple organisms). Initially, this disease manifests as papules in the genital or inguinal regions that later ulcerate. The lesions coalesce and form large ulcers and lymphatic obstruction; genital distortion may result.

Treponema pallidum is a microaerophilic spirochete that causes **syphilis**. Syphilis is an STD that is divided into primary, secondary, and tertiary stages. The **primary stage** presents about 3 weeks after contact with an infected individual as a single, painless, red lesion (chancre) on the cervix, vaginal wall, or anus. Using silver stains, dark-field examination, or immunofluorescence, spirochetes can be visualized within the chancre. The chancre heals in 3 to 6 weeks with or without treatment. Transplacental transmission occurs easily, and congenital syphilis is a serious sequela. Serology is used for diagnosing syphilis. Serologic tests include nontreponemal antibody and antitreponemal antibody tests. Both tests do not become positive until 4 to 6 weeks after infection.

Nontreponemal **tests** are used for screening and include the rapid plasma reagin (RPR) and Venereal Disease Research Laboratory (VDRL). The tests use cardiolipin, a phospholipid found in spirochetes and human tissue and can be falsely positive in other conditions, such as acute infection, collagen vascular disorders, drug addiction, pregnancy, and hypergammaglobulinemia of any etiology.

Treponemal **antibodies tests** are highly specific and are used as confirmatory tests. These tests include the fluorescent treponemal antibody absorption test (FTA-ABS) and the microhemagglutination assay for *T. pallidum* antibodies (MHATP).

Human papillomavirus (HPV) is a DNA virus that has not only been implicated in sexually transmitted vulvar **condyloma accuminatum** but is the most important agent in cervical carcinogenesis. Moreover, Specific HPV types have also been isolated in vulvar and vaginal squamous cell carcinomas. High-risk types associated with cervical cancer include: 16, 18, 31, 33, 35, 39, 45, 51, 52, 56, 58, 59, and 68. Low-risk types associated with condylomata include: 6, 11, 42, 44, 53, 54, 62, and 66.

Mycotic and yeast (Candida) infections are common and are found in patients with diabetes, in those who use oral contraceptives, are immunocompromised, or are pregnant. Typically patients will present with leukorrhea and pruritis. The presence of organisms on wet mounts is diagnostic *(Slide 10.5)*.

Trichomonas vaginalis (Slide 10.6) is a large, flagellated, and motile protozoan that can be identified on wet mounts of vaginal discharge. On vaginal examination, there is a yellow and foul-smelling vaginal discharge. The cervix is fiery red; hence, the term "**strawberry cervix.**"

Mycoplasma hominis accounts for some cases of vaginitis and cervicitis. This organism has been associated with spontaneous abortions and chorioamnionitis.

Gardnerella is a gram-negative bacillus that may cause vaginitis when other causes (*Trichomonas* and fungi) are excluded.

Pelvic Inflammatory Disorder (PID) is an acute suppurative reaction that ascends from the vagina to involve the cervix, endometrial mucosa, fallopian tubes, and ovary. It is characterized by pelvic pain with adnexal tenderness, fever, and vaginal discharge. PID is acquired in one of two ways: either sexually, or following parturition or a surgical procedure. When acquired sexually, it commonly is due to *N. gonococci, chlamydia* and enteric bacteria. When acquired after parturition or from a surgical procedure, it is due to polymicrobial infection commonly from staphylococci, streptococci, coliform bacteria, or *Clostridium perfringens*.

Common sequelae of PID include acute suppurative salpingitis, salpingo-oophoritis, tubo-ovarian abscesses, **pyosalpinx** (pus within the tube), or **hydrosalpinx** (serous fluid within the tube as a result of the purulent exudate undergoing proteolysis). Complications of PID include peritonitis, intestinal obstruction from adhesions between the intestine and pelvic organs, bacteremia (endocarditis, meningitis, suppurative arthritis), and infertility.

THE VULVA

Because the vulva is hair-bearing, many diseases of the skin are also found in the vulva, e.g., psoriasis, eczema, and allergic dermatitis. The entities discussed herein are specific to the vulva.

Bartholin Cyst *(Slide 10.7)* results from obstruction of the Bartholin duct. Bartholin's glands are paired and normally produce a clear and mucoid secretion, which functions to provide continuous lubrication of the vestibular surface. The cysts the result of obstruction and can be large (3 to 5 cm in diameter) They are lined by either transitional or squamous epithelium. Clinically, these cysts cause pain and discomfort. If the cyst becomes infected, acute inflammation of the gland (**adenitis**) or an abscess may form. Bartholin abscess may be associated with *Neisseria gonorrhea* infection. Treatment includes excision or permanent opening (marsupialization).

Vulvar Vestibulitis is defined as inflammation of the surface mucosa and vestibular glands of the vulvar vestibule. Small painful ulcerations may form. Vestibulitis is one common cause of **vulvodynia** (chronic vulvar pain). The etiology is unknown. Surgical removal of the inflamed tissue is the only current treatment modality.

Inflammatory epithelial disorders are characterized clinically as white, opaque, plaquelike thickenings that cause pruritis (itching). Collectively, this description is called **leukoplakia**. Leukoplakia is a non-specific vague term that may encompass benign lesions, e.g., vitiligo (pigment loss), or inflammatory lesions (psoriasis, chronic dermatitis) as well as malignant diseases like vulvar intraepithelial neoplasia, Paget disease, melanoma, or even invasive carcinoma. Thus, an astute clinician should always biopsy these types of lesions.

When non-specific inflammatory changes occur that cannot be definitively diagnosed either clinically or microscopically, they are categorized as **lichen sclerosis** (chronic atrophic vulvitis) or **lichen simplex chronicus** (previously called hyperplastic dystrophy). "Lichen" is a Greek term that is used to describe either a single papule or aggregate of papules that resembles a patterned configuration that resembles lichen growing on rocks.

Lichen sclerosis occurs most commonly in postmenopausal women but may be seen in prepubescent females as well. The skin is gray and wrinkled and looks like wrinkled parchment paper. This entity is diagnosed microscopically by the presence of 4 histopathologic features *(Slide 10.8)*:

1. Atrophy, which is characterized by thinning of the epidermis and loss of the rete ridges (the deep projections of the epidermis).
2. Hydropic degeneration of the basal cells.
3. The underlying dermis is replaced by dense collagenous fibrous tissue (very pink).
4. Bandlike dermal lymphocytic infiltrate in the dermis. The etiology is unknown but may be autoimmune related.

Lichen simplex chronicus is a non-specific condition that results from rubbing and scratching secondary to pruritis (itching). Irritants may be due to specific infections caused by fungal organisms or chemical exposures.

Microscopically, the squamous epithelium in lichen simplex chronicus is **acanthotic** (epidermal hyperplasia) with **hyperkeratosis** (thickening of the anucleated stratum corneum) with some inflammation in the dermal layer.

Benign Neoplasms

Two common benign neoplasms of the vulva include **papillary hidradenoma** and **condyloma accuminatum**. **Papillary hidradenoma** is identical to its counterpart in the breast, intraductal papilloma. Both are derived from apocrine sweat glands. The lesion presents as a small nodule on the labia majora or interlabial folds. The nodule may ulcerate, which is why it may be mistaken for carcinoma. Microscopically, the neoplasm is composed of tubular ducts lined by columnar cells. Beneath the columnar epithelium is a layer of myoepithelial cells.

Condyloma acuminatum, also referred to as **venereal warts**, are caused by the sexually transmitted human papillomavirus (HPV) types 6 and 11. Clinically, these lesions are raised and wartlike (**verrucous**) and usually occur in groups, which may coalesce *(Slide 10.9)*. Typically, they may also involve the perianal, perineal as well as vulvar areas.

Microscopically *(Slide 10.10)*, the lesion in condyloma acuminatum shows acanthosis, parakeratosis, hyperkeratosis, and koilocytotic atypia (nuclear atypia and perinuclear vacuolization) in the mature surface epithelial cells. This latter finding is termed a viral cytopathic effect and is a distinctive change present in the mature superficial cells of the epithelium as a result of viral life cycle completion. Generally, these lesions regress in immunocompetent patients and are not premalignant.

Malignant Neoplasms

Most of the malignant tumors of the vulva are squamous cell carcinomas, which are divided into two groups based on the presence or absence of HPV infection.

Vulvar Intraepithelial Neoplasia (VIN) comprises the first group of squamous cell carcinoma and is associated with high-risk (cancer-related) HPV types 16 and 18 as well as other high-risk types. Such patients have precancerous changes termed **vulvar intraepithelial neoplasia (VIN)**. VIN is defined as the presence of nuclear atypia in the epithelial cells, increased mitoses, and lack of surface differentiation. Based on the aforementioned criteria, VIN is divided into three grades:

1. VIN I – mild dysplasia
2. VIN II – moderate dysplasia
3. VIN III – severe dysplasia.

Other terms, like **Bowen disease** and carcinoma in situ are also used to describe VIN III, which all imply "full thickness dysplasia." Clinically, these lesions are slightly raised and are either flesh-colored or pigmented and may be ulcerated.

On histological exam, vulvar intraepithelial neoplasia may be well-differentiated and appear as "invasive warts" or poorly differentiated and consist of blue (**basaloid**) cells.

Squamous cell hyperplasia and lichen sclerosis comprise the second group that is associated with squamous cell carcinoma. Unlike the first group, the etiology of this association is not known. However, mutations of the p53 gene with increased p53 protein accumulation have been found in these tumors. These lesions manifest with nodules in areas of vulvar inflammation. In fact, they may be mistaken for dermatitis, eczema, or leukoplakia because they may cause local discomfort due to itching or secondary infection.

Histologically, squamous cell hyperplasia and lichen sclerosis show invasive nests of well-differentiated keratinized epithelial cells.

Once invasion occurs, distant metastatic spread is linked to tumor size and regional lymph node involvement (inguinal, pelvic, iliac, and periaortic). The lungs are the primary site for such metastatic spread. Treatment involves a vulvectomy (partial or radical) and lymph node dissection.

Extramammary Paget Disease is unlike its counterpart in the breast because Paget disease of the vulva is not always associated with an underlying carcinoma. In fact, Paget disease of the vulva is frequently confined to the epidermis and appendages. When Paget disease of the vulva occurs, it may persist in the epidermis for years without invasion. Clinically, this neoplasm manifests as an itchy, red and crusted lesion on the labia majora.

Microscopic examination of the vulvar Paget disease neoplasm is characterized by clusters of "Paget cells" — large tumor cells with clear separation (halo) from the surrounding epithelial cells. These cells are believed to arise from primitive epithelial progenitor cells.

Surgical resection is the mode of treatment of vulvar Paget disease; however, recurrence is common since the Paget cells extend beyond the clinically visible lesion.

THE VAGINA

Congenital and Benign Neoplasms

Congenital anomalies that occur in the vagina are Gartner duct cysts and mucous cysts, which arise from Wolffian duct rests and Müllerian epithelium, respectively. Furthermore, endometriosis is also Müllerian derived. Other benign lesions include rhabdomyomas, stromal polyps, leiomyomas, and hemangiomas. Typically, they occur in females of reproductive age.

Malignant Neoplasms

Primary malignancies of the vagina are uncommon. Important malignancies that are discussed herein are vaginal intraepithelial neoplasia (VAIN), squamous cell carcinoma, adenocarcinoma, and embryonal rhabdomyosarcoma.

Vaginal intraepithelial neoplasia (VAIN) is like VIN because it is also associated with HPV infection. A previous history of carcinoma of the vulva or cervix confers the greatest risk of VAIN and possible invasive carci-

noma. These lesions are commonly found in the upper posterior portion of the vagina near the ectocervical junction. Clinically, the patient will present with irregular spotting and eventual leukorrhea. Occasionally, these neoplasms are clinically silent and will present in advanced disease with urinary or rectal fistula formation.

Clear cell adenocarcinoma may present in young women (15-20 years old) whose mothers were treated with **diethylstilbestrol (DES)** for a threatened abortion during pregnancy. Fortunately, the majority of these DES-exposed young women present with vaginal adenosis (persistence of Müllerian type columnar epithelium) that grossly appears as red granular foci on the vaginal mucosa. Adenosis may be a precursor to adenocarcinoma; however, the incidence of malignant transformation is less than 1%. With early detection, most patients are managed successfully with irradiation and surgery.

Embryonal rhabdomyosarcoma is also termed **sarcoma botryoides**. Why this name, you ask? Grossly, these tumors resemble small grapes *(Slide 10.11)*; hence, the term "botryoides," which means grapelike. These tumors grow expansively and may project out from the vagina. These tumors are uncommon. They affect female infants and children less than 5 years old. Metastasis is uncommon if detected early. Management includes surgery and chemotherapy.

Histologically, sarcoma botryoides consists of a myxomatous stroma and round undifferentiated cells, which look like tennis rackets with the racket portion being a bleb of cytoplasm and the webbing being the oval nucleus. Interestingly, the tumor cells like to crowd around the vessels and form a cambium layer (think of the cambium layer of a tree).

THE CERVIX

The cervix, which is the lower portion of the uterus, connects the vagina to the rest of the uterus via the endocervical canal. The cervix is divided into ecto- and endocervix components. The ectocervix can be visualized on vaginal examination. This portion of the cervix is covered by **stratified, nonkeratinizing squamous epithelium** *(Slide 10.12)* that continues up to the external os (small central opening). The external os is connected to the internal os by the endocervical canal. The canal is lined by columnar mucus-secreting glands. The **squamocolumnar junction** is where the squamous and columnar cells meet. This junction migrates during life. At birth, the junction is within the endocervix; however, in young adulthood, it migrates caudally into the exocervical region. In the mature female, the junction is usually found in the exocervix, which is why it is visible on colposcopic examination. Within the junction, some of the columnar epithelium is replaced by squamous epithelium and is termed the **transformation zone**. This region is unstable and consequently changes; in fact, this region can be thought of as a battlefront where the opposing forces, squamous warriors and the glandular warriors, are fighting to gain territory. The battlefront represents the transformation zone since it is constantly changing within the junction. This zone as well as the squamocolumnar junction *(Slide 10.13)* is where precancerous lesions develop.

Non-Neoplastic Disorders

Cervicitis is invariably present in all women of reproductive age, albeit most cases are sub-clinical. Cervicitis is diagnosed by the combination of clinical exam, culture, and Papanicolaou smear. Cervicitis may be classified as either acute or chronic.

Acute cervicitis is defined by the presence of acute inflammatory cells that consist of mainly neutrophils *(Slide 10.14)*. Grossly, the cervix is erythematous and swollen. The patient may complain of purulent vaginal discharge and dysparenuria (pain during intercourse). Acute cervicitis is caused by trauma (childbirth or surgical manipulation) or from organisms that are either endogenous or are related to STDs.

Although inflammation is a key histopathologic component of acute cervicitis, additional histologic findings can be associated with particular organisms. For example, epithelial ulcers with intranuclear inclusions are associated with HSV infection. Moreover, a plasmacytic infiltrate and lymphoid germinal centers are associated with *C. trachomatis* infection.

Chronic cervicitis is very common in adult females. The pathogenesis is related to estrogen (from the ovary) stimulating maturation of the cervical and vaginal mucosa, which involves the takeup of glycogen. When these cells are shed, they serve as a nutritive substrate for bacterial organisms (endogenous vaginal aerobes and anaerobes, streptococci, enterococci, *Escherichia coli*, and staphylococci). Bacterial growth causes a decrease in pH. As a response to these changes, the reserve cells in the endocervical mucosa proliferate and "toughen up" to become squamous; hence, the term squamous metaplasia. As the epithelium proliferates, the glandular openings (crypts) become blocked and mucous secretions accumulate. **Nabothian cysts** *(Slide 10.15)* and inflammation result.

Histologically, chronic cervicitis is defined by the presence of (1) chronic inflammatory changes that consist of macrophages, plasma cells, and lymphocytes *(Slide 10.16)*, (2) granulation tissue with possible necrosis, and (3) reparative changes that resemble atypia or dysplasia. If the inflammatory response is brisk, erosion marked by the loss of the epithelial lining and ulcerative changes may be seen.

Endocervical polyps are benign inflammatory proliferations of cervical mucosa that result from chronic inflammation. The polyps are usually small but may reach several centimeters in size. Microscopically, they consist of dilated endocervical glands within an edematous, inflamed, and fibrotic stroma. Patients may present with irregular bleeding especially postcoital. Curettage or excision is curative.

Dysplasia and Carcinoma In Situ

Cervical dysplasia is disordered cell growth that is characterized by the loss of polarity and nuclear hyperchromasia that involves part or all of the cervical epithelium. Moreover, dysplasia is more likely to occur at the transformation zone because it is an unstable region. Dysplasia encompasses a spectrum of morphologic alterations and accordingly is classified into grades. There are many classification systems; however, the cervical intraepithelial neoplasia (CIN) classification is discussed herein. Lesions are graded 1, 2, or 3, which corresponds to mild, moderate, or severe dysplasia (carcinoma in situ), respectively.

1. **CIN 1** is used when the proliferation is confined to the **lower third** of the epithelium. The cells in the upper two thirds are mature, yet abnormal, with nuclear enlargement, hyperchromasia, and koilocytotic atypia. These cytological changes are associated with productive viral infection; hence, condyloma accuminata frequently fall into this grade. Generally, these lesions regress and do not transpire to malignancy.
2. **CIN 2** denotes moderate dysplasia of the parabasal cells where the atypia is limited to the **inner two-thirds** of the epithelium, i.e., the atypical proliferation involves more than one-third but not greater than two-thirds of the thickness of the squamous epithelium. Koilocytosis may be present; however, this finding is more common in CIN 1 lesions. The atypical cells show a higher nuclear to cytoplasmic (N/C) ratio, increased mitotic activity as well as abnormal mitotic figures and variation in nuclear size and nuclear hyperchromasia. These cells correspond to high-risk HPV types. Nevertheless, there is still some notion of maturation toward the prickle and keratinizing cell layers.
3. **CIN 3** *(Slides 10.17, 10.18, 10.19)* is also called carcinoma in situ (the lesion is still confined to the epithelium and has not broken through) and represents **full thickness** atypia where differentiation is absent, i.e., the entire thickness of the epithelium is replaced by immature atypical cells.

Fig. 10-4. Cervical dysplasia, seen in CN1, 2, and 3.

Lesions that are classified as CIN 1 or 2 are unpredictable. They may regress or progress to cancer, but have a lower risk of doing so compared to lesions clas-

CERVICAL DYSPLASIA

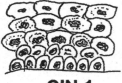

CIN 1

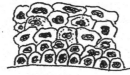

CIN 2

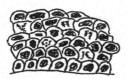

CIN 3

Figure 10-4

sified as CIN 3, which confer the greatest risk for cancer. Similarly, progression from dysplasia to malignancy is unpredictable and may span months to years.

Cervical Carcinoma and Disease Prevention

The Pap Test

Disease prevention and reduction of cervical cancer is due to screening techniques like the Papanicolaou cytologic test (Pap test), which screens for malignant and premalignant changes of the cervix. Screening is recommended for all women beginning at either age 18 or at the onset of sexual activity. The screening interval is every year. If a woman of reproductive age has had two normal Pap tests one year apart, then she may only need a Pap smear every three years.

The Pap test consists of scraping cells from the squamocolumnar junction and smearing them on a slide (conventional Pap) or suspending them in a liquid based media (thin prep). The cells (glandular and squamous) are examined for the presence or absence of atypia under a microscope. Non-neoplastic findings are reported as well. Examples of the latter include infections, e.g., herpes, *trichomonas vaginalis*, candida, inflammation, and changes associated with radiation. Common and important diagnostic cytological terms used, i.e., terms on the pathology report include the following:

- **"Negative for SIL"** (squamous intraepithelial lesion): denotes no cellular atypia.
- **ASC-US**: "atypical squamous cells of undetermined significance" is used to describe the cells on a Pap test that show features suggestive of a squamous intraepithelial lesion, CIN 1 or CIN 2. However, the features are either qualitatively or quantitatively insufficient to give a definitive diagnosis.

- **ASC-H**: "atypical squamous cells, cannot exclude HSIL" is used when these atypical cells are sparse.
- **LSIL**: "low-grade squamous intraepithelial lesion" corresponds to changes associated with HPV infection and denotes CIN 1.
- **HSIL**: "high-grade squamous intraepithelial lesion" denotes either CIN 2 or 3.
- **AGUS**: "atypical glands of undermined significance.
- **Squamous cell carcinoma**
- **Adenocarcinoma**

How does the clinician manage the above diagnoses?
"Negative for SIL": Patient should have a routine yearly screening.

ASC-US: The clinician may either choose to repeat the Pap test in 4-6 months or perform a colposcopy with biopsy. HPV DNA testing using either Polymerase Chain Reaction (PCR) or In-situ hybridization (ISH) methods should be performed since it is now considered standard of care. Because high-risk types of HPV are more commonly associated with progression to malignancy, HPV testing and typing is useful in determining which patients are at risk for cervical cancer. Patients who are HPV positive for the high-risk types should have a colposcopy with biopsy performed.

ASC-H: colposcopy with biopsy.
LSIL: colposcopy with biopsy.
HSIL: colposcopy with biopsy.
AGUS: colposcopy and endometrial biopsy.

HPV vaccines may prevent HPV infection and subsequent development of cervical cancer. Thus, HPV vaccines may also have a significant impact like the Pap test in the reduction of cervical cancer in the future.

Cervical carcinoma is associated with HPV infection (high-risk types) and is implicated in the pathogenesis of cervical cancer. Risk factors associated with HPV exposure include early age at first intercourse, multiple sexual partners, increased parity, male partner with a previous history of multiple sexual partners, presence of high-risk HPV and persistent detection of high viral load concentration, genital infections, oral contraceptives, and exposure to nicotine. Furthermore, the host's immune status, e.g., nutrition and HIV status, is also important.

Although the majority of cervical cancers are detected when the lesion is still precancerous, infiltrative disease still occurs. Morphologically, cervical cancer presents as a fungating, ulcerative, or invasive neoplasm that invades contiguous structures (urinary bladder, ureters, rectum, peritoneum, or vagina). The majority of cervical cancers are squamous carcinomas that consist of large cells, either keratinizing (well-differentiated) or non-keratinizing (moderately-differentiated) forms. Other types of cervical cancer include: **poorly differentiated squamous cell, small cell**, (looks similar to small cell/oat cell carcinoma of the lung), **adenocarcinoma** *(Slide 10.20)*, adenosquamous (mixed glandular and squamous differentiation), as well as **undifferentiated** carcinomas. These tumors are also associated with high-risk HPV infection, especially type 18.

Invasive squamous cervical cancer spreads first to contiguous organs; distant metastasis occurs in the liver, lungs, and bone marrow. Treatment and subsequent outcome depend on staging, where there is a 95% 5-year survival for patients with stage IA disease, 75% 5-year survival with stage IB, and less than 50% 5 year-survival with Stage III disease.

THE UTERUS

Fig. 10-5. Basic anatomy of the female reproductive organs. The female genital tract consists of the uterus, fallopian tubes, and ovaries.

In a nulliparous woman of reproductive age, the uterus weighs about 50 grams and measures 8.0 x 6.0 x 3.0 cm. The uterus following pregnancy (gravid) is slightly larger (70 grams). Following menopause, it diminishes to half its size and weight. The uterus is divided into three anatomic and functional regions: the **corpus**, the **lower uterine segment**, and the **cervix**.

The uterine cavity is lined by the glandular **endometrium**. Beneath this lining is the **myometrium**, which consists of smooth muscle cells

Pathology of the uterus can arbitrarily be divided by disorders that relate either to the endometrium or to the myometrium.

Endometrial Pathology

Bleeding is the most common manifestation of endometrial pathology. Functional disturbances of the menstrual cycle are the most common cause of bleed-

ing. Other causes of bleeding may be due to intrinsic abnormalities like endometritis, leiomyomas, (submucosal i.e., just beneath the endometrium), endometrial polyps, or endometrial neoplasms.

Functional endometrial disturbances manifest as bleeding during or between menstrual cycles, and are more commonly referred to as **dysfunctional uterine bleeding (DUB)**.

DUB encompasses many etiologies, but only the most common ones are discussed herein. Common etiologies include **anovulation**, **hormonal imbalances**, especially in perimenarchal and perimenopausal women, and **luteal phase defects**.

Anovulation results in prolonged estrogen stimulation in conjunction with an absent or weakened progestational phase. Histologically, the endometrium shows cystic dilatation of the endometrial glands as a result of prolonged estrogenic stimulation of the glands. Moreover, there may be focal stromal breakdown that is seen in menstruation; hence, "anovulatory menstruation."

Examples of diseases where anovulation may occur include endocrine disorders, (pituitary tumor, adrenal disease, or thyroid disease), primary estrogen-producing ovarian lesions (granulosa-theca cell tumor, polycystic ovarian disease), or a metabolic disorder (obesity, malnutrition, chronic disease).

Luteal phase defects occur when the corpus luteum is weak and does not produce enough progesterone. This disorder manifests infertility, irregular menstrual cycles with excessive bleeding, or amenorrhea. Luteal phase defects are diagnosed when the expected date (based on the secretory characteristics on biopsy) lags with respect to the patient's cycle day.

Oral contraceptives are used to treat DUB once organic and structural abnormalities have been ruled out. The endometrial changes seen with oral contracep-

FEMALE REPRODUCTIVE ORGANS

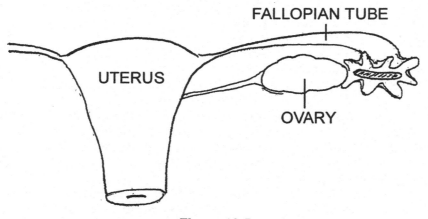

Figure 10-5

tive use show a discordant pattern. The endometrial glands are inactive and small; yet the stroma is decidualized as is seen in pregnancy. These changes are reversed once oral contraceptives are discontinued.

Acute endometritis is relatively uncommon and results from bacterial infection from retained products of conception after delivery or miscarriage and from *Chlamydia* infection. The pathogenic bacteria include group A hemolytic streptococci and staphylococci species. Polymorphonuclear (PMN, or neutrophils) are present on endometrial biopsy.

Chronic endometritis presents as abnormal bleeding, pain, discharge, or infertility. The most common etiologies include chronic PID (which may include *Chlamydia* infection), retained gestational tissue, intrauterine contraceptive devices, and tuberculosis infection. Tuberculosis is uncommon in the Western countries, but it is common in the rest of the world.

On biopsy, the cycle phase (secretory, proliferative, or menstrual) is difficult or impossible to discern and is often a good clue to endometritis. On closer inspection of the stroma, lymphocytes and plasma cells are present. Curettage or eliminating the cause of the endometritis, e.g. antibiotic therapy, are the modalities of treatment.

Endometriosis is defined by the presence of endometrial glands or stroma in locations that are outside the uterus. The most common sites include ovaries, uterine ligaments, rectovaginal septum, and pelvic peritoneum. Endometriosis manifests in women in their third or fourth decade as infertility, dysmenorrhea, dyspareunia, pain on defecation when the rectal wall is involved, dysuria when the bladder serosal wall is involved, or intestinal disturbances when the small intestine is involved.

Grossly, endometriosis appears as yellow-brown or red-blue nodules on or beneath the serosal surface of the involved organ. When the ovary is involved, endometriotic cysts containing necrotic blood, hence, the term "**chocolate cysts**," are present.

Histologically, the presence of endometrial glands and stroma is diagnostic of endometriosis. If the stroma is absent, Müllerian epithelium with adjacent hemosiderin-laden pigment is sufficient to make the diagnosis.

The pathogenesis relates to three theories:

1. **Regurgitation theory** suggests that there is retrograde menstruation and spread of the endometrial tissue through the fallopian tubes to the ovaries and peritoneal cavity.
2. **Metaplastic theory** suggests that the endometrium directly arises from the coelomic epithelium.
3. **Vascular or lymphatic dissemination theory** suggests that endometrial tissue spreads via the veins or lymphatics to distant organs like the lungs or lymph nodes.

Endometrial polyps are sessile masses that range from 0.5 to 3.0 cm and project into the endometrial cavity. They may be asymptomatic or present with bleeding, especially if they undergo necrosis or ulcerate. Polyps are composed of either 1 of 2 histological types:

- endometrial glands and stroma identical to the endometrium or
- hyperplastic (cystic type) endometrial glands.

The latter type is more common. Endometrial polyps may arise in the background of endometrial hyperplasia, tamoxifen use, or genetic alterations.

Fig. 10-6. Endometrial polyps. These may arise from prolonged estrogen stimulation.

BENIGN ENDOMETRIAL POLYP

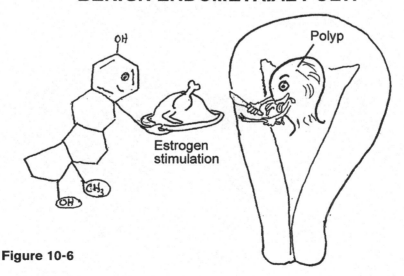

OH

Estrogen stimulation

Polyp

Figure 10-6

Endometrial Neoplasia and Carcinoma

Fig. 10-7. Endometrial hyperplasia. This entity is defined as an increased gland to stroma ratio and abnormalities in glandular growth.

The pathogenesis of endometrial hyperplasia relates to prolonged or unopposed estrogenic stimulation of the endometrium. Conditions that promote hyperplasia include anovulation due to menopause or polycystic ovarian disease, granulosa cell tumors, and estrogen replacement therapy. Another important factor in the development of hyperplasia is inactivation of the PTEN (phosphatase and tensin homolog deleted on chromosome 10) tumor suppressor gene which, when inactivated, makes the endometrial cells more sensitive to estrogenic stimulation.

Hyperplasia is divided into simple non-atypical and complex atypical (endometrial intraepithelial neoplasia or EIN) types:

1. **Simple non-atypical hyperplasia** is also known as cystic or mild hyperplasia and includes hyperplasia associated with anovulation. This entity is characterized with irregularly shaped glands with cystic alteration *(Slide 10.21)*. The glandular growth pattern is similar to that of proliferative type endometrium; however, the mitoses are not as prominent.

Simple non-atypical hyperplasia usually evolves into cystic atrophy where the epithelium and stroma become atrophic. It is uncommon for this type of hyperplasia to progress to adenocarcinoma.

2. **Complex atypical hyperplasia** (or **EIN**) shows hyperplasia marked by an increased number of glands; however, the glands are irregular and scalloped due to increased cell stratification and nuclear enlargement. Thus, there are both architectural and cytological atypia *(Slide 10.22)*. Nevertheless, the glands remain distinct and non-confluent. If the latter were not the case, then it would be adenocarcinoma! This type of hyperplasia is associated with loss of PTEN expression and more likely to progress to adenocarcinoma. For this reason, management is hysterectomy. In younger women, progestin therapy with close follow-up can be done; yet, the uterus should eventually be removed since these lesions usually do not regress with progestin.

Endometrial Adenocarcinoma may manifest grossly as an isolated polypoid mass or diffusely involve the entire endometrial surface. The route of spread involves extension into and through the myometrium involving contiguous structures (e.g., the bowel, bladder, and ovaries, and regional lymph nodes with eventual spread to lung, liver, and bone). There

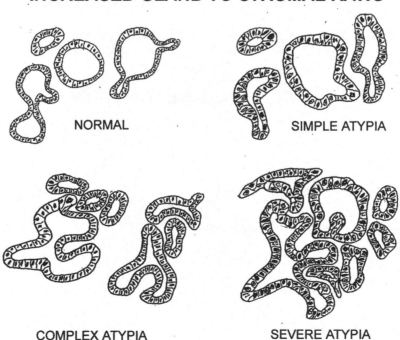

ENDOMETRIAL HYPERPLASIA: INCREASED GLAND TO STROMAL RATIO

NORMAL

SIMPLE ATYPIA

COMPLEX ATYPIA

SEVERE ATYPIA

Figure 10-7

are many subtypes of endometrial adenocarcinoma. The most common is the well-differentiated endometrioid type, which recapitulates normal endometrium. Other subtypes, which are more aggressive, include clear cell and papillary serous. *(Slides 10.23, 10.24)* The papillary serous type has a propensity to seed peritoneal structures.

In general, endometrial tumors are graded based on the presence of glandular formation and solid areas. Those tumors that consist of mostly glandular structures are well-differentiated and are Grade 1. Tumors that have glands but also solid areas composed of malignant cells are Grade 2, and those that consist of mostly solid areas are poorly differentiated and are Grade 3.

THE FALLOPIAN TUBES

The fallopian tubes consist of a patent lumen surrounded by delicately plicated mucosa composed of 3 cell types: **ciliated and nonciliated columnar cells**, **columnar secretory cells**, and **intercalated cells** (inactive secretory cells). Tumors of the fallopian tubes are uncommon. Adenomatoid tumor is the most common benign tumor; and adenocarcinoma, which usually arises from direct extension or metastasis is the most common malignant tumor. Primary adenocarcinoma of the tube is rare, but aggressive. Cysts containing a clear, serous fluid are frequently encountered. Small cysts (0.1-2.0 cm) are termed **paratubal** (cysts along the tube) and larger ones located near the fimbria are termed **hydatids of Morgagni**. They are incidental findings and usually clinically insignificant. Inflammation like suppurative salpingitis that is encountered in PID, ectopic pregnancy,

and endometriosis are the more common disorders that occur in the fallopian tubes.

THE OVARIES

Fig. 10-8. Normal histology of a functioning ovary.

Each ovary measures about 4.0 x 2.5 x 1.5 cm in dimension during the female reproductive years. It is composed of a cortex and medulla. Follicles in various stages of maturation are found within the cortex. The medulla consists of loosely arranged mesenchymal tissue that contains vessels, nerves, remnants of the Wolffian duct (**rete ovarii**), and steroid-producing hilar cells, which resemble interstitial cells of the testis.

Ovarian disease can be classified into non-neoplastic cysts and tumors.

Non-Neoplastic Cysts

Follicular cysts are expanded (greater than 2.5 cm) maturing or atretic follicles whereas **cystic follicles** are less than 2.5 cm and are actually considered physiologic rather than pathologic. Follicular cysts contain a clear serous fluid and are lined by a glistening gray membrane. A granulosa cell lining may be appreciated microscopically.

Luteal cysts (corpus luteum cysts) may develop at the end of the menstrual cycle or during pregnancy. Grossly, the cyst wall is yellow-orange and represents the luteinized granulosa cells. The luminal content is hemorrhagic.

Polycystic ovarian disease (PCOD, also called Stein-Levinthal Syndrome) is characterized by numerous subcortical cystic follicles or follicular cysts

NORMAL OVARY

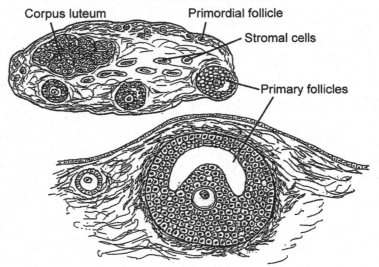

Corpus luteum   Primordial follicle

Stromal cells

Primary follicles

Figure 10-8

arranged like a "string of pearls." The ovaries are large and appear fibrotic in between the cystic areas. This latter feature is due to hyperplasia of the theca interna (**follicular hyperthecosis**). Corpora lutea and albicantia are usually absent. Patients with PCOD have persistent ovulation, obesity (40%), hirsutism (50%), and sometimes virilism. The pathogenesis is believed to stem from poor regulation of the enzymes involved in the synthesis of androgens and excess luteinizing hormone. Moreover, there is an association between insulin resistance and PCOD where patients who take insulin mediators like metformin resume ovulation.

Ovarian Tumors

Classification of ovarian tumors helps understanding their benign or malignant nature.

The ovary contains 4 major types of tissues:

1. surface (coelomic; germinal) epithelium
2. germ cells
3. sex cords and
4. ovarian stroma.

A neoplasm can arise from any of these tissues.

Surface epithelial tumors are the most important group because the majority of ovarian tumors arise from here. Benign disease is more common in women 20-40 years old, while malignant disease is common in women older than 40 years.

Fig. 10-9. Silent ovarian cancer. Ovarian cancer commonly remains clinically silent in the early stages and manifests as advanced disease with abdominal pain, abdominal enlargement, and ascites when the tumor has seeded the peritoneal cavity.

Fig. 10-10. Risk factors for ovarian cancer. These include: nulliparity, early menarche, late menopause, obesity, tobacco use, family history, and heritable mutations like BRCA 1 and 2. Important biomarkers for disease and especially for monitoring recurrence include CA-125 and newly identified osteopoetin. The pathogenesis of these tumors is believed to stem from transformation of coelomic epithelium.

Coelomic epithelium becomes invaginated into the cortex by the formation of surface adhesions or repair of ovulation sites. Once incorporated, cysts lined by mesothelial cells result. The coelomic epithelium within these inclusion cysts undergoes Müllerian differentiation and recapitulates epithelial types present in the normal female genital tract: serous (tubal), endometrioid (endometrium), and mucinous (cervix) as well as urinary bladder with transitional epithelium.

Transformation of coelomic epithelium into the various cell types may be a benign or malignant process. Because this categorization is cumbersome, surface epithelial tumors are classified by the following:

1. cell type – serous, mucinous, endometrioid (including clear cell), transitional
2. pattern of growth – cystic, solid
3. presence of fibrous stroma
4. benign, borderline, malignant

Serous tumors account for about 30% of ovarian tumors. Three types comprise this group:

- benign serous cystadenoma,
- "borderline" serous cystadenoma, and
- malignant serous cystadenocarcinoma. Benign and borderline tumors are the most common (70%).

Serous cystadenoma is a benign cyst lined by tall, ciliated, columnar cells (*Slides 10.25, 10.26*). The growth pattern is cystic, filled with a clear fluid (serous). The epithelial cyst wall is smooth and glistening.

"Borderline" serous cystadenoma has the same cell types as the benign variant, but there are focal papillary projections and epithelial thickening of the cyst wall (solid portions). Microscopically, these areas demonstrate a complex growth pattern with nuclear stratification and nuclear atypia (*Slides 10.27, 10.28*).

Serous cystadenocarcinoma (*Slides 10.29, 10.30*) shows even more complex papillary growth with invasion into the underlying stroma. These areas grossly correspond to solid areas within the cyst wall. There is abundant nuclear atypia. Concentric calcifications (**psammoma bodies**) may also be present.

Mucinous tumors are similar to serous tumors but are less common. These tumors consist of a spectrum that ranges from the **benign mucinous cystadenoma,** intermediate "borderline," also known as **mucinous tumor of low malignant potential**, and the malignant entity termed **mucinous cystadenocarcinoma.** Unlike serous tumors, mucinous tumors may become very large (25 kg), are multiloculated, and contain gelatinous fluid rich in glycoproteins, much like snot.

SILENT OVARIAN CANCER

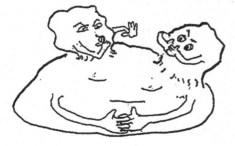

Figure 10-9

RISK FACTORS FOR OVARIAN CANCER

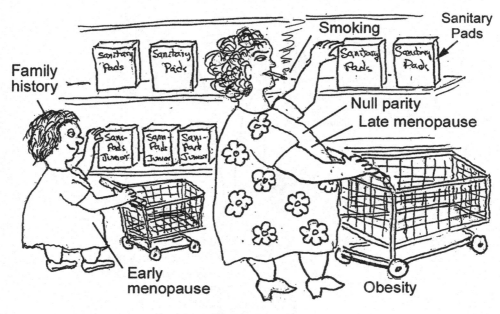

Figure 10-10

Microscopically, the epithelial lining of mucinous tumors consists of tall columnar cells and looks like cervical or intestinal epithelium; however, cilia are absent *(Slides 10.31, 10.32, 10.33)*. Like serous tumors, abundant papillary growth that corresponds to solid growth, nuclear stratification and atypia are criteria used to differentiate benignity from malignancy.

Pseudomyxoma peritonei is a disorder that consists of ovarian mucinous tumors and mucinous ascites. The primary site of disease is usually appendiceal with secondary ovarian and peritoneal involvement.

Endometrioid tumors are the third most common tumor type of the epithelial class. Most are malignant. Grossly, these tumors consist of solid and cystic components. These are differentiated from the serous and mucinous types by the presence of tubular glands, which resembles endometrium. One variant of this entity is **clear cell adenocarcinoma**, which is characterized by large epithelial cells with clear cytoplasm *(Slides 10.34, 10.35)*. Solid and cystic types exist where the neoplastic cells form sheets of tubules in the former or line the cystic spaces in the latter. These tumors tend to be aggressive.

Cystadenofibroma is similar to a serous cystadenoma except there is a benign stromal fibrous proliferation beneath the cyst wall epithelium. The cyst wall lining epithelium may be composed of serous mucinous, endometrioid, or transitional (**Brenner**) cell types.

Adenofibroma is like a cystadenofibroma where there is a fibrous stromal proliferation and an epithelial component; however, cyst formation is either small (< 1cm) or absent. It's a matter of semantics! An important example of an adenofibroma is a Brenner tumor, where the epithelial component consists of nests of transitional cells (resembles urinary bladder) within a fibrous stroma. Most Brenner tumors are benign.

Germ cell tumors basically consist of 4 tumors:

1. **Teratomas**
2. **Endodermal sinus (Yolk sac) tumor**
3. **Dysgerminoma**
4. **Choriocarcinoma**

Fig. 10-11. Germ cell tumors. Because you still may be overwhelmed from the last section, this mnemonic may help you remember the germ cell tumors: **Children should leave their germy** (germ cell tumors) **"tedy" bears** (t=teratoma, e=endodermal sinus tumor, d= dysgerminoma, and y= yolk sac tumor (same as endodermal but alternate name) **in the car** (car= choriocarcinoma).

Teratomas are further divided into 3 types: (1) mature, (2) immature, and (3) monodermal types.

Mature teratomas are important to know since they are **the most common germ cell tumor**. These are benign cysts that are lined by epidermis. They are sometimes referred to as **dermoid cysts**. Mature teratomas tend to arise in young women. They are derived from totipotential cells of ectodermal origin; however, structures from

GERM CELL LAYER TUMORS

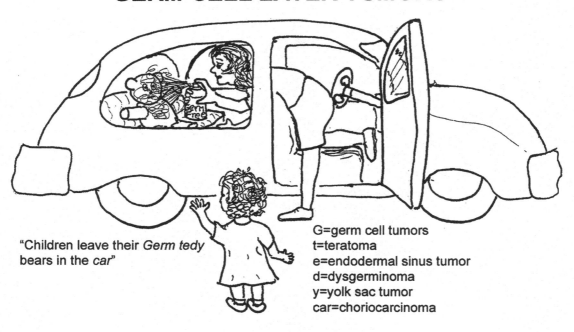

"Children leave their *Germ tedy* bears in the *car*"

G=germ cell tumors
t=teratoma
e=endodermal sinus tumor
d=dysgerminoma
y=yolk sac tumor
car=choriocarcinoma

Figure 10-11

other germ layers are commonly seen. Thus, these cysts may harbor hair, sebaceous contents, teeth, bone, cartilage, or even brain tissue.

Monodermal teratomas are a specialized type of benign teratoma which contains a single tissue, either thyroid or intestinal epithelium. These tumors are almost always unilateral. When thyroid tissue is present, it is termed **struma ovarii**. Hyperfunctional states may result. For example, hyperthyroidism may result from struma ovarii. Carcinoid syndrome may occur if the intestinal epithelium produces 5-hydroxytryptamine.

Immature teratomas are malignant! These occur in either adolescent females or young women (mean age is 18 years old). These tumors, like mature teratomas, may contain hair, bone, and teeth, but they also have areas of hemorrhage and necrosis. These tumors grow rapidly and metastasize. Metastatic potential is related to the proportion of immature neuroepithelial present in the tumor.

Dysgerminomas make up half of all malignant germ cell tumors. Like testicular seminomas, which they resemble, they are malignant, usually unilateral, and present in the second to third decades of life. Moreover, they are also very sensitive to radiation treatment.

Microscopically, dysgerminomas are composed of large vesicular cells with central nuclei. These cells are clustered in large groups and are separated from other groups by a lymphocytic-rich fibrous stroma *(Slide 10.36)*.

Fig. 10-12. Dysgerminomas. They are identical to seminomas of the testis. Mnemonic: **the dysgerminoma "dissed" the testis and went to the ovary.**

Endodermal sinus (yolk sac) tumor is the second most common malignant germ cell tumor. This tumor is derived from malignant germ cells that form yolk sac structures, which produce alpha-fetoprotein. It contains **Schiller-Duval bodies** *(Slide 10.37)*, which can be reminiscent of a renal glomerulus.

Fig. 10-13. Yolk sac tumors. This mnemonic is perhaps useful for those who rotate in pathology: **Everybody was chilled (Schiller-Duval bodies) on the Easter egg (yolk sac) hunt.**

Yolk sac tumor occurs in children or young women and is aggressive. (In general, tumors with embryonal or extraembryonal differentiation tend to be aggressive.)

Choriocarcinoma of the ovary looks and behaves just like the placental type. Again, this tumor is formed from malignant germ cells that recapitulate the placenta. The neoplastic cells comprise syncytiotrophoblastic and cytotrophoblast types *(Slide 10.38)*. The malignant cells neighbor dilated vascular sinusoids just like in the placenta, which explains why these tumors are hemorrhagic. Furthermore, the malignant syncytiotrophoblastic cells may also produce human chorionic gonadotropin (hCG), which may cause pseudoprecocity in pre-pubertal girls.

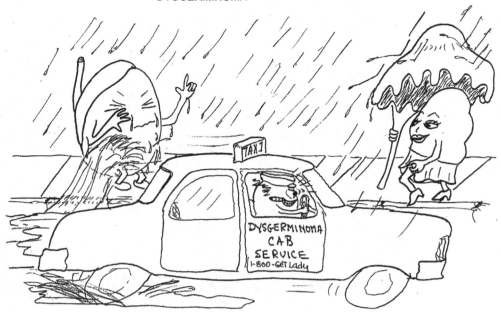

Dysgerminoma "disses" the testis and goes straight for the ovary.

Figure 10-12

When choriocarcinomas occur in young females, they mimic a tubal pregnancy. Unlike placental choriocarcinomas, these tumors are unresponsive to chemotherapy.

Sex-Cord (stromal) tumors are the last group of ovarian tumors. These ovarian tumors arise from primitive sex-cords during embryogenesis. These cords give rise to gonadal and stromal elements and include **Sertoli** and androgen-producing **Leydig** cells that are found in the male gonads, and **granulose** and estrogen-producing **theca cells** found in the female gonad as well as fibroblasts.

Fibroma-Thecomas *(Slide 10.39)* are rarely pure and usually consist of a mixture of fibroblasts (fibroma component) and theca cells, which are large cells with abundant lipid vacuoles (thecoma component). These benign tumors are usually unilateral. These are important to know because they are part of **Meigs' Syndrome**, which is characterized by fibroma-thecoma, ascites, and hydrothorax (usually right-sided).

Granulosa-Theca cell tumors also are a mixture of granulose and theca cells (cuboidal); however, pure granulose cells tumors do exist. These tumors tend to occur more commonly in post-menopausal women but are mostly benign.

Histologically, granulosa-theca cell tumors may form small follicle-like structures that contain eosinophilic material like a Graafian follicle. These structures, termed **Call-Exner bodies** *(Slide 10.40)* are important. These tumors may produce estrogen and cause precocious puberty, endometrial hyperplasia or even carcinoma. Moreover, serum inhibin levels may also be elevated in these tumors.

Fig. 10-14. Granulosa-Theca cell tumors. Mnemonic: **Granny (granulose) called Fed-Ex (Call-Exner bodies) to return her estrogen (produced by tumor) supplements.**

Sertoli-Leydig cell tumors may occur in women, most commonly in the second and third decades of life even though the cells constitute the male gonad. These tumors may produce androgens like testosterone or androstenedione and thus cause masculinization or defeminization (baldness, facial hair, amenorrhea, breast atrophy).

Histologically, Sertoli-Leydig cell tumors are composed of Sertoli cells, which form tubules *(Slide 10.41)*, and Leydig cells, which secrete testosterone. Most of these tumors are unilateral and well-differentiated; however, the poorly differentiated types appear sarcomatous.

Metastatic ovarian disease is most commonly of Müllerian origin and consists of primary tumors arising within the genital tract and metastasizing to the ovaries. Other extramüllerian types that metastasize to the ovary and are important include: **pseudomyxoma peritonei** and **Krukenberg tumor**, which is characterized by replacement of both ovaries with malignant mucin-secreting signet cells from a primary gastric carcinoma.

YOLK SAC TUMOR
SCHILLER-DUVAL BODIES

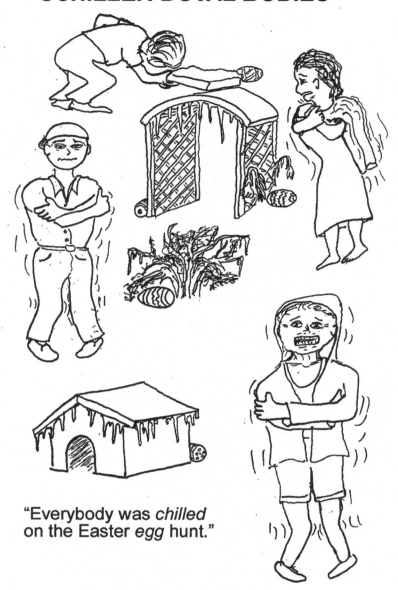

"Everybody was *chilled* on the Easter *egg* hunt."

Figure 10-13

PREGNANCY DISORDERS AND TROPHOBLASTIC PATHOLOGY
Disorders of Pregnancy

These disorders can arbitrarily be divided into gestational and placental pathologies.

Gestational disorders consist of spontaneous abortion and ectopic pregnancy.

Spontaneous abortion is pregnancy loss for "natural" reasons. Genetic abnormalities including acquired ones are most commonly implicated in pregnancy loss.

Other causes of abortion include infection due to *Toxoplasma, Mycoplasma, Listeria*, or viruses, uterine abnormalities (including leiomyomas, which may interfere with implantation), as well as trauma.

Ectopic pregnancy *(Slides 10.42, 10.43)* means that fetal implantation occurs outside the uterus. The most common site of extrauterine implantation is the fallopian tubes. Other sites include the abdominal cavity and cornu (where the fallopian tube enters the uterine cavity). The most important risk factor for an ectopic pregnancy is PID.

GRANULOSA-THECA CELL TUMOR

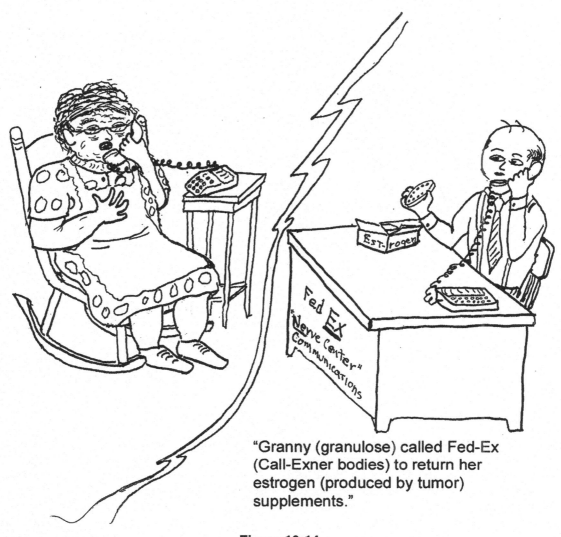

"Granny (granulose) called Fed-Ex (Call-Exner bodies) to return her estrogen (produced by tumor) supplements."

Figure 10-14

Fig. 10-15. Tubal ectopic pregnancy. This may be caused by tubal inflammation and scarring, usually due to cervitis.

Other risk factors for ectopic pregnancy include surgery, leiomyomas, peritubal adhesions, endometriosis, and intrauterine devices (IUDs). Patients often present with severe abdominal pain, amenorrhea, vaginal bleeding, and a positive beta-hCG. Tubal rupture may result in serious hemorrhage and is a medical/surgical emergency.

Placental disease may result from abnormal formation, inflammation, and infections. Below are important terms that pertain to the placenta that are clinically significant.

Placenta accrete occurs when the decidua (placental membrane tissue, seen in hyperprogesteronic condi-

tions) is partial or absent and results in placental villi interdigitating superficially with the myometrium. Patients who have had a previous Cesarean section are more predisposed to having this condition due to uterine scar formation.

Placenta increta occurs when the chorionic villi insert deep into the myometrium.

Placenta excreta occurs when the chorionic villi extend through the myometrium.

Placenta previa is a condition when the placenta inserts in the lower uterine segment or cervix.

Abruptio placentae (placental abruption) means complete premature separation of the placenta, which is an obstetric emergency for the mother and fetus.

Placental inflammation and infection can involve the placenta (**placentitis**), villi (**villitis**), umbilical cord

TUBAL ECTOPIC PREGNANCY

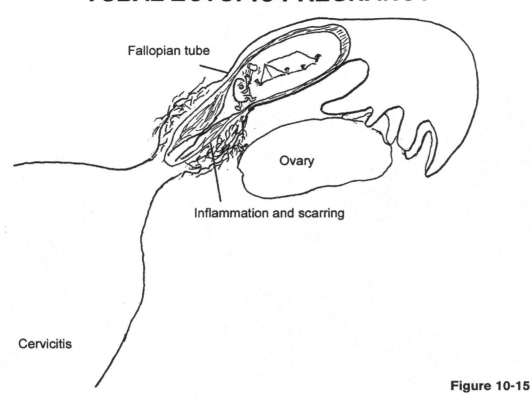

Figure 10-15

(**funisitis**), and chorion (**chorioamnionitis**). Infections that are most commonly implicated in placental disease either by transplacental transmission or via the birth canal are toxoplasmosis, syphilis, tuberculosis, listeriosis, rubella, cytomegalovirus, and herpes simplex. These infections are better known collectively as "**TORCH**" where each letter represents a disease except "O", which means others – syphilis, tuberculosis, and listeriosis.

Toxemia of pregnancy is defined by the presence of **hypertension, proteinuria**, and **edema**. It occurs more commonly during the third trimester of a women's first pregnancy. Preeclampsia is a mild form of toxemia, whereas eclampsia is a severe form of toxemia that includes convulsions and disseminated intravascular coagulation (DIC). The pathogenesis is not clearly understood but relates to shallow placental implantation, which results in placental ischemia. Eclampsia can be fatal, but usually resolves once the fetus is delivered.

Trophoblastic disease

Proliferation of trophoblastic tissue is usually associated with pregnancy. The types of trophoblastic disease consist of a spectrum that ranges from benign, non-invasive disease (e.g., the **hydatiform mole** to the **invasive mole**, and to **malignant choriocarcinoma**).

Hydatiform mole consists of cystic and swollen chorionic villi that grossly look like bunches of grapes. These moles are more prevalent in the Far East compared to the United States where they are generally uncommon. Teenagers and women in their fourth and fifth decades are more commonly affected. Women typically present with bleeding in their fourth to fifth month of gestation with a larger uterus than expected for their gestation. There are 2 variants: (1) complete (classic) and (2) partial. Although these moles are benign and non-invasive, they may progress to choriocarcinoma, especially the complete type.

Complete (classic) mole is more likely to become choriocarcinoma. Like its name implies, all of the villi are edematous, and there is diffuse (as opposed to focal in the partial mole) trophoblastic proliferation *(Slide 10.44)* that is associated with very elevated levels of hCG. Some of the trophoblastic cells show atypia. These types result from fertilization of an egg whose chromosomes have been lost. The karyotype is paternally derived and is diploid, either 46XY or 46XX. There is no embryo formation, and therefore no fetal parts are present in this type of mole.

Partial mole is less likely to become choriocarcinoma. Like its name implies, some of the villi are edematous, and there is just focal trophoblastic proliferation without atypia. Partial moles result from fertilization of an egg by two or more spermatazoa; thus, the karyotype is triploid (69XXY) or tetraploid (92XXXY), respectively. The fetus is viable for only a few weeks and thus fetal parts are present in this type of mole.

Invasive moles have hydropic chorionic villi that invade into the myometrium. They manifest with vaginal bleeding, uterine enlargement, and elevated hCG levels. These moles may transform into choriocarcinoma. They respond well to chemotherapy.

Choriocarcinoma is a malignant trophoblastic neoplasm that arises from a hydatiform mole (complete type) 50% of the time or following a normal or ectopic pregnancy 20-30% of the time. These are rapidly invasive tumors that, once discovered, have already metastasized to the lungs. They present with irregular spotting, and very high levels of hCG. The tumor does not produce uterine enlargement.

Grossly, choriocarcinomas are hemorrhagic with intermixed pale areas that have undergone ischemic necrosis.

There is a higher incidence of choriocarcinoma in African countries like Nigeria compared to the United States. Unlike choriocarcinoma of the ovary, gestational choriocarcinomas are very responsive to chemotherapy even in patients with pulmonary and bone metastasis.

11

Breast Pathology

OVERVIEW

Breast pathology, in particular breast cancer, is so important both medically and culturally that it deserves its own chapter. In North America, breast cancer is the **most common type of malignancy in women**, and the **second most common cause of death from cancer** in women. The differential diagnosis of breast pathology also includes a variety of inflammatory lesions and benign tumors, in addition to carcinoma. The key to understanding breast pathology is realizing that breast lesions correspond to a woman's age and hormonal status. We begin with a review of the anatomy and histology.

ANATOMY AND HISTOLOGY

Fig. 11-1. Normal female breast structure. The female breast is composed of 6-10 major duct systems, each of which is subdivided into lobules. Every duct opens at the nipple through a lactiferous sinus and ends proximally as a lobule. Under the influence of estrogen and progesterone at puberty, the ducts proliferate proximally and branch to form more lobules. The **terminal duct** and its ductules (**acini**) collectively form the **terminal duct lobular unit**, the functional portion of the mammary gland. *(Slide 11.1)*

Histologically, the nipple and areola are covered by stratified squamous epithelium. Entering the ducts, the lining becomes cuboidal epithelium with an underlying layer of myoepithelial cells, which aid in the expression of milk. Two distinct types of stroma are present within the breast. The **interlobular** stroma (which separates different lobules) is composed of relatively dense fibrous tissue with admixed adipose tissue. The **intralobular** stroma closely surrounds the lobules, consisting of hormonally responsive fibrous tissue with scattered lymphocytes.

NORMAL BREAST ANATOMY

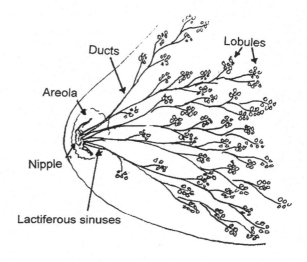

Figure 11-1

HORMONAL RESPONSE

With each ovulation, the increasing levels of estrogen and progesterone stimulate cellular proliferation, resulting in an increased number of acini per lobule. Stromal edema also occurs, which may cause tenderness and swelling. Due to the fall in hormonal levels during menstruation, epithelial cell atrophy occurs, causing regression of lobular size and return to the preovulatory state.

During pregnancy, there is a marked increase in lobular proliferation with a noticeable increase in breast size and volume and an increased lobule:stroma ratio. In the third trimester, a large number of secretory vacuoles appear in acinar cells, preparing the breast for lactation.

At the completion of lactation, lobular regression and atrophy occur secondary to the reduction in hormonal levels. Increasing atrophy and lobular regression occurs in post-menopausal women, resulting in a greater proportion of adipose tissue in the breast.

CONGENITAL ANOMALIES

Fig. 11-2. Supernumerary nipples or breasts. These are the most common congenital anomaly, occurring in both males and females. They arise along the mammary ridge (the "**milk line**"), and they are variably developed.

Another congenital anomaly is **inversion** of the nipples. This condition typically occurs in larger breasted women and may cause difficulty with breast feeding. **Acquired inversion** may occur secondary to scarring from inflammatory conditions or **may signify an underlying malignancy**.

INFLAMMATORY DISORDERS
Acute Mastitis

Mastitis almost always occurs during **breast feeding**, usually in the early stages. Cracks and fissures in the areola allow entry of skin flora, creating an infection typically caused by *Staphylococcus aureus* and less commonly, *Streptococcus*. The condition presents as a localized area of redness, tenderness, warmth and swelling. The infection may progress to an abscess, or may spread diffusely. Treatment is with continued drainage of breast milk (typically using a breast pump) and appropriate antibiotics.

Duct Ectasia

Fig. 11-3. Duct ectasia. This is an uncommon condition typically found in multiparous women of the 5th or 6th

decade. Women typically present with a palpable sub-areolar mass, which **may mimic malignancy**.

Histologically, duct ectasia shows dilated ducts with inspissated eosinophillic secretions and necrotic debris. A periductal chronic inflammatory infiltrate is present, containing lymphocytes and foamy macrophages.

Fat Necrosis

Fat necrosis typically occurs after **repetitive trauma** and is localized to the affected area. The tissue damage causes early hemorrhage with acute inflammation. This is replaced by chronic inflammation and lipid-laden macrophages, with surrounding necrotic debris. Resolution involves progressive fibrosis and calcification to form scar tissue. *(Slides 11.2, 11.3)*

DUCT ECTASIA

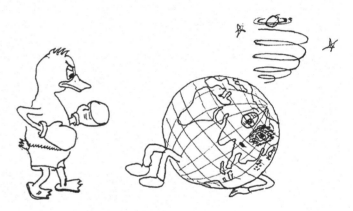

No, no, not Duck Decked Asia....

THE CONGENITAL MILK LINE

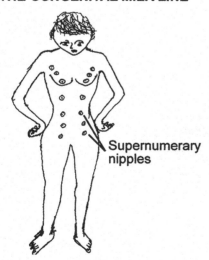

Supernumerary nipples

Figure 11-2

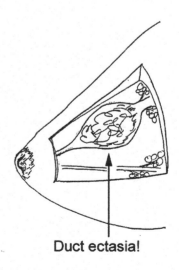

Duct ectasia!

Figure 11-3

Fibrocystic Changes

Fig. 11-4. Normal breast tissue with different types of fibrocystic changes. Fibrocystic change is the **most common disorder of the breast** and encompasses a range of morphologic changes. This used to be called "fibrocystic disease," but it is so common and of such little clinical consequence that it would be like calling brown hair a disease — no comments from you blondes!)

Women typically present between 20 and 40 years of age, usually after menarche and prior to menopause. It commonly is present in multiple areas of **both breasts**. Patients may complain of **midcycle sensitivity and tenderness**, and multiple lumps may be noted on palpation. Hormonal imbalance with a high estrogen/ progesterone ratio is the proposed mechanism, supported by improvement of symptoms in patients taking combined oral contraceptive pills ("balanced" hormones). Histologic features include some or all of the following *(Slides 11.4, 11.5, 11.6)*:

1. **Cysts:** These range in size from microcysts to large, grossly evident cysts. They are formed via cystic dilatation of ducts and lobules containing proteinaceous fluid. They may be lined with flattened epithelium or cuboidal-columnar epithelium with distinctly granular eosinophilic cytoplasm (**apocrine metaplasia**). Large cysts may appear blue (**"blue-**

domed" cysts); they disappear on drainage by fine needle aspiration.

2. **Fibrosis:** An increased amount of fibrous tissue is seen secondary to cyst leakage, causing chronic inflammation with scarring.

3. **Adenosis:** Adenosis refers to an increased number of acinar units per lobule. When extensive adenosis is combined with intralobular fibrosis, creating numerous small, variably flattened and dilated glands, it is called **sclerosing adenosis (Slide 11.7)**. This may create firm, palpable areas which also may have microcalcifications. Unlike adenosis or fibrosis, **sclerosing adenosis confers a slightly increased risk of carcinoma.**

PROLIFERATIVE BREAST DISEASE

Fig. 11-5. Normal ductal tissue compared with ductal hyperplasia. Epithelial proliferation, or **hyperplasia**, occasionally accompanies fibrocystic change, and it carries a higher risk of carcinoma. It results in an increased number of cells in the duct or lobule. Benign hyperplasia confers a slightly increased cancer risk. The proliferating cells form sheets with heterogeneous fenestrations (slit-like lumina) at the duct periphery, and the cells appear to overlap.

Atypical ductal or lobular hyperplasia refers to cellular proliferation with atypical ductal or lobular cells or

NORMAL BREAST TISSUE WITH DIFFUSE FIBROCYSTIC CHANGES

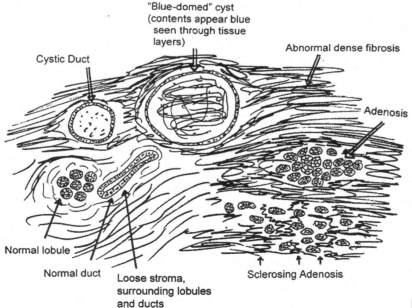

"Blue-domed" cyst (contents appear blue seen through tissue layers)

Cystic Duct

Abnormal dense fibrosis

Adenosis

Normal lobule

Normal duct

Loose stroma, surrounding lobules and ducts

Sclerosing Adenosis

Figure 11-4

DUCTAL HYPERPLASIA

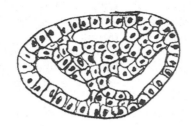

DUCTAL HYPERPLASIA

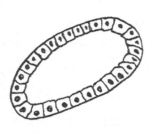

NORMAL DUCT

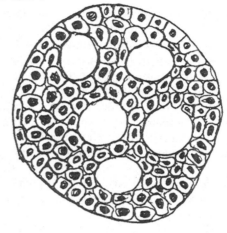

ATYPICAL DUCTAL
HYPERPLASIA
(Continuum to ductal
carcinoma-in-situ)

Figure 11-5

cellular architecture respectively, approaching carcinoma in situ, discussed later. Both types of atypical hyperplasia confer a **significantly increased risk of carcinoma** of up to 5x normal.

BENIGN TUMORS
Fibroadenoma

Fibroadenoma is the **most common benign tumor of the breast**, occurring predominantly in females in the 2nd or 3rd decade. Patients typically present with a **singular, painless, firm mass** clinically noted to be **mobile and well circumscribed**.

Histologically, fibroadenoma is composed of benign proliferation of stroma and glands. The ducts are compressed and distorted, surrounded by dense fibrous tissue. *(Slides 11.8, 11.9, 11.10)*

Both the glandular and stromal elements proliferate under the influence of estrogen and progesterone, and the rapid growth compresses the surrounding tissue into a thin fibrous "pseudocapsule." The tumor may increase in size late in the menstrual cycle. Over the course of time, fibroadenomas may hyalinize and develop calcifications. Surgical removal (excisional biopsy) is curative.

Intraductal Papilloma

These neoplasms result from papillary proliferation of ductal epithelium, creating multiple branching papillae protruding into the ductal lumen supplied by a fibrovascular core *(Slides 11.11, 11.12)*. They typically occur in a large lactiferous duct or sinus and are **solitary** and **unilateral**. Patients present with a small, palpable subareolar mass, typically with a **bloody nipple discharge**. Surgical excision is curative.

MALIGNANT TUMORS
General Overview

Breast cancer is the most common cause of cancer in women, occurring in **one out of every nine women** in the United States during their lifetime. It is the second most common cause of death from cancer, second only to lung cancer. Approximately **one in every three women who develop breast cancer will die from this disease**. Carcinoma of the breast is the most common variety of breast cancer, and the following discussion relates chiefly to this type.

Risk Factors

The risk factors for breast carcinoma should be known by heart! They include the following:

1. **Age.** The incidence of breast cancer rises with increasing age. It is rare before age 25, and the average age of diagnosis is 65. **Postmenopausal** women have the greatest increase in risk, leading to recommendations for yearly mammograms after age 50.
2. **Genetics.** The risk for breast cancer is increased in patients who have first degree relatives (e.g., mother, sister) with a history of breast cancer. This is increased further in patients with multiple relatives affected. Some genes (**BRCA1, BRCA2, p53**) have been associated with a greatly increased risk for breast cancer. Familial breast cancer typically presents at an earlier age (<40 years), and early screening examinations should be encouraged. African-American women develop breast cancer less often than Caucasian women, but they are more likely to present with more advanced disease.
3. **Proliferative Breast Disease.** Patients with biopsies showing sclerosing adenosis and/or epithelial hyperplasia, and particularly atypical ductal or lobular hyperplasia, are at increased risk for developing carcinoma of the breast.
4. **Environmental Influences.** Though of unknown etiology, the **U.S. and Northern European** populations have much higher rates of breast cancer than other countries. Immigrants to the U.S. develop gradually increased risk for breast cancer with each subsequent generation.

   High-dose local radiation is known to increase the risk for future breast cancer. Dietary influences have been suggested but lack substantial evidence, though **heavy alcohol consumption** appears to increase the risk.
5. **History of Contralateral Breast Cancer or Endometrial Cancer.**
6. **Parity.** Breast cancer occurs more frequently in nulliparous women due to unopposed estrogen effects.
7. **Length of Reproductive Life.** The risk for breast cancer increases in patients with **early menarche and/or late menopause.**
8. **Age at First Child.** The risk is increased in women who give birth for the first time after age 30.
9. **Obesity.** Postmenopausal, obese women have an increased risk for breast cancer due to increased estrogen synthesis in peripheral adipose stores.
10. **Exogenous Estrogens.** A theoretical increased risk with hormone replacement therapy has been proposed. However, this is predominantly thought to occur in estrogen-alone supplements, and **combined estrogen-progesterone supplements pose a small risk, if any**.

Both endogenous and exogenous estrogen are believed to promote growth factor induction with potential dysregulation of growth. For this reason, **estrogen receptor blocking agents commonly are used in treatment regimens**.

Epithelial proliferation and progression to carcinoma may involve overexposure to estrogen and underexposure to progesterone, expression of oncogenes (c-erb-B2, Her2/neu, c-ras), decreased expression of tumor suppressor genes, altered cell structure, loss of cell adhesion and integrins, increased expression of angiogenic factors, and increased expression of proteases.

Clinical Features

Women should be encouraged to perform self-breast examinations each month following menstruation, as the patient is most likely to notice a change before a clinician will. Common presenting features include:

1. Palpable breast mass
2. Skin changes (redness or dimpling)
3. Nipple retraction or inversion
4. Enlarged axillary lymph nodes

Mammographic Features

Increasing use of screening mammograms in recent years has resulted in earlier detection of lesions. If a lesion is found, core needle biopsies or an excisional biopsy can be obtained for a definitive diagnosis. For cystic lesions, ultrasound can be used to determine the nature of the cyst and guide a fine needle aspiration. Significant mammographic features include:

1. Densities
2. Architectural distortion
3. Calcifications
4. Change over time. Always compare with previous mammogram!

Types and Distribution

The breast can be divided into 4 quadrants based on upper, lower, inner, and outer regions. The **majority of lesions occur in the upper outer quadrant.** *Table 11.1* shows the types of breast cancer and their relative fre-

Table 11.1. Types of breast cancer

Breast cancer type	% of breast cancers	Points to remember
Ductal carcinoma in situ (DCIS)	10 - 20%	DCIS is contained by the basement membrane of the duct
DCIS, comedocarcinoma type	4 - 8%	Only high-grade pattern of DCIS, central necrosis
Invasive ductal carcinoma, no special type	79%	Most common type of breast cancer
Invasive ductal carcinoma, inflammatory type	2%	Caused by invasion/blockage of dermal lymphatics, peau d'orange, poor prognosis
Invasive ductal carcinoma, medullary type	2%	Rare cancer in premenopausal women, better prognosis
Invasive ductal carcinoma, mucinous type	2%	Rare cancer in women 65+, mucinous lakes, better prognosis
Invasive ductal carcinoma, tubular type	6%	Rare cancer in women 40 – 50, excellent prognosis
Invasive ductal carcinoma, papillary type	1%	Rare cancer, subareolar mass, clinical findings like intraductal papilloma, surgical resection is curative
Lobular carcinoma in situ (LCIS)	1 - 6%	LCIS is contained by the basement membrane of the intralobular ductules and acini
Invasive lobular carcinoma	10%	Often multicentric, may be bilateral
Paget's disease of the breast	1 - 2%	Ulcerating, inflamed nipple or areola, large cancer cells in the epidermis, look for underlying invasive ductal carcinoma
Phyllodes tumor	<1%	Rare cancer in women 60+, locally aggressive, rarely metastasizes
Primary angiosarcoma of the breast	<1%	Extremely rare, secondary to radiation
Metastatic cancer to the breast	<1%	Extremely rare, caused by leukemia, lymphoma, melanoma

quency. Ductal adenocarcinoma is the most common, and **different subtypes confer different prognoses**.

Ductal Carcinoma

Fig. 11-6. "Inside" location of carcinoma in situ. Intraductal Carcinoma, Ductal Carcinoma in situ (DCIS) is a proliferation of atypical ductal cells **contained by the basement membrane of the duct**, though the cells can spread intraductally. It can be low-grade or high-grade based on nuclear features, and 5 patterns are recognized—**comedocarcinoma, solid, papillary, cribriform** and **micropapillary**.

Fig. 11-7. Comedocarcinoma, the only high-grade pattern of DCIS, involves solid sheets of highly atypical malignant cells within a duct and **central necrosis** *(Slide 11.13)*. It is a highly aggressive form of ductal carcinoma in situ. The central necrotic area frequently calcifies, which can be detected by mammography.

Infiltrating/Invasive Ductal Carcinoma is the **most common kind of breast cancer**, in which malignant cells invade the stroma, often producing a brisk fibrous connective tissue reaction known as **desmoplasia**. Grossly, a palpable mass may be present, and sectioning reveals a gritty consistency with interspersed calcifications. Microscopically, the cancer cells are arranged as cords and nests that invade the surrounding tissue *(Slide 11.14)*. **Invasion of lymphatics** and peri-neural spaces is common.

CARCINOMA IN SITU

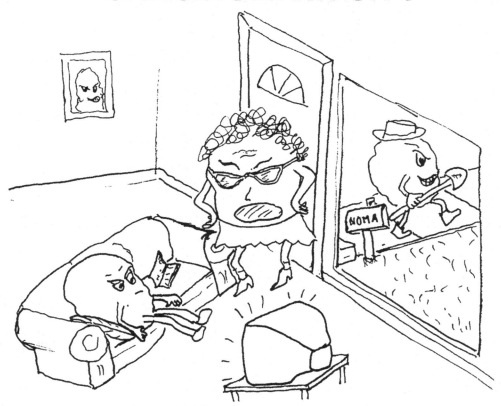

"Carci, why don't you go out invading and metastasizing
with your father instead of sitting around *in situ* all day?"

Figure 11-6

Inflammatory Carcinoma is most commonly caused by infiltrating ductal carcinoma. It represents rapid and diffuse involvement of the breast with **invasion of dermal lymphatics**. Blockage of dermal lymphatics results in **acute redness, swelling and tenderness**, and grossly appears as **peau d'orange** (skin thickening and dimpling that resembles an orange peel. This form involves a high incidence of metastasis and carries a **poor prognosis**.

Medullary Carcinoma presents as a well-circumscribed mass in younger women (premenopausal), representing less than 5% of breast carcinomas. Histologically, large cells form solid sheets with a non-infiltrating border, surrounded by a marked lymphocytic infiltrate *(Slide 11.15)*. This form carries a slightly better prognosis than infiltrating ductal carcinoma.

Mucinous Carcinoma is a rare form of cancer typically presenting in women over 65 years, and it also has a better prognosis than infiltrating ductal carcinoma. The islands of neoplastic cells float within large muci-

nous lakes, which dissect across fibrous tissue planes *(Slides 11.16, 11.17)*.

Tubular Carcinoma usually affects young women aged 40-50 and often is multifocal. The lesion involves well-formed tubules lacking a myoepithelial layer *(Slides 11.18, 11.19)*. This form carries an excellent prognosis.

Papillary Carcinoma, a rare form, frequently presents as a subareolar mass with findings typical of an intraductal papilloma. Histologic examination, however, reveals papillary architecture *(Slides 11.20, 11.21)* with pleomorphic cells, mitoses, and areas of necrosis. Local excision is curative.

Lobular Carcinoma

Lobular Carcinoma in situ (LCIS), a rare form, typically is found in premenopausal women. It usually is an incidental finding on biopsy and rarely is associated with calcifications.

Histopathologically, the lesion in LCIS consists of monomorphic acinar cells *(Slides 11.22, 11.23)* with

COMEDOCARCINOMA

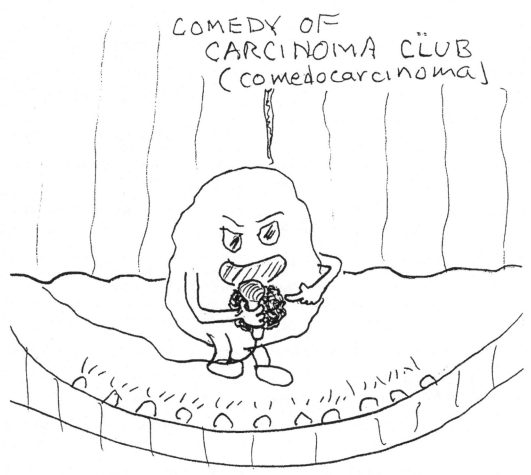

....so she says: "That's not a belly button it's central necrosis" (heh-heh) I got a million of 'em!

Figure 11-7

intracytoplasmic mucin filling the acini. By definition, the clonal proliferation is **confined by a basement membrane.** It usually is multifocal in the affected breast, and it is **often bilateral.**

Invasive Lobular Carcinoma represents about 5-10% of breast malignancies. It usually is multicentric and can be bilateral. Involved portions of the breast typically show strands of invasive cells, often in single file (known as **"Indian filing"**). Strands of cells often encircle normal ducts, referred to as a **"targetoid"** pattern. **(Slides 11.24, 11.25)**

Paget's Disease

Paget's disease of the nipple usually presents as an ulcerating, inflamed lesion of the nipple or areola.

Histologically, malignant cells **("Paget's cells")** are found scattered throughout the epidermis, both singly and in groups. The cells have large nuclei with abundant, mucinous cytoplasm *(Slides 11-26, 11-27)*. Almost all cases herald an **underlying infiltrating ductal carcinoma.**

Sarcoma

Phyllodes tumor (malignant cystosarcoma phyllodes) is a rare tumor found in women over age 60. Phyllodes tumors arise from intralobular stroma. They are low-grade malignancies with a capacity to invade locally, but they **rarely metastasize.** Grossly, they may look similar to a fibroadenoma, but the mass grows much more rapidly.

Histologically, the phyllodes stroma is very cellular with nuclear pleomorphism and increased mitoses. The ductal epithelium appears benign, but the ducts are compressed into slit-like spaces by the stromal overgrowth (Slide 11.28).

Though locally aggressive, surgical excision is curative. Phyllodes tumors tend to metastasize through the bloodstream, so lymph node dissection is unnecessary.

Angiosarcoma. As a primary neoplasm, angiosarcoma is rare. It usually is secondary to chest wall radiation (e.g., for breast cancer, lymphoma, etc.).

Metastatic Tumors

Metastasis to the breast is rare. Some of the more common causes are lymphoma, melanoma, and **leukemia.**

Staging and Clinical Course

Staging of breast cancer primarily is performed **surgically.** Generally, breast cancer presents in one of two ways—as a painless, clinically palpable mass or as mammographic findings that prompt a biopsy. As age increases, the chances of clinical or mammographic findings representing cancer increase. Clinically detected masses average 2-3 cm in size, and 30% of these patients have positive lymph nodes at the time of diagnosis. Mammographically detected cancer averages 1 cm in size, and less than 20% of patients have positive lymph nodes.

Breast cancer typically **spreads via lymphatics,** most commonly to **axillary nodes** or to **internal mammary** and **supraclavicular nodes,** based on the site of the primary lesion. Spread through the bloodstream most commonly produces metastases in the lungs, bones, liver, adrenals, brain, and meninges.

Prognostic Factors and Treatment Options

Multiple prognostic factors for breast cancer have been identified, many of which affect treatment strategies. Treatment varies according to staging, but most treatment modalities involve surgical excision (lumpectomy, modified radical mastectomy, radical mastectomy) with or without chemotherapy and/or local radiation. Axillary node dissection usually is performed for staging purposes, regardless of the size of the primary neoplasm. The most important prognostic factors include:

Lymph node metastases is the **most important prognostic factor.** Without lymph node involvement, 70%-80% of patients live longer than 10 years. This figure falls to 40% when 1-3 lymph nodes are involved, and if more than 10 nodes are involved, only 10% of patients live for 10 years. For this reason, lymph node resection is performed for almost every invasive cancer and directly affects staging.

Locally advanced disease with invasion of the overlying skin or underlying skeletal muscle suggests metastatic disease.

Tumor size directly affects staging; larger primary tumors carry a worse prognosis.

Certain histologic subtypes, as mentioned above, carry a better prognosis, particularly tubular and mucinous subtypes.

Tumor grade typically is denoted as grade 1-3, based on the modified **Scharff-Bloom-Richardson** grading system. The system takes into account differentiation (tubule formation) and mitotic rate, with grade 3 representing a poorly differentiated tumor and numerous mitoses.

Estrogen and progesterone receptors, with tumors containing estrogen and progesterone receptors, demonstrated immunohistochemically, carry a **better prognosis** because they are treatable by **hormonal suppressive therapy**. The majority of these tumors respond to anti-estrogen chemotherapy, and many patients remain on anti-estrogen therapy for many years after surgical resection.

In breast carcinoma, expression of oncogenes, or loss of expression of tumor suppressor genes indicates genetic alteration in these genes. This is associated with a good prognosis. Though many oncogenes and tumor suppressor genes have been identified, **Her2/neu** commonly is tested for in breast cancer workups. Presence of Her2/neu in the tumor cells indicates an overexpression of this epidermal growth factor receptor due to amplification of its oncogene. This is associated with poor prognosis and is also helpful in predicting response to certain chemotherapy.

Lymphovascular invasion found in histologic specimens correlates with positive lymph node metastases and a worse prognosis.

Proliferative rate is usually estimated by mitotic rate and represented by tumor grade. Increasing mitoses support a more invasive neoplasm with a worse prognosis.

THE MALE BREAST
Gynecomastia

Gynecomastia involves **enlargement of the male breast** due to an **imbalance** between **estrogens,** which stimulate growth of breast tissue, and **androgens,** which counteract estrogenic stimulation. It typically presents as unilateral or bilateral painless subareolar swelling. Prepubertal and elderly males may develop mild gynecomastia with no definable etiology or significance. Pathologic conditions which may cause gynecomastia include Klinefelter syndrome, a functioning testicular tumor (estrogen-producing), hyperestrogenic states, and certain drugs.

The **most common cause of gynecomastia,** especially in older men, is **cirrhosis of the liver.** The liver metabolizes estrogen, and destruction of liver parenchyma results in higher levels of circulating estrogens. In **younger males**, however, **obesity** is considered to be the most common etiology of this disease. Drugs causing gynecomastia include alcohol, marijuana, heroin, and anabolic steroids. Histologically, the breast tissue shows micropapillary hyperplasia of ductal epithelium surrounded by hyalinized, myoid intralobular connective tissue *(Slide 11.29)*.

Carcinoma

Breast cancer in males is **very rare** (less than 1% of all tumors), though the risk factors are thought to be the same as in women. The prognosis usually is poor because male patients tend to present at advanced stages, and infiltration occurs rapidly due to the smaller amount of breast tissue. Due to the absence of lobular tissue in males, men only develop **ductal cancer**.

12

Endocrine Pathology

OVERVIEW

The organs of the endocrine system are some of the smaller organs in our body, but do not confuse size with simplicity. The endocrine glands secrete hormones in the bloodstream, and these hormones help to regulate various body functions. This system can be one of the most challenging systems for students due to the many regulatory pathways involved in controlling the secretions of these glands. Remember when studying this system, that an increase in gland size does not necessarily mean a gland will secrete excess hormone.

DEFINITIONS

A **hormone** is a chemical substance produced in one organ or group of cells that controls/induces the activity of a different organ, or group of cells.

Primary dysfunction occurs when a problem **originates** in a particular gland. For example: hyperplasia, hypoplasia, neoplasia, or destruction.

Secondary dysfunction occurs when a **problem outside** the gland of choice causes an effect to another gland or tissue.

THE PITUITARY GLAND
Anatomy and Histology

The pituitary is the main regulatory gland of the endocrine system. It is located at the base of the brain where it is attached to the hypothalamus via the pituitary stalk. Nesting here, it can receive the close neuronal control required for proper functioning. Also, the pituitary gland is granted a large blood flow to help regulate the endocrine feedback mechanisms.

The anterior pituitary, or **adenohypophysis**, makes up a clear majority of the gland, and contains a portal system of blood flow. The anterior pituitary produces and stores its own hormones, but the posterior pituitary serves only to store hormones that are made in the hypothalamus. Also, the posterior pituitary, or **neurohypophysis**, is smaller and releases fewer hormones than the anterior lobe.

Anterior Pituitary

Hormones produced by the anterior pituitary include:

Growth Hormone (GH): promotes growth.

Prolactin: initiates milk production.

Adrenocorticotropic Hormone (ACTH): stimulates steroid synthesis/secretion.

Follicle-Stimulating Hormone (FSH): acts on ovaries to promote progesterone secretion and growth of the Graafian follicle.

Leutinizing Hormone (LH): acts on ovaries to promote progesterone secretion and induce the formation of the corpus luteum.

Thyroid-stimulating Hormone (TSH): stimulates thyroid hormone synthesis and secretion.

The anterior pituitary cells are categorized on histological staining, as **acidophils** and **basophils.** Further subdivision can occur, but are mostly self explanatory (for example, Thyrotrophs secrete TSH, Somatotrophs secrete GH, etc.).

Fig. 12-1. The anterior pituitary hormones. Mnemonic: **GPA is B FLAT:**

G = Growth hormone
P = Prolactin
A = **A**bove produced by **A**cidophil cells
B = **B**elow produced by **B**asophil cells
F = FSH
L = LH
A = ACTH
T = TSH

THE PITUITARY HORMONES

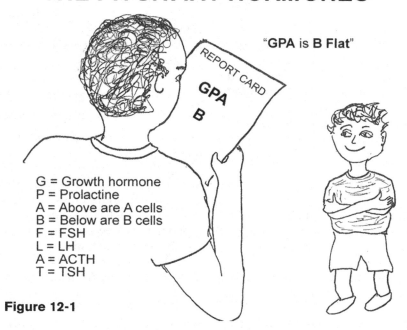

"GPA is B Flat"

G = Growth hormone
P = Prolactine
A = Above are A cells
B = Below are B cells
F = FSH
L = LH
A = ACTH
T = TSH

Figure 12-1

Hyperpituitarism and Adenomas

Hyperplasia and malignant carcinomas are rarely seen. Adenomas are the most common lesions of the pituitary gland. They may be associated with headaches, visual field defects, increased secretion of a certain hormone (**hyperpituitarism**) or, when the tumor has a destructive mass effect, decreased secretion (**hypopituitarism**). The hormonal symptoms correspond to the type of cell involved.

Adenomas are the **most common** cause of hyperpituitarism and are usually monoclonal, secreting a single hormone. They may be hormone negative (non-secretory), but still give rise to symptoms through compression of the optic chiasm, erosion of the sella turcica, or destruction of the pituitary gland.

Fig. 12-2. Growth Hormone Adenomas secrete excess growth hormone, which results in **gigantism** in children and **acromegaly** in adults. In acromegaly, there are large hands and feet, jutting jaw, large tongue, and prognathism). It is associated with diabetes, hypertension, congestive heart failure, gonadal dysfunction, and increased risk for gastrointestinal cancers.

Prolactinomas are the **most common** pituitary adenoma. In men this adenoma can result in hypogonadism and infertility. In women it can also cause **hypogonadism, amenorrhea,** and **galactorrhea.**

Corticotroph Adenomas can secrete excess ACTH, which causes bilateral adrenal hyperplasia, thus causing an increase in cortisol.

Other Anterior Adenomas are rare. They include those that secrete FSH, causing hypogonadism in males (not in females), or adenomas secreting TSH, causing hyperthyroidism.

Hypopituitarism

The main pathology seen in hypopituitarism depends on the hormone that is depleted. Hypopituitarism

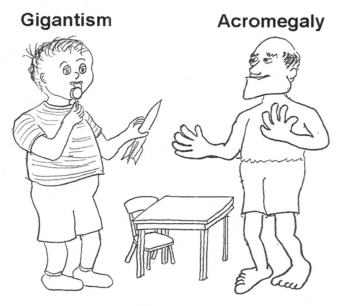

Gigantism   Acromegaly

Figure 12-2

results from decreased secretion or decreased releasing factors.

- A decrease in TSH causes hypothyroidism
- A decrease in ACTH causes adrenal cortical insufficiency, malaise, weight loss and hypoglycemia.
- A decreased in GH, causes dwarfism, decreased growth rate, increased body fat mass, and impaired cardiac function.
- A decreased in FSH/LH causes hypogonadism and poor libido.
- A decreased in prolactin causes absent lactation.

Causes for Hypopituitarism:

- **Non-secreting adenomas** are the **most common** cause of hypopituitarism. They result in visual field defects, and a decrease in all hormones through pituitary destruction.
- **Sheehan's syndrome** (post partum pituitary necrosis). The most prominent decreases are seen in TSH and ACTH.
- **Empty sella syndrome** is uncommon, but may have different causes. Most cases are due to herniated arachnoid, causing pressure atrophy of the pituitary gland.
- **Other tumors. Craniopharyngiomas** are derived from Rathke's cleft, the embryonal precursor of the anterior pituitary

Posterior Pituitary

Anatomy and Histology

The posterior pituitary is composed of modified glial cells, named pituicytes, and axonal processes that extend from the hypothalamus to the posterior lobe. The posterior pituitary secretes 2 hormones: Anti-Diuretic Hormone (ADH), which causes the kidneys to resorb water, and Oxytocin, which causes uterine/lactiferous smooth muscle to contract.

Posterior Pituitary Syndromes

Diabetes insipidus, which is caused by an ADH deficiency, presents as excess urination. It can have several causes, including tumor, inflammation, surgery, or head injury. Serum lab testing for ADH is not readily available, so urine and serum osmolarity are measured when diabetes insipidus is suspected. (Low urine osmolarity, low urine specific gravity, high serum osmolality, and hypernatremia are seen.)

The **Syndrome of Inappropriate ADH (SIADH) secretion** is caused by excess ADH, which results in excess water retention and hyponatremia. SIADH is most often caused by malignant neoplasms that secrete ADH (**paraneoplastic syndrome**, which most often occur in small cell carcinomas of the lung). Symptoms include confusion, weakness, lethargy, convulsions and/or coma.

Tumors that originate in the hypothalamus may cause hyper- or hypofunction of the anterior pituitary, including diabetes insipidus. Most often these tumors are gliomas.

THE THYROID GLAND
Anatomy and Histology

The thyroid gland has two lateral lobes connected by a midline isthmus. The glandular tissue contains colloid-filled follicles lined by cuboidal epithelial cells (*Slide 12.7*). The colloid is composed of thyroglobulin, which is converted to triiodothyronine (T3) and thyroxine (T4) by the follicular epithelial cells. The stroma between the follicles contains blood vessels and parafollicular cells (**C cells**), which secrete **calcitonin**.

A developmental abnormality can occur when the thyroid migrates from its embryological origin to its mature resting spot. These abnormalities, **thyroid cysts**, are always located in the midline between the thyroid isthmus and hyoid bone.

Thyroid Function

The main function of the thyroid is to make TH, which increases the basal metabolic rate via increasing oxidative phosphorylation and protein synthesis. Also, the "C cells" manufacture calcitonin, which aids in the deposition of calcium in the bones.

Diagnosing thyroid gland pathology has a lot to do with its regulation mechanisms. Thyroid Releasing Hormone (TRH) induces the release of Thyroid Stimulating Hormone (TSH), which then causes the thyroid to release Thyroid Hormone (TH). TH comes in two forms, T3 and T4. Most of this is T4, but T3 is 3 times more potent.

Today, the best screen test for hyper/hypothyroidism is a TSH screen. This test is pretty straightforward if you understand the TH feedback mechanisms. In primary hyperthyroidism TSH is undetectable, since the thyroid hormone has negative feedback on TSH production. In primary hypothyroidism TSH is high, since there is no negative feedback.

To determine a secondary (pituitary origin) versus a tertiary (hypothalamic origin) hypothyroidism, a TRH stimulation test is used. When TRH is injected into a patient, TSH will rise in tertiary (hypothalamic) hypothyroidism, since the pituitary gland is responsive. However, TSH will remain the same in secondary (pituitary) hypothyroidism, where the pituitary gland is damaged.

Hyperthyroidism

Fig. 12-3. Hyperthyroidism. Patients with hyperthyroidism present with heat intolerance, insomnia, diarrhea,

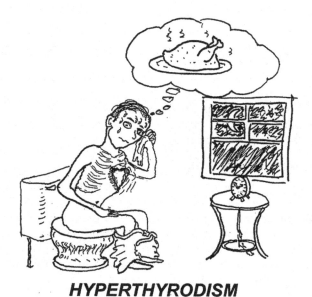

HYPERTHYRODISM

Figure 12-3

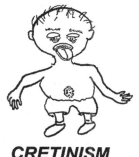

CRETINISM

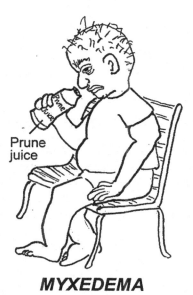

Prune
juice

MYXEDEMA

Figure 12-4

weight loss despite a good appetite, heart palpitations, rapid pulse and nervousness.

Pathologic causes of hyperthyroidism include diffuse toxic hyperplasia, toxic multinodular goiter, toxic adenoma, and rarely a TSH secreting pituitary tumor/carcinoma.

Graves' disease *(Slide 12.1)* is also a clinically important cause of hyperthyroidism, but the pathology differs from that above. This disease is caused by antibodies (via autoimmunity) to the TSH receptors in the thyroid gland. The antibodies are termed thyroid-stimulating immunoglobulins (TSIs). This disease typically occurs in 20 – 40 year-old women. The triad of symptoms is the above-mentioned symptoms of hyperthyroidism, as well as proptosis and dorsal leg edema.

Hypothyroidism

Fig. 12-4. Hypothyroidism. In children, TH deficiency results in **cretinism**: coarse features, large protuberant tongue, short stature, umbilical hernias, and mental retardation. Adults present with **myxedema**: overweight, cold intolerance, dull mentation, coarse facial feature, hair loss, constipation, dry skin, periorbital edema, and sometime psychosis (myxedema madness).

Microscopically, myxedema presents as mucopolysaccharides in the soft tissue.

Chronic Lymphocytic Thyroiditis (Hashimoto's thyroiditis) is characterized by lymphocytic infiltrate *(Slides 12.2 - 12.3)* with germinal centers surrounded by atrophic thyroid follicles. This is an autoimmune

disease and is more common in women. Antimicrosomal antibodies and antithyroglobulin antibodies can be obtained from these patients. This disease is also associated with a small increased risk of lymphoma.

De Quervain's subacute granulomatous thyroiditis is histologically characterized by granulomas and giant cells. Clinically it presents with fever, pain, thyroid enlargement, and transient hypofunction.

Reidel ligneous thyroiditis clinically presents as a dense fibrous thyroid. It can fix the thyroid to the trachea, thus mimicking carcinoma.

Diffuse and multinodular goiters are due to a decreased T4 output, which causes an increase in TSH production, thus causing thyroid enlargement to try to compensate for the low TH levels. Clinically goiters can present as masses that can cause dysphagia or tracheal compression. **Diffuse non-toxic goiters** are colloid distended follicles, caused by iodine- deficiency or goitrogens. **Multinodular goiters** are clinically important if they are toxic (hormone-secreting), because they are diagnostic of **Plummer disease**.

Other causes of hypothyroidism include surgery, radiation and some drugs.

Thyroid Tumors

An important concept to know is that "hot" tumors take up radioactive iodine and use it to make TH, whereas "cold" tumors do not take up radioactive iodine or make TH. This is prognostically important in determining the patient's outcome. Hot nodules are more likely to be benign, while cold nodules are more likely to be malignant.

Hurthle cell adenomas are adenomas with bright eosinophilic cytoplasm.

Thyroid Cancer

Papillary Carcinoma is the most common type of thyroid cancer. It has local lymphatic spread, with a good prognosis.

Histologically, papillary carcinoma is characterized by clear or empty-appearing nuclei with "Orphan Annie eyes," intranuclear inclusions, nuclear grooves, and psammoma bodies (laminated calcifications). It is correlated with the genetic defect of RET/PTC gene fusion.

Follicular Carcinoma has no Orphan Annie nuclei, or psammoma bodies. There is vascular invasion with distant metastases. The prognosis depends on the stage. The most common genetic mutation is in a RAS gene or PAX8-PPARgamma1 fusion.

Medullary Carcinoma derives from the calcitonin secreting cells of the thyroid; thus, calcitonin can be used as a tumor marker. It consists of an amyloid stroma. It has a bad prognosis, and is associated with multifocal tumors, RET mutations, and MEN2 syndrome.

Anaplastic Carcinoma is the least common type of thyroid cancer. It is highly aggressive, with almost a 100% mortality rate. Morphologically, it consists of highly anaplastic cells with many histological patterns.

THE PARATHYROID GLAND
Anatomy and Histology

The parathyroid consists of 4 pea-sized glands that are located on the posterior aspect of the thyroid gland. Each of the 4 glands occupies one of the 4 corners of the posterior thyroid. These glands release parathyroid hormone (PTH). (*Slide 12.6*)

PTH Function

Parathyroid hormone **elevates serum calcium**, through 3 mechanisms. First, through a complex renal mechanism, PTH minimizes phosphate loss; thereby maximizing tubular calcium reabsorption. Second, PTH mobilizes bone calcium. Third, PTH increases Vitamin D production, which increases intestinal calcium absorption.

Key Causes of Hypercalcemia

- Cancer (squamous lung, breast) that spreads to bone
- Hyperthyroidism
- Iatrogenic (antacids, milk, thiazides)
- Multiple Myeloma
- Primary Hyperparathyroidism
- Sarcoidosis
- Vitamin D intoxication

Primary Hyperparathyroidism

Primary hyperparathyroidism occurs when the parathyroids release too much PTH, which leads to hypercalcemia. Clinically it is seen most often in adult women. Most often it is due to an adenoma, manifest as gland hyperplasia, least often as a carcinoma. Lab values for this disease shows high serum calcium, low phosphate and markedly increase serum PTH.

Fig. 12-5. Primary hyperparathyroidism. Patients with primary hyperparathyroidism present with "Moans, groans, bones and stones." Moans are caused by the psychiatric symptoms of depression, anxiety and fatigue. Groans are due to the abdominal pains caused by peptic ulcers and pancreatitis. Bone symptoms include osteoporosis and osteitis fibrosa cystica. Stones include the multiple kidney stones these patients get.

Secondary Hyperparathyroidism

Secondary hyperparathyroidism is due to renal failure, which causes phosphate retention and calcium loss. This then causes parathyroid gland hyperplasia. Lab values show increased serum phosphate, decreased serum calcium, and again increased PTH.

Lab table			
Ca	PTH	Condition	Cause
High	High	Primary hyperpara.	Adenoma, hyperplasia
High	Low	Non-para.	"CHIMPS" No-P
Low	High	Secondary hyperpara.	Chronic renal failure, low vitamin D
Low	High	Secondary hyperpara.	Chronic renal failure, low vitamin D

Hypoparathyroidism

The main cause of hypoparathyroidism is an autoimmune disease, followed by congenital, then surgical (due to accidental removal during thyroid surgery) and lastly idiopathic causes. These patients produce low/no PTH, which causes low serum calcium. Low calcium can cause increased muscle excitability (**tetany**), prolonged QT intervals, and psychic problems.

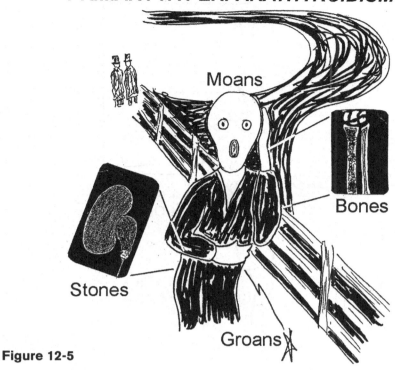

PRIMARY HYPERPARATHYROIDISM

Moans

Bones

Stones

Groans

Figure 12-5

Pseudohypoparathyroidism (Albright hereditary osteodystrophy)

Patients with pseudohypoparathyroidism are PTH resistant. Lab values show high PTH, low calcium, and high phosphate.

Pseudopseudohypoparathyroidism (Albright hereditary osteodystrophy without resistance)

Patients with pseudopseudohypoparathyroidism present with the somatic abnormalities as pseudohypoparathyroidism without the biochemical findings. To distinguish this disease from pseudohypoparathyroidism, lab values are needed, which show normal PTH, normal calcium and normal phosphate levels.

THE ADRENAL GLAND
Anatomy and Histology

The adrenal glands are 2 egg-sized glands that sit atop either kidney. Each gland is composed of 4 layers. Three layers make up the cortex; 1 layer is the medulla. The outermost layer of the cortex is the **Zona Glomerulosa**, which secretes aldosterone (a mineralocorticoid regulated by renin-angiotensin and potassium). The next layer is the **Zona Fasciculata**, which is responsible for secreting cortisol (a glucocorticoid that helps regulate blood sugar). The innermost layer is the

Zona Reticularis, which secretes sex hormones. Mnemonic: **GFR (G=glomerulosa; F=fasciculate; R=reticularis; GFR also = glomerular filtration rate, and the adrenal sits atop the kidney)** (*Slide 12.5*)

The **medulla** is the innermost layer of the adrenal gland. Its main function is to secrete epinephrine upon stimulation.

The Adrenal Axis

The hypothalamus creates and secretes CRH (corticotrophic-releasing hormone), which stimulates the pituitary to secrete ACTH, which then acts on the adrenals, causing them to secrete cortisol. Intravenous (IV) drugs can disrupt the adrenal axis, leading to adrenal hypertrophy or atrophy. For example, IV cortisol causes a rapid decrease in circulating ACTH, which can then lead to adrenal atrophy.

Hyperadrenalism causes an increase in circulating cortisol or aldosterone.

Cushing's Syndrome (Hypercortisolism)

Fig. 12-6. Cushing's Syndrome is characterized by: truncal obesity, buffalo hump, skin striae, moon facies, osteoporosis, hypertension, glucose intolerance, muscle weakness and neuropsychiatric changes.

The **main cause** of Cushing's Syndrome is exogenous glucocorticoids.

CUSHING'S SYNDROME

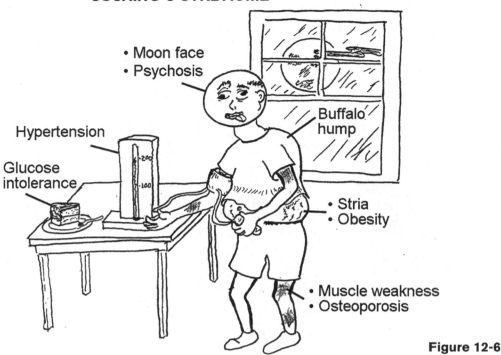

- Moon face
- Psychosis

Buffalo hump

Hypertension

Glucose intolerance

- Stria
- Obesity

- Muscle weakness
- Osteoporosis

Figure 12-6

Endogenous causes include:

1. **Cushing's Disease:** A pituitary ACTH secreting tumor causes an increase in cortisol, along with bilateral adrenal hypertrophy.
2. **Cushing's Syndrome, due to adrenal dysfunction:** An adrenal adenoma/carcinoma secretes cortisol in spite of decreased serum ACTH.
3. **Cushing's Syndrome, not due to adrenal dysfunction:** An ectopic tumor (most often small cell carcinomas of the lung) secretes ACTH. This causes an increase in ACTH and bilateral adrenal hyperplasia.

Diagnosing Cushing's Syndrome

A 24-hour urine cortisol test is an excellent screening test for Cushing's syndrome, but the Dexamathasone (a potent synthetic glucocorticoid) suppression test can help diagnose the specific cause of the disease. The test administers a high dose of dexamethasone in the evening and measures morning cortisol levels. The kinds of results are as follows:

ACTH	Cortisol	Cause
High	Suppressed	Pituitary Cushing's
High	Not suppressed	Ectopic ACTH tumor
Low	Not suppressed	Adrenal Cushing's

Aldosterone Regulation

Aldosterone helps to regulate serum sodium, potassium, and blood pressure. Aldosterone is regulated by the renin-angiotensin system. Basically, an increase in renin causes an increase in angiotensin, which then causes an increase in aldosterone, which increases blood pressure.

Primary Hyperaldosteronism: Conn's Syndrome

In Conn's syndrome, the adrenal glands produce too much aldosterone, **most often from an adrenal adenoma**. Patients present with weakness and hypertension. Lab values show increased sodium, increased water retention, and hypertension with low potassium and renin.

Secondary Aldosteronism

Secondary aldosteronism is due to an increase in serum renin. It is most commonly due to renal ischemia or renin secreting tumors.

Congenital Adrenal Hyperplasia (Adrenogenital Syndrome)

Adrenogenital syndrome is a congenital disease caused by an autosomal recessive defect in the adrenal enzymes. It should be suspected in any newborn that has ambiguous genitalia with refractory dehydration. The enzyme defects cause defective cortisol synthesis, thus causing increased ACTH release and gland hyperplasia. The cortisol precursors spill over to produce excess androgens, thus causing ambiguous genitals in females (female virilization). **It is most commonly** caused by **21-hydroxylase deficiency**. It results in renal salt wasting, characterized by low serum sodium, low blood pressure, and high serum potassium.

Hypoadrenalism

Hypoadrenalism causes a decrease in cortisol and aldosterone. Eighty percent of cases are due to autoimmune disorders (**autoimmune polyendocrine syndrome APS1 and 2**), while 20% are due to tuberculosis. In adults, it is seen in people with disseminated intravascular coagulation (DIC), amyloidosis, and sarcoidosis (AIDS can also affect the adrenals but it is uncommon). In infants, it is seen after meningococcemia with DIC and Waterhouse-Friderichsen syndrome.

Primary Acute Adrenocortical Insufficiency (Adrenal Crisis)

Patients with adrenal crisis present with hypotension, shock, fever, dehydration, weakness, and hypoglycemia. The condition is treated with IV cortisol.

Primary Chronic Adrenocortical Insufficiency (Addison's Disease)

Increased skin pigmentation (ACTH and melanin have the same chemical precursor) distinguishes Addison's disease from an acute disease. As in adrenal crisis, labs show low serum glucose and sodium, low blood pressure, and high potassium with increased ACTH.

Secondary Adrenocortical Insufficiency

Secondary adrenocortical insufficiency is due to pituitary or hypothalamic lesions or prolonged exposure to exogenous glucocorticoids. These patients have low ACTH, but do not have increased skin pigmentation.

Adrenal Cortical Tumors

Most adenomas are silent, but others can produce Cushing's or Conn's syndrome. Virilizing tumors are likely to be carcinomas.

Adrenal Medulla Tumors

Adrenal medulla cells, which are embryologically derived from neural crest cells, and are responsible for secreting epinephrine. Two main pathological conditions involve the medulla:

1. **Pheochromocytomas** *(Slide 12.4)* : These tumors secrete catecholamines (norepinephrine and epinephrine). Thus, they cause paroxysmal hypertension, tachycardia, anxiety, cardiomyopathy and diaphoresis. They follow the **Rule of 10's** — 10% are familial, 10% are extra-adrenal, 10% are malignant and 10% occur in childhood. They may be associated with MEN2, von Hippel-Lindau, von Recklinghausen or Sturge-Weber diseases. Laboratory analysis reveals increased urine catecholamines, vanillylmandelic acid (VMA) and metanephrine.

2. **Neuroblastoma (ganglioneuroblastoma, ganglioneuroma):** These are small round blue cell tumors that typically present in children less then 2 years of age. They present with an abdominal mass, fever and weight loss. These tumors are interesting in that they may spontaneously mature or regress.

Histologically, neuroblastomas are characterized by **Homer-Wright rosettes** (tumors cells wrapped around a central space filled with fibrillary cytoplasm).

Fig. 12-7. Homer-Wright rosettes in neuroblastoma.

THE PINEAL GLAND

This gland, which plays a role in the regulation of the various biorhythms of the body, very rarely presents any significant pathology. However, when tumors do arise, they are typically germinomas. Pineoblastomas (children) and pineocytomas (adults) are rare. When large, pineal tumors may compress adjacent structures, such as the trochlear nerve.

THE ENDOCRINE PANCREAS
Anatomy and Histology

The endocrine pancreas contains islet cells that are nested on the surface of the pancreas. These include alpha, beta and gamma cells, each of which secretes it own unique hormone (alpha cells — glucagon; beta cells — insulin; gamma cells — somatostatin).

Diabetes Mellitus

Insulin aids in the uptake of glucose by the cells of the body. **Hyperglycemia** results from a deficiency or defective insulin production, or lack of response to it. There are two main types of diabetes, insulin dependent diabetes mellitus (IDDM) or non-insulin dependent diabetes mellitus (NIDDM). Characteristics of the two include:

Type 1 IDDM	Type 2 NIDDM
Young onset	Old at onset
Normal weight	Obese
Autoimmune islet destruction	Decreased secretion, peripheral resistance
Polyuria, polydipsia, hyperphagia	Weakness, asymptomatic
Ketosis prone	Ketosis rare

Long term complications of diabetes include:

• Nephropathy: glomerular sclerosis
• Retinopathy: non-proliferative and proliferative

HOMER-WRIGHT ROSETTES

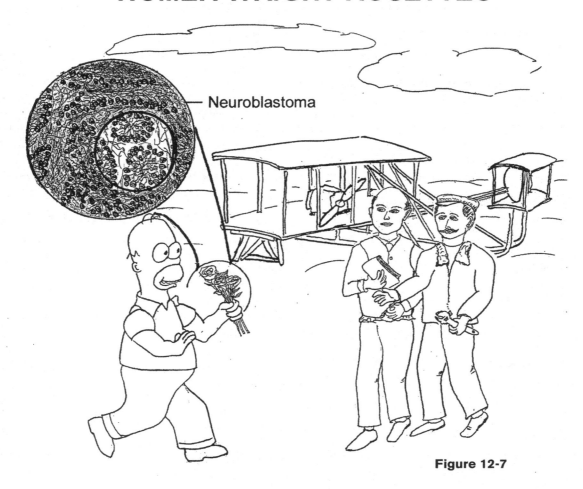

Neuroblastoma

Figure 12-7

- Neuropathy: motor and sensory
- Microangiopathy and accelerated atherosclerosis

The mechanism of these long term manifestations is believed to be due to non-enzymatic glycosylation end products of hyperglycemia and to glucose being converted to sorbital (which causes osmotic cell injury).

Diagnosing Diabetes

Three main tests are used to diagnose diabetes:

- fasting plasma glucose test
- a casual plasma glucose test and
- an oral glucose tolerance test.

Islet Cell Tumors

Islet cell tumors come in 2 forms:

1. **Insulinomas** (mostly benign): Patients present severely hypoglycemic with CNS signs (confusion, stupor). The hypoglycemic attacks are relieved by glucose.
2. **Gastrinomas** (mostly malignant): Patients secrete excess gastrin, which creates an intractable peptic ulcer disease.

MULTIPLE ENDOCRINE NEOPLASMS (MEN)

MEN is the last topic to be considered in this chapter, because it deals with tumors that affect multiple endocrine glands.

MEN1 (Wermer's syndrome) is associated with "P" lesions. These neoplasm's affect the Parathyroid, Pituitary, and Pancreas (causing Peptic ulcers).

MEN2a (Sipple's syndrome) is associated with medullary carcinoma of the thyroid, pheochromocytomas and parathyroid hyperplasia. It is familial and is due to a mutation in the RET proto-oncogene.

MEN2b is the same as MEN2a above, but without the parathyroid hyperplasia.

13

Dermatopathology

OVERVIEW

Inflammatory dermatoses are quite common and can cause significant morbidity. Neoplastic skin conditions are particularly important because they are easily identifiable via a thorough physical examination, and do not require invasive procedures in order to discover the lesion. Although morbidity is a problem with non-melanoma skin cancers, high death rate is the most feared problem with melanoma skin cancers. Fortunately, both non-melanoma and melanoma skin cancers have the potential for complete cure if diagnosed early.

ANATOMY AND HISTOLOGY

Fig. 13-1. Layers of the skin. The skin is composed of multiple layers of epithelium and connective tissue. The most superficial layer, the **epidermis,** consists of stratified squamous epithelium, which is well-suited to resist external trauma, yet allows elasticity and adaptability (ability to regenerate itself).

The most superficial layer of the epidermis is a non-vital **stratum corneum,** which is composed of anucleated **keratinocytes** that form a tough protective coating. It is relatively impermeable to water and provides some prevention against the absorption of toxic materials into the bloodstream.

Beneath this is the **stratum granulosum** (granular cell layer), so-called due to the presence of abundant keratohyalin granules within the cytoplasm of keratinocytes.

Underneath this layer is the bulk of the epidermis, known as the **stratum spinosum** (spinous layer or prickle cell layer), in which keratinocytes are connected to one another via desmosomal intercellular attachments, which on routine hematoxylin and eosin (H&E) stains, appear as intercellular "spikes" separating each cell from one another.

The deepest layer of the epidermis is the germinative (reproductive) layer, called the **stratum basalis** or **germinativum** (basal or germ cell layer). This layer contains the least differentiated keratinocytes, which undertake a dynamic journey through each of the more superficial layers of the epidermis, changing into the cells of those layers, until they are ultimately sloughed off of the stratum corneum.

Also present in the stratum basalis are non-epithelial cells, particularly **melanocytes,** which produce melanin for protection from the damaging effects of ultraviolet light upon the skin. Additionally, **Langerhans cells** reside in the epidermis and react to exposure to external antigens, by alerting the immune system to recognition of foreign material.

Beneath the epidermis is the **dermis** *(Slide 13.1),* which is composed of 2 layers: the **papillary** dermis and the **reticular** dermis. The papillary dermis lies in the zone of connective tissue between the rete ridges, which are deep projections of the epidermis. It contains loosely woven collagen, fibroblasts, blood vessels, and abundant mucopolysaccharides.

The reticular dermis is the bulk of the dermis. It lies beneath the papillary dermis and above the subcutaneous fat. Here, the collagen is thicker and more tightly packed, elastic fibers are abundant, and mucopolysaccharides are less plentiful. More blood vessels and peripheral nerves are present, as well as the bulk of the adnexal structures, including hair follicles, sebaceous glands, and eccrine and apocrine ducts. Like the epidermis, this layer of skin resists damage, yet provides flexibility and elasticity.

The subcutaneous fat is simply composed of mature lobules of fat and a generous vascular framework. A small portion of this fat also surrounds the regenerative portions of the glandular adnexae, including the eccrine coil and apocrine coil. This layer of fat allows some cushioning against trauma, particularly the blunt form, and it also serves as a source of energy storage and insulation.

NORMAL SKIN

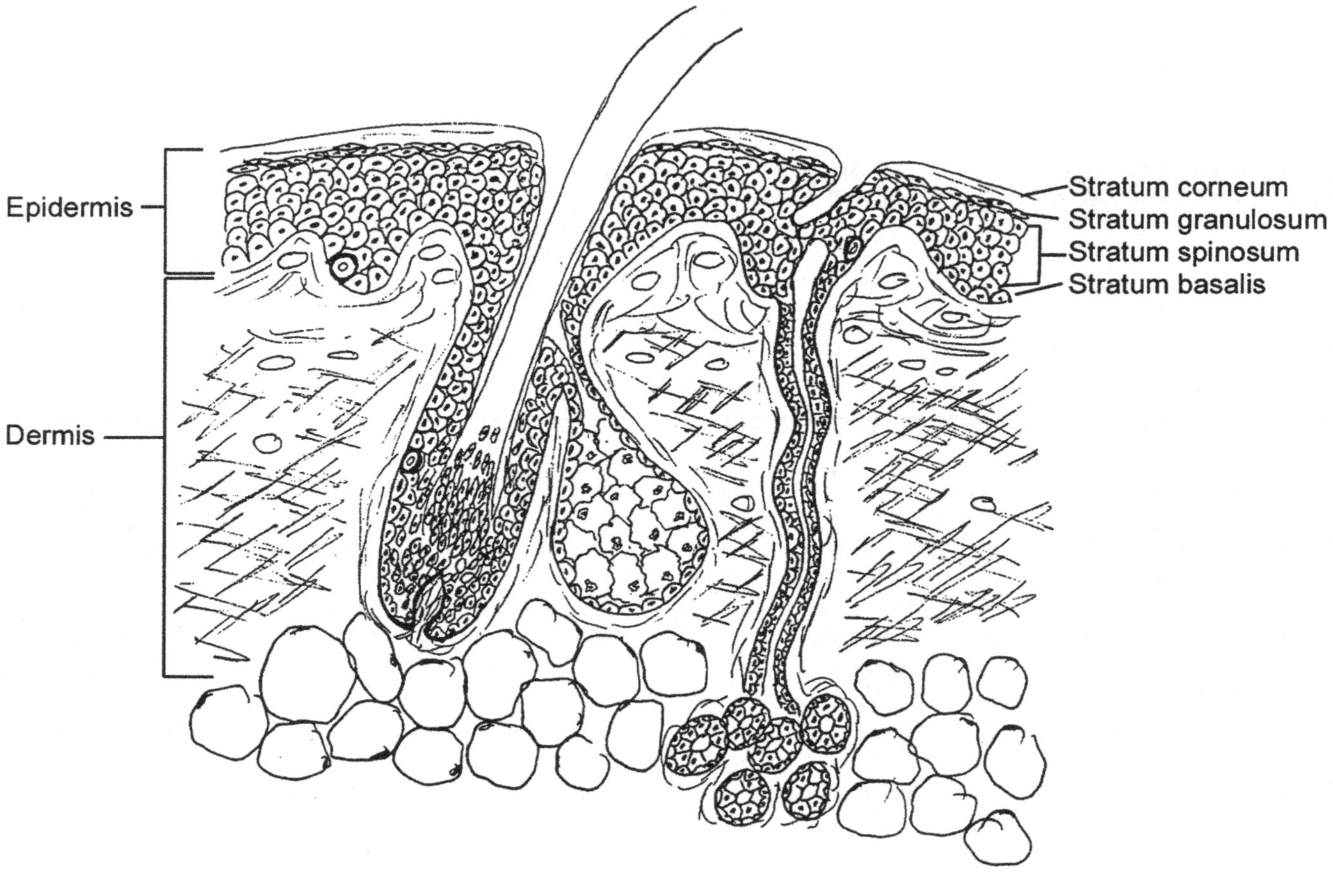

Epidermis —

Dermis —

— Stratum corneum
— Stratum granulosum
— Stratum spinosum
— Stratum basalis

Figure 13-1

DESCRIPTIVE TERMINOLOGY

Because of the vast variety of skin disease manifestations, dermatopathology relies heavily on precise descriptive terms. Below are definitions of several gross and histological findings, which will significantly aid the discussions of specific disease processes throughout the rest of this chapter.

Macroscopic Terms

Fig. 13-2. Macroscopic terms.

Macule: a well-circumscribed, flat area with difference in color from the surrounding skin

Papule: an elevated solid area less than 5 mm in diameter

Nodule: an elevated solid area more than 5mm in diameter

Plaque: an elevated, flat-topped area greater than 5mm in diameter; may represent coalescence of multiple papules

Vesicle: an elevated fluid-filled area less than 5mm in diameter

Bulla: an elevated fluid-filled area more than 5mm in diameter

Pustule: an elevated pus-filled area

Wheal: transient elevated area with blanching and erythema, and little if any surface epidermal change

Scale: dry, plate-like excrescence on skin surface, resulting in abnormality of stratum corneum

Lichenification: thickened, roughened skin with prominent skin markings

Excoriation: trauma-induced linear raw area of skin, resulting from loss of epidermis due to scratching

Microscopic Terms

Fig. 13-3. Microscopic terms.

Hyperkeratosis: thickening of anucleated stratum corneum

Parakeratosis: thickened stratum corneum, with abnormal retention of nuclei

Acanthosis: epidermal hyperplasia

Dyskeratosis: abnormal keratinization of individual keratinocytes beneath the granular cell layer

MACROSCOPIC TERMS

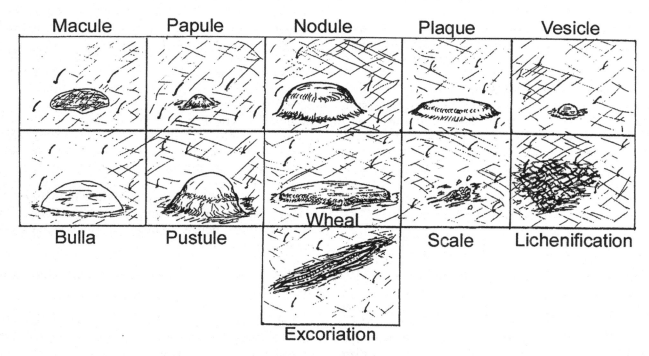

Figure 13-2

MICROSCOPIC TERMS

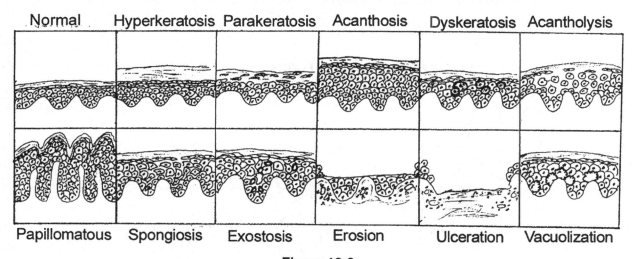

Figure 13-3

Acantholysis: loss of cohesion between keratinocytes in granular or spinous layer

Papillomatosis: hyperplasia of epidermis and papillary dermis, resulting in undulating and "warty" surface

Spongiosis: intercellular edema between keratino-cytes

Exocytosis: infiltration of epidermis by inflammatory cells (usually lymphocytes)

Erosion: superficial loss of epidermis

Ulceration: complete loss of epidermis, with or without loss of underlying dermis

Vacuolization: vacuoles within or adjacent to keratinocytes along the basal layer

INFLAMMATORY DERMATOSES

Generally speaking, inflammatory conditions of the skin can be divided into those resulting in acute dermatoses (lasting days to weeks) and those resulting in chronic dermatoses (lasting months to years).

Acute Dermatoses

Dermatoses in this category are short-lived, lasting only days to weeks. Most of these are the result to a hypersensitivity reaction to some transiently present hapten. After cessation of exposure, the dermatoses resolve without sequelae. The most common conditions presenting as acute dermatoses are **urticaria** (hives), **eczematous dermatitis** (most commonly, contact or irritant), and **erythema multiforme**.

Urticaria (Hives)

Fig. 13-4. Hives. Urticaria (hives) is typified by the numerous wheals, which are erythematous and edematous dermal nodules that are extremely pruritic (itchy). Individual wheals last less than 24 hours, although new lesions can form in the interim. The pathogenesis is a Type I hypersensitivity reaction of IgE to an antigen in the bloodstream, via external or internal sensitization (e.g. a bug bite vs. oral medication). IgE recognizes the antigen, resulting in the release of mast cell granules, particularly histamine. Histamine release results in an increase in local vascular permeability, swelling, and pruritis.

Histologic features of urticaria are usually subtle: mild papillary dermal edema, telangiectasia (tortuous, dilated blood vessels visible through the skin), with or without a prominent lymphocytic or neutrophilic inflammatory infiltrate. Eosinophils may be present, but often are not. If the causative antigen is identified and removed, urticaria will resolve.

Eczematous Dermatitis

Eczema is a type of spongiotic dermatitis, in which the patient develops papulovesicular, erythematous lesions with some oozing and crusting that, over time, may develop into plaques with secondary lichenification from scratching. Therefore, depending on the duration of antigen exposure and development of secondary changes of epidermal reactive thickening and lichenification, there are 3 main types of eczema: **acute, subacute**, and **chronic**.

Fig. 13-5. Acute, subacute, and chronic eczematous dermatitis.

Acute eczema is typified by juicy, moist papules that are extremely itchy. **Poison ivy** (Rhus dermatitis) is the classic example of an acute eczematous dermatitis, mediated by direct contact with the antigen.

Many types of eczema fit into the **subacute** category, in which some secondary scale and plaque formation develops; typically, the causative stimulus cannot be identified. Examples of this include **atopic dermatitis**,

URTICARIA (HIVES)

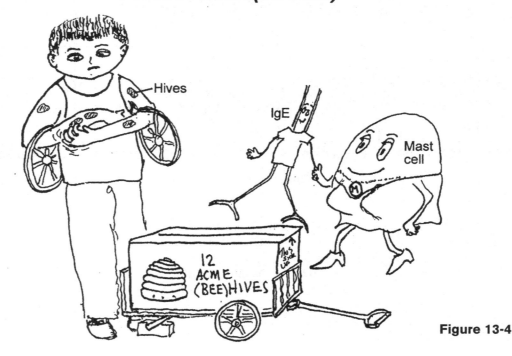

Figure 13-4

3 TYPES OF ECZEMATOUS DERMATITIS

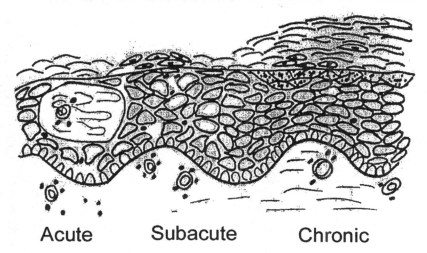

Figure 13-5   Acute   Subacute   Chronic

seborrheic dermatitis, contact (irritant) dermatitis, and **nummular eczema**. Many of those go on to metamorphose into a **chronic** eczematous dermatitis, in which lichenification is the predominant appearance clinically. Nummular eczema, seborrheic dermatitis, and atopic dermatitis are more common examples of this.

Histologically *(Slides 13.2, 13.3)*, acute eczematous lesions have large intraepidermal spongiotic vesicles, subacute lesions show parakeratosis and mild spongiosis, while **chronic** lesions show marked hyperparakeratosis and acanthosis, with little spongiosis.

Erythema Multiforme

Erythema multiforme (EM) is an uncommon reaction to certain viral agents or medications. Clinically, it may range from mild to life threatening. The "target" lesion is classic, manifested as a maculopapule with a central bulla/necrotic zone, surrounded by a slightly pale, then outermost erythematous halo. Lesions may be widespread, but are most frequent on the extremities. If involvement is extensive with mucous membrane involvement and systemic manifestations of fever, the condition is referred to as **Stevens-Johnson syndrome**. Further involvement of the epidermis may result in total body skin sloughage, known as **toxic epidermal necrolysis**. These latter conditions are complicated by extensive fluid loss and sepsis secondary to superinfection of skin, much as can occur in a burn patient.

Fig. 13-6. Erythema multiforme. It may be due to medications or certain viruses. It is called Stevens-Johnson syndrome with fever and widespread involvement of skin and mucous membranes.

Histologically, *(Slide 13.4)* EM is a lichenoid or bullous inflammatory process, which results in a central subepidermal separation of the epidermis from the dermis, with secondary necrosis and ulceration. The dermis is quite edematous and contains an infiltrate of lymphocytes, which are homing in on the epidermis to cause necrosis and blister formation. Causative agents include herpes simplex virus, *Mycoplasma pneumoniae*, and certain medications, such as **sulfonamides**, penicillin, antiepileptics, and antimalarials.

Chronic Dermatoses

Chronic dermatoses are those that typically have no known etiologic agents and do not usually spontaneously regress. The archetypical diseases are **lichen planus**, **cutaneous lupus erythematosus**, and **psoriasis vulgaris**, although there are many other less typical and common types of chronic dermatoses.

Lichen Planus

Pruritic, polygonal, purple papules are the hallmark of lichen planus. The lesions involve oral and genital mucosa, as well as skin. Although the disease is usually self-limited, it nevertheless can take years to resolve. Patients develop the condition at any age. Oral lesions may be quite debilitating, with inability to eat or drink due to the painful ulcerations. Trauma may induce lesions to form on previously normal skin (**Koebner phenomenon**). Healed lesions are typically hyperpigmented.

The histologic pattern in lichen planus is that of "lichenoid dermatitis." *(Slides 13.5, 13.6)* There is destruction of the basal cell layer by lymphocytes along with the formation of necrotic keratinocytes (**eosinophilic necrosis, cytoid bodies, colloid bodies, Civatte bodies**) and a band-like lymphocytic infiltrate in the superficial dermis. This destruction of the basal cell layer also results in the dispersal of melanin directly

ERYTHEMA MULTIFORME

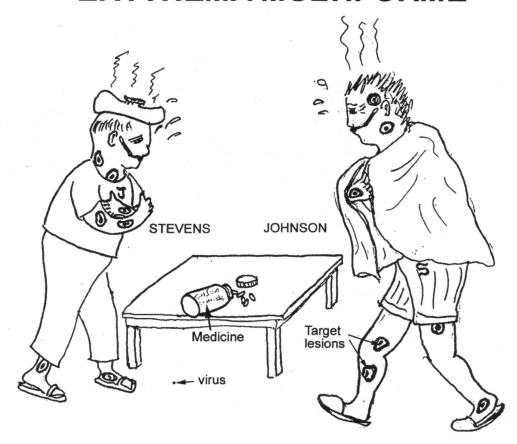

STEVENS   JOHNSON

Medicine

Target
lesions

← virus

Figure 13-6

into the dermis, giving rise to the clinical hyperpigmentation, which may be permanent.

Fig. 13-7. Lichenoid dermatitis. Bands of lymphocytes destroy the basal cell layer.

Although the pathogenesis is not known, most theories postulate that some antigen in the basal layer or dermal-epidermal junction elicits an abnormal cell-mediated immune response, resulting in the rash.

Cutaneous Lupus Erythematosus

One of the most obvious manifestations of cutaneous lupus is its classic skin rash. In acute systemic lupus (SLE), the "malar rash" is an erythematous maculopapular rash on the face. In subacute cutaneous lupus (SCLE), the skin rash may be annular or maculopapular and diffuse. In discoid lupus (DLE), the rash presents as scaly, sharply demarcated erythematous plaques, most prevalent on the face. Lesions are photosensitive, meaning that they are prone to develop on sun-exposed areas.

The histologic picture *(Slide 13.7)* depends on the subtype of lupus. Discoid lupus shows marked hyperkeratosis with keratinous plugging of hair follicles. The dermis contains a lichenoid infiltrate of lymphocytes in the upper dermis, associated with destruction of basal layer cells. Different than lichen planus, the infiltrate also extends along the vessels and skin appendages. Extension to the subcutaneous fat may evolve into a lupus panniculitis. Subacute and acute cutaneous lupus manifest with a less dense inflammatory infiltrate and subtle basal layer damage. Follicular plugging is also absent.

Direct immunofluorescence testing of a skin biopsy from lupus patient with DLE will show a granular band of IgG and C3 along the dermal-epidermal junction. Non-lesion skin is negative. In SCLE and SLE, lesional and non-lesional skin are positive for IgG and C3.

Psoriasis Vulgaris

Psoriasis may develop at any time from childhood through adulthood, with a predilection for those with a Nordic ancestry. Elbow, knee, scalp, lumbosacral, and

LICHENOID DERMATITIS

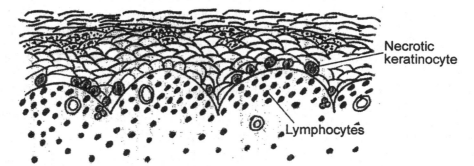

Necrotic keratinocyte

Lymphocytes

Figure 13-7

gluteal involvement are common. Nail abnormalities are also frequent.

The lesions in psoriasis are quite distinct: well-demarcated, pink to purplish plaques with silvery, loosely adherent scales. Clinically, gently scratching off the scale results in pinpoint bleeding, known as the **Auspitz sign**. The **Koebner phenomenon** is also common. Total body involvement (**erythroderma**) can develop, while systemic involvement can include **arthritis**, myopathy, or enteropathy. Psoriatic arthritis, in particular, can be quite debilitating.

Fig. 13-8. Histological appearance of psoriasis (Slides 13.8, 13.9). The picture is distinctive, demonstrating regular epidermal hyperplasia (psoriasiform), with elongation of the rete ridges and dermal papillae; parakeratosis; diminished granular cell layer; intracorneal (**Munro's**) microabscesses (not shown in figure), and intraepidermal neutrophils.

Patients with certain HLA types are genetically predisposed to develop the disease. New research seems to indicate that lymphocytes play a role in the activation of disordered growth of the epidermis.

Vesiculobullous Disorders

Vesiculobullous disorders form a group of dermatoses in which blistering is the primary manifestation of injury. All of these disorders are the result of immunologic damage to some component of the epidermis, resulting in separation and blister formation. There are many different types, and, although fairly uncommon, they are important to recognize due to their associated morbidity and connection with other systemic conditions.

Blistering disorders are categorized according to the level of separation within the epidermis: **subcorneal** (such as impetigo, considered under bacterial infection), **suprabasal**, or **subepidermal**.

Pemphigus Vulgaris

Pemphigus presents in patients in their 50-70s, affecting both sexes equally. They develop flaccid bullae with an erythematous or non-erythematous base on

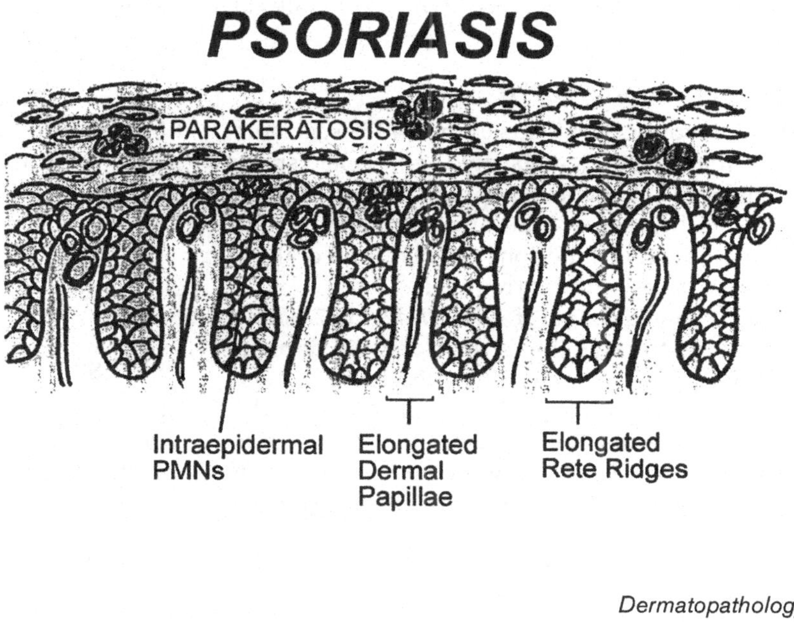

PSORIASIS

PARAKERATOSIS

Intraepidermal PMNs

Elongated Dermal Papillae

Elongated Rete Ridges

Figure 13-8

pressure points and areas of trauma (face, scalp, etc.). Oral involvement may be the presenting symptom.

The bulla is caused by suprabasal acantholysis of the keratinocytes *(Slide 13.10)*, which become discohesive and result in blister formation. The spinous keratinocytes lose their desmosomal attachments due to IgG antibodies directed at desmoglein 3, which is a principle component of desmosomes. The **basal layer remains intact**, because it is attached to the basement membrane via hemidesmosomes, which do not contain this protein. Because the blister forms within the epidermis, it is fragile and prone to rupture, making intact lesions difficult to identify. Erosions are commonly seen and are the cause of secondary infection, which is one of the reasons this disease has a high mortality rate if left untreated. Direct immunofluorescence of a skin biopsy shows positive staining with IgG between keratinocytes in the **spinous layer**.

Bullous Pemphigoid

Pemphigoid presents in an older age group than pemphigus. Blister formation is primarily at points of friction (axilla, groin, forearms, lower abdomen, and medial thighs). These lesions are quite itchy, and are tense bullae with or without an erythematous base. Oral involvement may occur. Since the blister is firmer than in pemphigus, rupture is not as common, resulting in fewer secondary infections.

The bulla is firm because the level of separation is deeper. Histologic sections show a **subepidermal** separation *(Slide 13.11)*, with or without eosinophils and lymphocytes in the blister cavity. The split occurs between the epidermis and dermis due to antibodies against two antigens, named bullous pemphigoid 1 and 2, which are now known to be normal constituents of hemidesmosomes. Immunofluorescence studies show deposition of IgG and C3 in a linear pattern along the dermal-epidermal junction.

Remember that pemphigu**S** separates at a more **S**uperficial layer than pemphigoi**D**, which separates at a **D**eeper layer.

Dermatitis Herpetiformis (DH)

DH is found in younger patients in their 40-50s, is more common in males, and is associated with celiac sprue (gluten sensitivity). Patients complain of itchy, urticarial plaques and vesicles that often occur in crops (hence, "herpetiformis"). Lesions are distributed along the extensor surfaces of the extremities.

Histologic characteristics of DH *(Slide 13.12)* show collections of neutrophils lining up along the dermal-epidermal junction, forming microabscesses, which eventually lead to separation of the epidermis from the dermis (**subepidermal bulla**). Immunofluorescence shows granular deposits of IgA at the tips of the dermal papillae, which appear to be targeting gliadin, present in anchoring fibrils responsible for holding the basement membrane to the dermis. Patients with the dermatitis may respond to the gluten-free diet, similar to patients with the enteropathy.

Inflammatory Disorders of the Skin Appendages

Acne Vulgaris

Common in both sexes at the time of puberty, and often lasting into early adulthood, acne vulgaris is felt to be a primary disorder of inflammation of the hair follicle. This inflammation may be triggered by hormones (testosterone, corticosteroids), occlusive conditions, and certain irritants.

Histology reveals keratin accumulation in hair follicles, with cystic expansion, rupture, and resulting granulomatous inflammation and abscess formation. *Propionibacterium acnes* has been a suspected culprit, thought to break down lipids in sebum, resulting in fatty acids that are irritative and cause an inflammatory reaction. Many different pharmacotherapeutics target the removal of the bacteria or their lipase-inducing activity, in order to lessen inflammation.

Panniculitis

Panniculitis is inflammation of the subcutaneous fat. As mentioned earlier, discoid lupus may have a concomitant panniculitis, called **lupus profundus,** or **lupus panniculitis**. Here, we will consider the other common panniculitis, **erythema nodosum**.

Erythema Nodosum

Patients with erythema nodosum typically have an acute onset of painful deep nodules in the skin along the anterior lower extremities. Lesions occur after **acute infections** (beta-hemolytic streptococcus, tuberculosis, histoplasmosis, leprosy), medications (**sulfonamides**), sarcoidosis or **inflammatory bowel disease**. Diagnosis requires a deep wedge biopsy to include subcutaneous fat.

Histologically, the sections will show widening of the septa between the fat lobules. In early lesions, the septa contain neutrophils and edema. Later, they are fibrotic and contain a granulomatous infiltrate. Importantly, there is no vasculitis, a feature that helps distinguish it from other panniculitides.

SKIN INFECTIONS

Bacterial Infections

Impetigo

Impetigo is a common, highly transmissible superficial skin infection, usually found in small children. The main causative agents are coagulase-positive Staphylococcus or beta-hemolytic Streptococcus. It usually infects the face or hands and begins as an erythematous macule, evolving into a vesicle and then a pustule. When the pustule breaks, a **honey-colored crust** is formed. Impetigo is spread by direct contact. Microscopically, a subcorneal pustule is present. It must be treated with topical and oral antibiotics.

Fungal Infections

Dermatophytoses

Fungal organisms that infect the superficial epidermis are known as **dermatophytes**. They are found within the stratum corneum, and form annular itchy plaques with an erythematous, scaly edge. These infections occur in children and adults. All dermatophyte infections are called "**Tinea**." Further classification is based on body site involved (for example, Tinea capitis= head; corporis= body; cruris=groin). A fungal nail infection is referred to as **onychomycosis**.

Typical organisms include *Trichophyton* and *Malassezia*. Diagnosis can be made by scraping the leading edge of the lesion and making a KOH slide preparation in the office, which will allow identification of the fungal hyphae in the skin scales. If a biopsy is performed, the fungal organisms are identified in the stratum corneum.

Viral Infections

Verrucae (Warts)

Warts are caused by different types of human papilloma virus (HPV). The names depend on the body site involved and the clinical appearance. **Verruca vulgaris** is the common wart, usually present on the hands, periungual (fingernails and toes) areas, and are papillomatous growths. Flat warts (**verruca plana**) occur on the face and are flat papules. **Verruca palmaris** and **verruca plantaris** occur on the palms and soles, respectively. These often grow into the underlying skin (endophytic) with an overlying plug of hyperkeratosis. **Condyloma acuminatum** occur on the genitalia and appear polypoid and cauliflower-like. In all types, cytopathic viral changes are found, usually in the form of perinuclear clearing of the keratinocytes (**koilocytosis**) or clumping of the keratohyalin granules in the granular cell layer. Infection is spread by autoinoculation or direct contact.

Molluscum Contagiosum

Molluscum is a poxvirus, commonly spread by direct contact. Children develop lesions on the face and body, while adults often develop lesions on the genitalia (via sexual contact). The lesions appear as flesh-colored papules with a central umbilication, which may extrude a "cheesy" material, containing the "molluscum bodies" (infected keratinocytes).

Histologically *(Slide 13.13)*, the lesions in molluscum contagiosum show a cup-shaped invagination of the epidermis, containing a central area of keratinocytes with large, eosinophilic intracytoplasmic viral inclusions.

Herpes Simplex

Herpes simplex types 1 and 2 infect the skin. Oral lesions usually are type 1, and genital infections are usually type 2 (**genital lesions "take 2 to tango!"**). However, depending on the method of inoculation, which only takes direct contact, either type could be a cause at any body site! The lesions are vesicles which rupture and cause painful ulcers.

Histologically, the lesions in herpes simplex show extensive acantholysis of the keratinocytes due to direct toxic effect of the virus. Keratinocytes contain intranuclear viral inclusions *(Slide 13.14)*, which, when adjacent infected cells form syncytium, become multinucleated keratinocytes. The nuclei appear homogeneous (like "ground-glass"), with the chromatin pushed to the periphery of the nucleus.

SKIN INFESTATIONS
Arthropods

Bites by arthropods may cause damage by 1) direct irritation, 2) hypersensitivity response to saliva or insect parts, 3) response to toxins in venom, 4) serving as mediators to transmission of bacteria.

Arthropod bites usually appear as urticarial lesions with a wedge-shaped inflammatory infiltrate containing eosinophils. Body or head lice simply show mites embedded in the stratum corneum, causing secondary inflammation in the underlying dermis.

NEOPLASIA

Skin growths may develop in the epidermis or dermis. Epidermal neoplasms are formed by proliferation of keratinocytes or melanocytes. Dermal neoplasms are formed by proliferation of fibroblasts, blood vessels, nerves, or inflammatory cells. As elsewhere, both benign and malignant tumors exist.

Epidermal Neoplasms – Keratinocytic

Benign Epidermal Tumors

Seborrheic keratosis develops on the face, trunk or extremities in middle-aged to elderly patients. It appears as flat/elevated, pigmented, papillomatous, well-circumscribed papules. Keratin plugs may be seen clinically. Many have a "stuck-on" appearance.

Histologically, seborrheic keratosis forms exophytic and papillomatous growths of basaloid keratinocytes. Pseudocystic spaces containing keratin are present and characteristic *(Slide 13.15)*. These actually represent downgrowths of the surface epithelium into the tumor, and correspond to the keratin plugs noted clinically. Some patients may develop hundreds over a short period of time, associated with an underlying malignancy (sign of **Leser-Trelat**).

Fibroepithelial polyps (acrochordon, skin tag) are seen in middle-aged to older patients at sites of irritation (neck, intertriginous areas). They appear as soft, polypoid, flesh-colored protrusions of skin and dermis. Histologically, they show squamous epithelium over a fibrovascular core.

Epithelial cysts (sebaceous cysts, pilar cysts) can form at any age. They are ingrowths/invaginations of squamous epithelium into the dermis. When arising from the surface epithelium or upper hair follicle, they contain a granular cell layer and loosely-woven keratin (**epidermal inclusion cyst**). When arising on the scalp, they often arise from the lower portions (isthmus) of the hair follicle, do not have a granular cell layer, and they contain compact keratin (**pilar cysts**). They commonly rupture, inciting a brisk foreign-body type granulomatous inflammatory response.

Adnexal Tumors

There are literally hundreds of adnexal tumors. They can arise from any or multiple parts of the skin appendages (hair shaft, sebaceous glands, etc.). They are not very distinctive clinically, other than **cylindromas**, which commonly occur on the scalp; **eccrine poromas**, which commonly arise on the sole of the foot; **syringomas**, which arise periorbitally; and **trichoepitheliomas**, which arise around the nose and mouth. Benign and malignant variants have been described.

Tumors of Intermediate Malignant Potential

Actinic keratosis (AK) usually develop in older individuals with a long history of sun exposure. They result from dysplastic changes in the keratinocytes from ultraviolet radiation over time. They appear as scaly papules to plaques, with a "sandpaper"-like texture.

Histologically, *(Slide 13.16)* there is crowding and atypia of the basal layer in AK, with disorganization of the epidermis. Surface parakeratosis is present. The dysplastic changes often spare the ostia of hair follicles and acrosyringeal ducts. Over a long time, they may evolve into invasive squamous cell carcinoma.

Keratoacanthoma is often found in older individuals, who develop a cup-shaped invagination of squamous epithelium with a central crater of keratin that arises over a period of weeks—much faster than most malignancies. Patients typically have a background of sun-damage and, other than the rapid growth, have other risk factors (e.g., genetics, fair skin) for non-melanoma skin cancer. They were originally thought to

be benign, because many regress without treatment. Many now believe they represent well-differentiated squamous cell carcinomas with the tendency for spontaneous regression.

Histologically *(Slide 13.17)*, keratoacanthoma demonstrates a cup-shaped invagination of squamous epithelium with abundant "glassy" cytoplasm, surrounding a central crater of parakeratotic and hyperkeratotic material. They may extend deep into the dermis. Current recommendations are to excise these completely.

Squamous cell carcinoma in situ (SCIS) resembles actinic keratosis, but is often larger, with areas of erosion or an overlying "cutaneous horn" of compact keratin. Sun-exposed areas are most commonly involved. Risk factors include ultraviolet radiation, burn scars, and a history of arsenic ingestion. Human papilloma virus may also play a role, as in other body sites.

Histologically *(Slide 13.18)*, SCIS demonstrates full-thickness dysplasia of keratinocytes, without extension into dermis. This may progress to invasive squamous cell carcinoma with time.

Malignant Tumors

Basal cell carcinoma is one of the most common non-melanoma skin cancers. It arises in middle-aged to elderly patients with a fair complexion and a history of chronic ultraviolet radiation. This results in defective DNA repair and uncontrolled proliferation of the basal cell component of the epidermis. These tumors show growths that resemble the basal layer of the normal epidermis.

Histologically *(Slides 13.19, 13.20)*, basaloid cells arrange themselves as well-circumscribed nodules (**nodular basal cell carcinoma**), or multifocal superficial growths (**superficial basal cell carcinoma**). All show a characteristic cleft-like space between the tumor cells and the surrounding stroma. A rare variant, known as the **morpheaform basal cell carcinoma**, is much more aggressive clinically, and shows infiltrative strands of tumor extending into a sclerotic dermis.

All types of basal cell carcinoma are cured by simple excision, with virtually no risk of metastasis.

Squamous cell carcinoma is the other common type of non-melanoma skin cancer. The risk factors are essentially the same as for actinic keratosis and squamous cell carcinoma in situ. Ultraviolet damage to DNA repair is the underlying defect, resulting in proliferation of dysplastic clones of keratinocytes.

Histologically, squamous cell carcinoma shows extension of atypical keratinocytes into the dermis. Lymphovascular invasion may occur, but is usually rare, so the risk of metastasis is usually small. Exceptions are those tumors arising at highly-vascularized sites, such as the oral cavity.

Epidermal Neoplasms – Melanocytic

Benign Epidermal Melanocytic Tumors

Lentigo consists of small, dark brown, well-circumscribed macules, usually occurring on adults on sun-exposed areas. Histologically, it consists of epidermal hyperpigmentation with some lentiginous melanocytic hyperplasia, but no nest formation or junctional confluence.

Junctional nevus is a small, dark brown to lighter brown macule that resembles a lentigo. Histologically, these are composed of small nests or clusters of benign melanocytes at the dermal-epidermal junction.

Fig. 13-9. Junctional nevus with nests of melanocytes in the dermal-epidermal junction.

Compound nevus consists of junctional and dermal nests of melanocytes. With time, a junctional nevus becomes less pigmented and slightly raised, corresponding to a compound nevus.

Intradermal nevus is usually a flesh-colored papule.

With senescence, the compound nevus loses its junctional component, so that it only maintains nests in the dermis and loses pigment. *(Slide 13.21).*

Tumors of intermediate Malignant Potential

Dysplastic nevi (atypical nevi, Clark's nevi) are nevi that have some atypia in their clinical appearance, which corresponds to atypical histologic findings. Namely, these lesions exhibit ABCD criteria: **Asymmetry, Border irregularity, Color variation within the lesion, Diameter over 6mm.** These same criteria are used in the diagnosis of melanoma.

Histologically *(Slide 13.22),* dysplastic nevi show atypia of both architectural and cytologic features. **Architectural atypia** is in the form of junctional nests which bridge to adjacent rete ridges, extension of junctional nests well beyond the boundaries of any dermal component (if the nevus is compound), lentiginous melanocytic hyperplasia, rare suprabasal spread of melanocytes, and lamellar fibrosis around rete ridges. **Cytologic atypia** may be visualized as enlarged nuclei with prominent nucleoli, or abundant eosinophilic cytoplasm. Many of these features are also present in melanomas, but the importance is that not all are present at once in a dysplastic nevus.

Dysplastic nevus syndrome occurs when literally hundreds of dysplastic nevi appear all over the body. These patients have a markedly increased risk of developing melanoma during their lifetime.

Sporadic dysplastic nevus is more common than the dysplastic nevus syndrome, but it is uncertain how significant sporadic dysplastic nevi are, and whether or not they have an increased likelihood of developing into a melanoma.

Melanoma in situ (Lentigo maligna, Hutchinson's freckle) usually arises in sun-exposed areas of fair-skinned adult patients with a history of chronic sun exposure, severe sunburns, or a history of a melanoma in a first-degree relative. Histologically, they show severe cytologic atypia and junctional confluence of marked pagetoid (suprabasal) scatter of melanocytes. The important thing to remember is that invasion is not yet present; therefore, this is entirely curable.

Malignant Epidermal Melanocytic Tumors

Malignant Melanoma

Malignant melanoma has the same risk factors as melanoma in situ, but now there has been invasion into the dermis. The atypical melanocytes are arranged as sheets or expansile nests extending into the dermis. Intraepidermal spread as suprabasal (pagetoid) melanocytes or confluent junctional melanocytes are common. Different types are categorized by clinical as well as histologic patterns:

JUNCTIONAL NEVUS

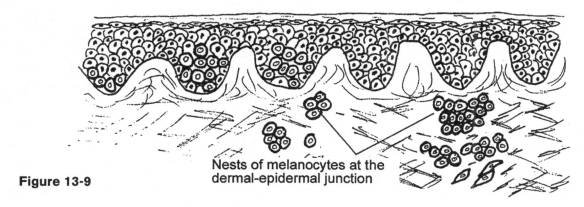

Figure 13-9

Nests of melanocytes at the dermal-epidermal junction

1. **Superficial spreading melanoma**—radial growth pattern of spread, many suprabasal (pagetoid) melanocytes microscopically.
2. **Nodular melanoma** *(Slide 13.23)* —no evidence of an in situ component extending beyond the dermal invasive component. This pattern is usually associated with deeper lesions with vertical growth invasion.
3. **Lentigo maligna melanoma**—large macular variegated lesion, typically on the face of an elderly patient and indolent growth in in situ phase for many years, until dermal invasion takes place. Histologically, there is junctional confluence as lentiginous melanocytic hyperplasia is seen.
4. **Acral lentiginous melanoma**—as the name implies, (acral - limb) this is a melanoma arising on the palms or soles, grows as lentiginous melanocytic hyperplasia along the junctional component. Melanomas are measured in thickness from the granular cell layer down to the deepest invasive cell (in millimeters).

Breslow thickness, the distance between the granular cell layer of uninvolved skin and the deepest point of invasion, is used to determine prognosis.

Melanoma can also be reported according to the tissue level of invasion (**Clark's level**):

1. Clark level I is melanoma in situ (localized to epidermis).
2. level II is invasion into the papillary dermis.
3. level III is invasion into the reticular dermis at the level of the vascular plexus.
4. level IV is well into the reticular dermis.
5. level V is into the subcutaneous fat.

Melanomas less than 1.0mm in thickness have a high rate of cure and usually correlate with Clark level I or II lesions. Melanomas over 4.0mm in thickness have an extremely poor 5 year survival, and usually correlate with Clark level IV and V lesions. Melanomas intermediate between these measurements and levels have an intermediate prognosis.

Other prognostically important histologic features include

- vertical (invasive) vs. radial (in situ) growth phase
- presence/absence of regression or ulceration
- lymphovascular or perineural invasion
- tumor mitotic rate/mm^2
- lymphocytic host response
- microscopic satellitosis (represents in-transit metastasis) and
- surgical margin status.

Intermediate prognosis melanomas may be offered an elective lymph node dissection, or a sentinel lymph node biopsy. Sentinel lymph node biopsy involves injecting the primary melanoma excision site with a radioactive tracer and dye, then determining which lymph node the tracer and dye first travel to, which is the "**sentinel node**". This is thought to be the first place a metastasis would be, if present at all. After removing this node, if it is negative, in theory, the rest of the lymph node basin can be assumed to be negative. If positive, the patient proceeds to complete lymph node dissection to determine if other metastases are present.

Dermal Neoplasms

Benign Dermal Tumors

Fibrocytic tumors include **dermatofibroma (benign fibrous histiocytoma)**. These are firm papules or nodules on the lower extremities of young adults. When the lesion is squeezed gently, it shows central dimpling ("**dimple sign**"). This is actually a non-encapsulated proliferation of histiocytes and fibroblasts in the dermis *(Slide 13.24)*. The overlying epidermis is often hyperpigmented and acanthotic. The etiology is uncertain, but often related to a history of trauma.

Vascular tumors include **hemangiomas**. These are common in infants and children ("**strawberry hemangioma**") and acquired in adulthood ("**cherry angioma**"). Variants in infants and children often spontaneously regress. Adult variants are often due to increased circulating estrogens (e.g., due to liver failure, pregnancy).

Histologically *(Slide 13.25)*, hemangiomas show increased numbers of capillary and venular-sized blood vessels.

Neural tumors include **neurofibromas**. Commonly sporadic lesions (on abdomen and extremities), neurofibromas resemble fibroepithelial polyps clinically. Multiple lesions may be present in syndromes, such as Von Recklinghausen's disease (Neurofibromatosis).

Histologically, neurofibromas show non-encapsulated proliferation of peripheral nerve fibers and surrounding fibroblasts.

Hematopoietic tumors include **mastocytosis.** While different forms of this disease exist, they most commonly arise in infancy and childhood (**urticaria pigmentosa**), resulting in itchy papules that urticate (produce hives) and heal with hyperpigmentation. These spontaneously resolve with time. There are also less common systemic forms of the disease, which may have bone marrow, liver, or lymph node infiltration. The latter forms are more difficult to manage and often do not resolve spontaneously.

Malignant Dermal Tumors

Malignant fibrocytic tumors include **typical fibroxanthomas.** They arise on solar-damaged skin and are usually found on the face of elderly individuals. Most pathologists feel they are a superficial variant of a malignant fibrous histiocytoma, which lack the ability to metastasize due to their superficial dermal location.

Histologically, fibroxanthomas consist of atypical spindle to pleomorphic cells in the dermis. Many mitotic figures, including atypical forms, are easy to identify. Local complete excision is curative.

Malignant vascular tumors include **angiosarcomas.** These typically occur on the head or neck of an elderly patient. An aggressive clinical course with metastases is the norm.

Histologically, angiosarcoma consists of pleomorphic endothelial cells that form recognizable, but irregular, vascular channels.

Kaposi's sarcoma in its classic form occurs on the lower extremities of elderly individuals. An epidemic form is present in Africa. There is also a form associated with immunodeficiency, particular HIV infection. Kaposi's sarcoma is more common in homosexual males with HIV. Retroviral therapy has decreased its incidence.

Histologically *(Slide 13.26)*, Kaposi's sarcoma shows a spindle cell proliferation with poorly formed vascular channels with hemosiderin and red blood cell extravasation. There is mild atypia of the endothelial cells of the blood vessels, but not marked pleomorphism as in angiosarcoma. It is thought to be due to infection with human herpes virus-8.

Malignant neural tumors include **malignant peripheral nerve sheath tumors (neurofibrosarcoma):** These rare neoplasms usually arise in patients with neurofibromatosis, within a pre-existing plexiform neurofibroma, or de novo. Histology is of a spindle cell sarcoma.

Hematopoietic tumors include **mycosis fungoides.** This cutaneous helper T-cell lymphoma is found in older patients. It is often thought to be a chronic eczematous dermatitis, which begins as erythematous macules/plaques, and develops into violaceous nodules to tumors. It is often difficult to diagnose this lymphoma clinically and histologically in its early stages.

Histologically *(Slide 13.27)*, mycosis fungoides shows hyperchromatic and irregular lymphocytes infiltrating the epidermis, sometimes as clusters, forming **Pautrier's microabscesses.** There is also a dermal perivascular lymphocytic infiltrate. The malignant lymphocytes are in the epidermis; reactive T-cells remain in the dermis. Gene rearrangement studies confirm the presence of a clonal proliferation of T-cells. Erythroderma (abnormal skin redness) may develop. Some patients also develop a leukemic phase, with circulating atypical lymphocytes (**Sézary cells**).

14

Soft Tissue, Bone, and Joint Pathology

SOFT TISSUE PATHOLOGY
Overview

The pathology of soft tissues primarily is the pathology of soft tissue tumors and the lesions that mimic them. The soft tissues can be defined as the nonepithelial supportive and specialized tissues, excluding the reticuloendothelial system (i.e. the lymph nodes and spleen), glial tissues and the supportive tissues of solid parenchymal organs. Soft tissue tumors attempt to recapitulate the normal mesenchymal tissues of the body, including fibrous, adipose, vascular, neural, and smooth and skeletal muscle tissue.

Occasionally, tumors of soft tissue are difficult to classify according to the lineage of differentiation (e.g., synovial sarcoma). This segment will review the most common of the soft tissue tumors and the tumor-like lesions that can cause diagnostic confusion.

Incidence of Soft Tissue Tumors

The incidence of the various soft tissue tumors varies considerably; however, the benign lesions far outnumber the malignant ones by nearly 100:1.

Fig. 14-1. The preponderance of benign versus malignant soft tissue tumors. The true incidence of these lesions is difficult to know since many benign tumors are overlooked or not biopsied. Malignant soft tissue tumors, compared to carcinomas of epithelial origin, are relatively rare and make up approximately 1% of all cancers in adults.

The age of the patient influences the incidence and the type of tumors encountered. The incidence of soft tissue tumors increases with age. Sarcomas remain as the 4th most common malignant neoplasm in the pediatric age group.

Pathogenesis of Soft Tissue Tumors

The pathogenesis of most soft tissue tumors is still unknown. Of the recognized causes of soft tissue tumors, environmental and genetic factors are the most understood.

Environmental Factors

1. **Trauma** is frequently implicated in the development of sarcomas. Most of the reports are likely coincidental but occasional sarcomas have arisen from sites of fracture, burns, scars, and surgical implants.
2. **Chemical carcinogens** such as asbestos (implicated in pleural and peritoneal mesotheliomas), phenoxyacetic acid herbicides, chlorophenols (e.g., dioxin in Agent Orange), and vinyl chloride (associated with hepatic angiosarcoma) are well-known as potent carcinogens in the development of various sarcomas.

SOFT TISSUE PROLIFERATIONS

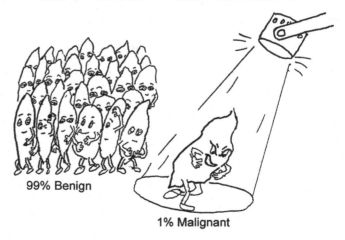

99% Benign

1% Malignant

Figure 14-1

3. **Radiation exposure** is well documented as a risk factor for the development of sarcoma, however, the incidence is very rare, ranging from 0.03% to 0.80%. Fibrosarcoma and angiosarcoma are the most commonly implicated in cases of radiation exposure.

Genetic Factors

The understanding of the various molecular mechanisms of soft tissue tumor development has progressed significantly over the past decade. A minority of the tumors that are encountered in everyday practice are related to well-defined genetic syndromes. Of these, mutations involving the TP53 gene (in **Li-Fraumeni syndrome**), the retinoblastoma gene, **NF1** and **NF2** (in **neurofibromatosis**), and APC gene (in **Gardner's syndrome**) are the best known.

Classification of Soft Tissue Tumors

The classification of soft tissue tumors and tumor-like lesions has gone through many changes over the past century. Currently, tumors of soft tissue are classified according to the presumed histogenetic tissue of origin. The general categories of tumors encountered most commonly recapitulate the following tissue types:

1. **Fibrous tissue** (fibroma, nodular fasciitis, myositis ossificans, fibromatosis and fibrosarcoma)
2. **Fibrohistiocytic tissue** (benign fibrous histiocytoma, malignant fibrous histiocytoma)
3. **Adipose tissue** (lipoma, liposarcoma)
4. **Smooth muscle tissue** (leiomyoma, leiomyosarcoma)
5. **Skeletal muscle tissue** (rhabdomyoma, rhabdomyosarcoma)
6. **Vascular tissue** (hemangioma, Kaposi's sarcoma, angiosarcoma)
7. **Peripheral nervous tissue** (neuroma, schwannoma, neurofibroma, malignant peripheral nerve sheath tumor)
8. **Other** (synovial sarcoma)

Tumors of Fibrous Tissue Origin

Fibroma

The majority of "fibromas" arise in the skin and oral cavity as tumor-like lesions consisting of abundant dense collagen and scant amounts of spindled fibroblasts. In general, most fibromas are considered to be reactive in nature and not neoplastic. These lesions need to be differentiated from the benign soft tissue neoplasms that have collagen as a significant component (e.g., **neurofibroma, nuchal fibroma, elastofibroma**).

Nodular Fasciitis

Nodular fasciitis is one of the most common of the reactive pseudosarcomatous fibroblastic proliferations. Nodular fasciitis typically arises in younger to middle-age adults, with a propensity to involve the forearm, chest, and back. A preceding history of trauma to the area of involvement is elicited in 15-20% of cases. Often the lesion is noted to grow rapidly over a period of weeks.

Nodular fasciitis most commonly involves the subcutaneous tissue; however, origin within the skeletal muscles can be seen rarely. The lesion is usually well circumscribed and consists of a uniform cellular growth of immature plump fibroblasts in a **storiform** (Latin, "**woven mat**") pattern resembling tissue culture.

Fig. 14-2. "Woven mat" appearance in nodular fasciitis. With the cellular growth accompanied by abundant mitotic activity and rapid growth, it is not difficult to appreciate why this reactive lesion can superficially resemble a sarcoma. *(Slide 14.1)* Treatment consists of simple excision. Recurrence is rare, consonant with the non-neoplastic nature of this lesion.

Myositis Ossificans

Myositis ossificans is a non-neoplastic proliferative process characterized by a cellular fibroblastic proliferation associated with variable degrees of metaplastic bone formation. The condition is most commonly seen in adolescents and young adults; often a history of trauma to the affected site can be elicited. Typically the patient will

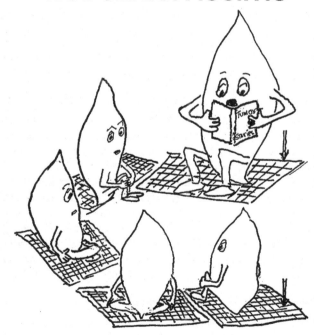

NODULAR FASCIITIS

"Woven mat" pattern

Figure 14-2

present with pain or discomfort in the affected area followed by progressive soft tissue swelling and eventual mass formation over a period of weeks.

Radiographically, myositis ossificans can vary from an area of vague soft tissue fullness early on to transformation to a well-defined mass containing varying degrees of calcification most concentrated at the periphery of the lesion.

Grossly, myositis ossificans is a well-circumscribed mass seen in the subcutis or underlying musculature. The zonal characteristics of the mass as seen on plain radiographs can usually be appreciated grossly. Microscopically, the central portions of the mass consist of a cellular proliferation of fibroblast-like cells with transition to an osteoblastic rim replete with active osteoid deposition and bone formation. The most peripheral aspects often consist of well-formed and completely ossified trabecular bone.

Myositis ossificans is cured by simple excision.

Fibromatosis

This group of lesions is characterized by a locally aggressive pattern of growth of benign fibroblasts arranged in fascicles. They are known to arise in just about every anatomic site; however the propensity to involve specific locations has been well characterized. Involvement of the palmar fascia with progressive flexion of the fourth and fifth digits of the hand has been coined "Dupuytren's contracture." Similar alterations occur in the plantar fascia of the foot, however flexion of the toes typically does not occur. **Peyronie's disease (penile fibromatosis)** is manifested as thickening of the dorsolateral aspect of the penile shaft, leading to painful curvature with erections and/or urethral stenosis.

Aggressive fibromatoses (**desmoid tumor**) typically present as ill-defined firm-rubbery soft tissue masses in young adults (20's to 40's). They can arise in the abdominal cavity with involvement of the abdominopelvic walls or mesentery in patients with Gardner's syndrome, or they can arise in the abdominal organs (e.g., the ovary). Extra-abdominal desmoid tumors have a propensity to arise in the shoulder girdle, back or thigh with a predilection for young women.

Pathologically, desmoid tumors have a similar fascicular growth pattern regardless of their site of origin and tend to locally infiltrate surrounding soft tissues. Due to this locally infiltrative growth pattern, desmoid tumors may be difficult to completely resect, leading to a significant rate of recurrence. Despite the propensity to recur, they do not have the capability to metastasize.

Fibrosarcoma

Fibrosarcomas arise most commonly in middle-aged and elderly individuals with a tendency to involve the retroperitoneum and deep soft tissues of the thigh and lower extremity.

Grossly, fibrosarcomas are fleshy neoplasms which may appear well circumscribed when small; larger neoplasms tend to appear less well defined and infiltrative. Microscopically, fibrosarcomas grow in a distinct fascicular pattern known as a herringbone pattern.

Fig. 14-3 (Slide 14-2). "Herringbone" pattern of fibrosarcoma. Areas of necrosis or hemorrhage are not uncommon.

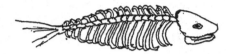

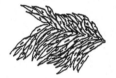

"Herringbone" pattern

Figure 14-3

Treatment consists of wide local excision, however recurrence is not infrequent and metastases occur in up to one-fourth of cases, most commonly to the lungs.

Fibrohistiocytic Tumors

Benign Fibrous Histiocytoma: This group of neoplasms arises most commonly in the dermis of the skin, with occasional examples seen in the subcutis. The most common entity, also known as a **dermatofibroma**, arises exclusively in the dermis and is often seen in young individuals, with a tendency toward female predominance.

Microscopically, dermatofibromas consist of an ill-defined proliferation of fibroblast-like cells in a storiform pattern *(Slide 14.3)*. This entity is uniformly benign and simple excision is curative.

Other variants of benign fibrous histiocytoma vary with the degree of inflammation seen, the presence of lipid-laden macrophages, the vascularity of the neoplasm and the varying proportions of epithelioid or spindle cells comprising the lesion.

Malignant Fibrous Histiocytoma: This is one of the most controversial neoplasms encountered in soft tissue pathology. The controversy involves the misclassification of certain sarcomas into this category, which has made the diagnosis of malignant fibrous histiocytoma appear as a "catch-all" for those difficult-to-classify tumors.

Clearly, malignant fibrous histiocytoma as a true entity has in general been agreed upon. The majority of these sarcomas are classified as the storiform-pleomorphic subtype consisting of anaplastic spindled cells arranged in a storiform growth pattern *(Slide 14.4)*. Other less common variants consist of the myxoid, inflammatory, giant cell and angiomatoid types. Regardless of the subtype, the majority of these sarcomas arise in the middle aged to elderly population with a predilection for the retroperitoneum or lower extremities. The only exception is the angiomatoid variant which tends to arise in a younger age group (adolescents and young adults).

In general, malignant fibrous histiocytoma is an aggressive neoplasm with a high rate of recurrence and distant metastasis despite wide local excision.

Adipose Tissue Tumors

Lipoma and Liposarcoma

Lipomas are benign neoplasms composed almost exclusively of mature adipose tissue surrounded by a thin membranous capsule. They are the most common soft tissue neoplasms seen in adults, typically arising in the subcutis of the back, neck, extremities, abdomen, chest, and buttocks. Variants of the conventional lipoma include **angiolipoma**, **fibrolipoma**, **spindle cell lipoma**, and **pleomorphic lipoma**. An uncommon condition where an abnormal collection of lipomatous tissue arises in various sites throughout the body is known as **lipomatosis**. Simple excision is curative.

Liposarcomas are the malignant counterpart of the adipocytic tumors and usually are seen in adults in their fifth to seventh decades of life. They commonly arise in the retroperitoneum as well as in the deep tissues of the extremities. Various subtypes have been identified. However they all have in common the presence of a characteristic cell type: the **lipoblast**. Lipoblasts are neoplastic cells which contain multiple cytoplasmic vacuoles of lipid that indent the nucleus and recapitulate the differentiation of adipose tissue seen in the fetus.

Fig. 14-4. Lipoma versus liposarcoma.

Histogenetically, the different subtypes of liposarcoma are the **well-differentiated type** *(Slide 14.5)*, the **myxoid type** *(Slide 14.6)*, the **round cell type**, and the **pleomorphic type**. In general these neoplasms are treated by wide local excision with prognosis depending on the subtype and resectability of the liposarcoma. The well-differentiated and myxoid types are relatively

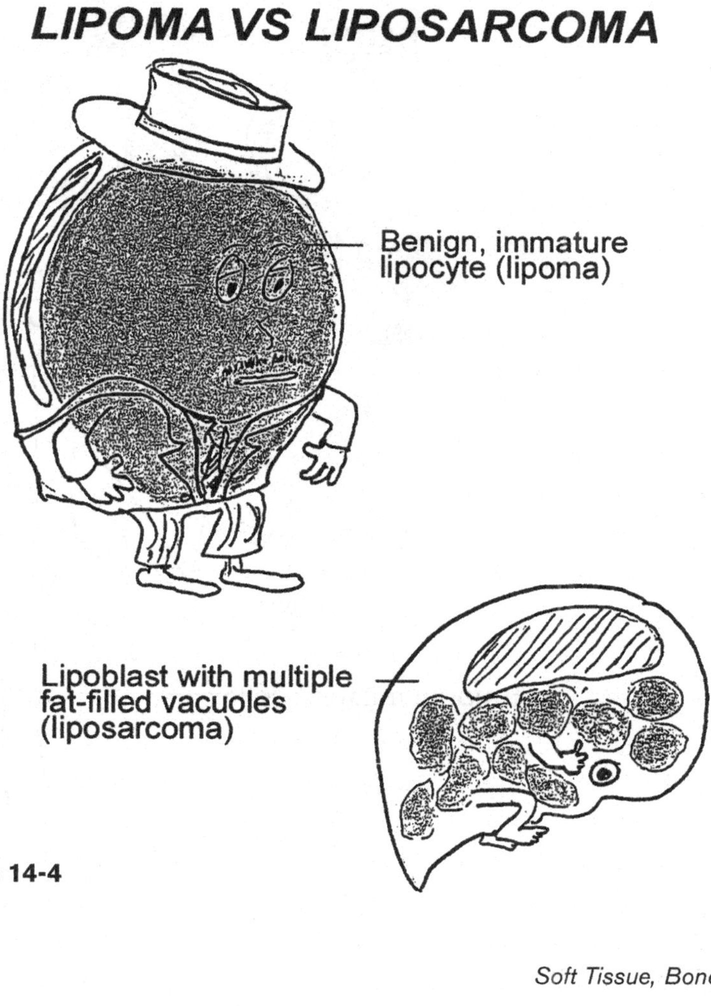

LIPOMA VS LIPOSARCOMA

Benign, immature lipocyte (lipoma)

Lipoblast with multiple fat-filled vacuoles (liposarcoma)

Figure 14-4

indolent, with the round cell and pleomorphic types behaving much more aggressively.

Smooth Muscle Tumors

Leiomyoma and Leiomyosarcoma

Leiomyomas are relatively common benign smooth muscle neoplasms. They are much more common in the uterine myometrium. When leiomyomas are identified in the soft tissues they are most commonly seen to arise from vessels or the arrector pili muscles of the skin in adolescents or young adults.

Microscopically, soft tissue leiomyomas resemble their uterine counterparts, consisting of intersecting fascicles of spindle cells closely resembling normal smooth muscle. Simple excision is curative.

Fig. 14-5 (Slide 14.7). "Smooth muscle" cells, characteristic of leiomyoma and leiomyosarcoma.

Leiomyosarcomas of soft tissue are much less common than leiomyomas and tend to develop in the retroperitoneum and deep tissues of the extremities. They typically arise in older patients in comparison with leiomyomas. Leiomyosarcomas are usually larger than leiomyomas and often contain grossly evident areas of hemorrhage and/or necrosis.

Histologically, leiomyosarcomas consist of pleomorphic spindle cells growing in intersecting fascicles reminiscent of mature smooth muscle. *(Slide 14-8)* The presence of hemorrhage and necrosis, pleomorphic nuclei, and excessive mitotic activity can be a strong clue to the malignant nature of this neoplasm. Prognostically, retroperitoneal tumors are more aggressive; However this appears most often related to their larger size and the greater difficulty in obtaining adequate resection margins.

Skeletal Muscle Tumors

Rhabdomyoma and Rhabdomyosarcoma

Unlike most soft tissue tumors, the majority of tumors of skeletal muscle are malignant. Rhabdomyomas are exceedingly rare, with the preponderance of cases

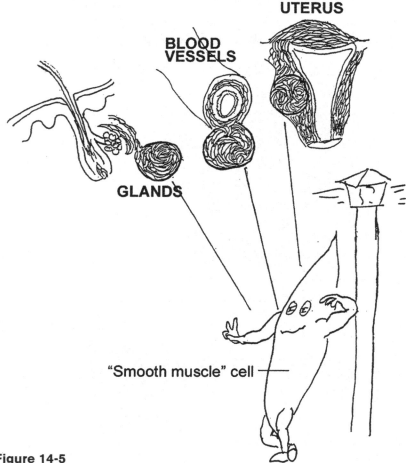

LEIOMYOMAS AND LEIOMYOSARCOMAS

UTERUS

BLOOD VESSELS

GLANDS

"Smooth muscle" cell

Figure 14-5

identified in the heart, often as a part of the tuberous sclerosis complex.

In contrast to rhabdomyomas, rhabdomyosarcomas are more common. In fact, rhabdomyosarcoma ranks as the most common soft tissue sarcoma of the pediatric age group. The most common anatomic sites for rhabdomyosarcoma are the head and neck, urinary bladder and genital tract. A smaller proportion of tumors are identified in the retroperitoneum and extremities.

Three variants of rhabdomyosarcoma have been described: **embryonal, alveolar,** and **pleomorphic.** Of the three, the embryonal variant is the most common, accounting for nearly two-thirds of all cases.

Histologically, **embryonal rhabdomyosarcoma** is characterized by a variable cellular growth of immature spindle cells and occasional cells that recapitulate skeletal muscle embryogenesis: **rhabdomyoblasts (Slide 14.9).** A variant of embryonal rhabdomyosarcoma, **sarcoma botryoides,** tends to arise in hollow organs, most commonly, the urinary bladder and vagina. It is typified by a grape-like cluster growth of tumor protruding into the hollow organ cavity.

Fig. 14-6. Sarcoma botryoides, "bunch of grapes" appearance.

Alveolar rhabdomyosarcoma typically arises in a slightly older age group than that associated with the embryonal type. This variant receives its name from the characteristic growth pattern which superficially resembles the histology of the alveoli of the lungs. The tumor cells grow in nests, but are so dyscohesive that they tend to separate from each other, forming spaces lined by tumor cells. *(Slide 14.10)*

Pleomorphic rhabdomyosarcoma is a very rare variant that is seen more often in adults in their 50's and 60's. Pleomorphic rhabdomyosarcoma consists of a haphazard growth of large, anaplastic tumor cells containing dense eosinophilic cytoplasm. Rare cross striations can be identified, giving a clue to the skeletal muscle histogenesis.

Fig. 14-7. Occasional cell cross striations in pleomorphic rhabdomosarcoma.

Rhabdomyosarcomas have a variable prognosis depending on the subtype as well as the extent of tumor spread and resectability. Embryonal rhabdomyosarcoma has the best prognosis with the botryoid variant having an especially good survival rate. The alveolar and pleomorphic variants have a significantly worse

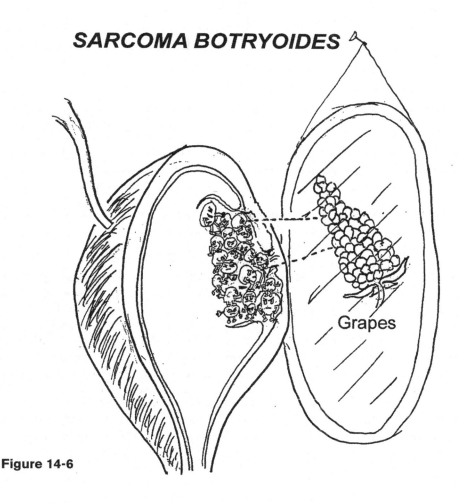

SARCOMA BOTRYOIDES

Grapes

Figure 14-6

PLEOMORPHIC RHABDOMYOSARCOMA

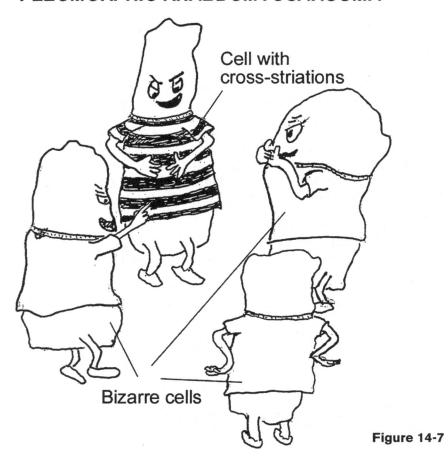

Cell with cross-striations

Bizarre cells

Figure 14-7

prognosis, with survival depending heavily on the stage at time of diagnosis.

Vascular Tumors

Hemangiomas are exceptionally common neoplasms, most often seen in the skin. They can be identified in any age group, but congenital varieties tend to be more significant cosmetically. The most common subtypes of hemangioma are characterized by either a growth of multiple small entangled capillaries or that of large dilated channels filled with blood. These patterns have been coined as the capillary and cavernous types *(Slides 14.11, 14.12).*

Capillary hemangiomas are the most common type and can vary tremendously in size and distribution. They are mostly identified in the skin; However they may also occur in the mucous membranes as well as in the viscera (e.g., the liver). A related variant of capillary hemangioma is the **pyogenic granuloma**. Pyogenic granulomas often have a polypoid growth pattern and usually arise from the skin and mucous membranes (most commonly around the oral cavity).

Histologically, pyogenic granuloma is characterized by a lobular growth pattern of small capillaries, giving rise to the other term used for this common tumor: **lobular capillary hemangioma**. This lesion has a propensity to arise in children as well as in pregnant women.

Cavernous hemangiomas are less common lesions, with a similar tendency to arise in children. They are most commonly seen in the skin, but occasional lesions occur in the viscera, e.g., the liver and brain.

Regardless of the type of hemangioma, simple excision is curative.

Kaposi's Sarcoma

Prior to the appearance of the AIDS epidemic in the early 80's, Kaposi's sarcoma was a rare neoplasm occurring primarily in the distal lower extremities of elderly men of Eastern European descent (the classic form). With the emergence of HIV infection and AIDS, the incidence of Kaposi's sarcoma increased significantly. Unlike the classic form of Kaposi's, the AIDS-associated form can arise in both the skin and viscera (especially the lung and GI tract) and has the propensity to metastasize widely and cause death.

The etiology of Kaposi's sarcoma remains unknown, however evidence supports the role of human herpes virus 8 in the development of many cases.

Clinically, Kaposi's sarcoma can be identified in 1 of 3 stages from early to late: **patch, plaque** and **tumor** stages.

Histologically, the earliest stage of Kaposi's sarcoma is characterized by a proliferation of small anastamosing capillary-like vessels lined by plump endothelial cells. Later stages demonstrate an increasing number of vessels which begin to form slit-like spaces containing red blood cells (*Slide 14.13*). As lesions progress, the coalescence of vascular spaces intermixed with proliferating neoplastic endothelial cells forms nodular aggregates (tumor stage).

Prognosis of Kaposi's sarcoma depends heavily on the immunologic status of the patient, with AIDS-related cases demonstrating a far worse prognosis. Surgical resection can be curative for localized lesions, but radiation and chemotherapy is usually necessary in AIDS-related cases due to the multifocality of the neoplasm.

Angiosarcoma

A rare sarcoma, angiosarcoma most commonly arises in older adults, with a predilection to involve the skin and superficial soft tissues. In addition, angiosarcoma is the most common primary sarcoma of the liver. A number of well-defined risk factors are known for the development of angiosarcoma. Chronic lymphedema is one of the most commonly identified predisposing factors. The prototypical patient is that of a women who develops angiosarcoma in the upper extremity following axillary lymph node dissection for breast cancer (**Stewart-Treves syndrome**). In addition, radiation therapy and Thorotrast use (in cases of hepatic angiosarcoma) have been identified as predisposing factors.

Clinically, angiosarcoma usually presents as an ill-defined area of red-purple discoloration of the skin. They are typically hemorrhagic in appearance on cut section and often have a sponge-like consistency.

Histologically, angiosarcoma consists of variably sized anastamotic vascular channels lined by plump hyperchromatic, and often pleomorphic, endothelial cells (*Slide 14.14*). Hemorrhage is usually a prominent feature, and mitotic figures are usually easy to identify. Prognostically, angiosarcomas are highly aggressive neoplasms. Despite treatment, nearly 90% of patients succumb to their disease within 5 years of diagnosis due to local extension of their tumor or metastasis.

Tumors of Peripheral Nerve

Neurofibroma

Neurofibromas are relatively common, usually occurring as solitary sporadic lesions arising in the dermis of the skin. Less commonly, they can be identified in association with the genetic syndrome **Neurofibromatosis 1 (von Recklinghausen's disease).** They can be identified in any age group; However tend to appear at an earlier age in patients with Neurofibromatosis 1.

Grossly, neurofibromas cause fusiform expansion of the nerve and typically appear as small discrete skin nodules. However they may reach massive proportions and have a pedunculated growth pattern. Histologically, solitary neurofibromas consist of a mixture of "wavy" spindle cells (fibroblasts. Schwann cells and perineurial cells) and variable amounts of inflammation (lymphocytes, mast cells) embedded in a loose mucoid matrix (*Slide 14.15*).

Fig. 14-8. Wavy appearance to neurofibroma cells.

Treatment of solitary neurofibromas consists of simple excision. The risk of malignant degeneration into a malignant peripheral nerve sheath tumor has been described, but it is an extremely rare event.

A less common variety of neurofibroma, known as a **plexiform neurofibroma**, typically occurs within nerves of the deeper soft tissues. These are designated as plexiform lesions due to their expansion of nerve fibers within a single nerve trunk resembling a "bag of worms." The importance of noting this variant of neurofibroma is twofold:

1. The strong association with Neurofibromatosis 1
2. The increased risk of malignant degeneration.

Due to the larger size and deep nature of these lesions, surgical management can be challenging. In those unresectable lesions, close follow-up is necessary due to their increased propensity for malignant degeneration.

Schwannoma

Like neurofibromas, schwannomas are relatively common soft tissue tumors. (Slide 14.16) They are seen at all ages, but tend to predominate in young to middle aged adults. Most often, schwannomas arise in the superficial tissues (dermis and subcutis) of the head and neck and flexor aspects of the extremities. Occasionally, they can be identified in the deeper soft tissues, e.g., the retroperitoneum. A characteristic location is in the cerebellopontine angle where they are often called "acoustic neuromas."

Miscellaneous Soft Tissue Tumors

Synovial Cell Sarcoma

Synovial cell sarcoma, a relatively common sarcoma, accounts for nearly 10% off all sarcomas. It is of uncertain histogenesis. However, it has been named due to its frequent association within or near large joints and its resemblance to immature synovium. Synovial sarcoma has a propensity to arise in or around the knee and tends to involve middle-aged adults, with a male predominance.

NEUROFIBROMA CELLS

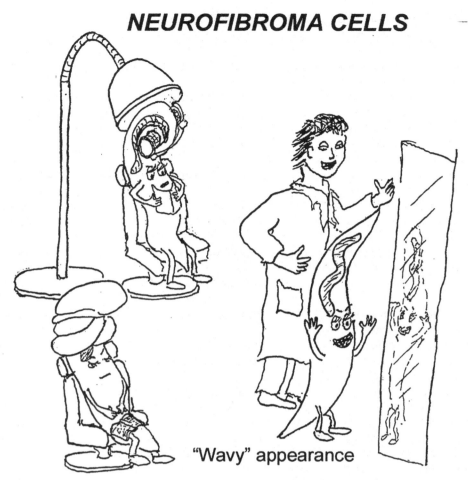

"Wavy" appearance

Figure 14-8

Histologically, synovial sarcoma is most commonly composed of an intimate admixture of fibroblast-like spindle cells and gland-forming epithelioid cells (the **biphasic pattern**). Occasionally, a pattern of growth consisting only of spindle cells or epithelioid cells can be seen (the **monophasic pattern**) *(Slide 14.17)*.

When exclusively spindled, the neoplasm can closely resemble a fibrosarcoma or malignant peripheral nerve sheath tumor.

In nearly all synovial sarcomas a characteristic chromosomal translocation can be identified: t(X:18) (p11.2;q11.2). In difficult cases, identification of this translocation can be very helpful.

In general, synovial sarcomas are aggressive neoplasms with 5-year survival rates of approximately 40-50% with amputation or limb-sparing surgery.

BONE PATHOLOGY

Congenital Abnormalities

Osteogenesis Imperfecta

Also known as "brittle bone disease," osteogenesis imperfecta is a group of disorders characterized by an abnormality in the synthesis of type I collagen fibrils. Mutations in the genes that code for the alpha-1 and alpha-2 chains of collagen are inherited in either an autosomal dominant or recessive manner. Depending on the type, affected patients typically present early in the postnatal period with skeletal fractures and deformities, blue sclerae, joint laxity, hearing abnormalities and abnormal tooth development.

Fig. 14-9. Features of osteogenesis imperfecta. Currently, no treatment exists, but early recognition is important for genetic counseling.

Achondroplasia

Achondroplasia is the most common cause of dwarfism. In the majority of cases (80%), a sporadic germline mutation in unaffected parents leads to the genetic abnormality. Depending on the genetic make-up of the parents, 2 major forms exist: a more common **heterozygote** form and a rare and more severe **homozygote** form. The heterozygote form occurs when one parent passes on a mutated gene in an autosomal dominant inheritance pattern. The heterozygote form presents in infancy as shortened proximal limbs with shortened

OSTEOGENESIS IMPERFECTA

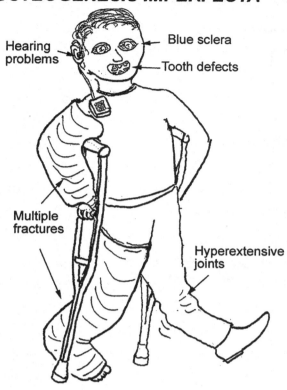

Hearing problems

Blue sclera

Tooth defects

Multiple fractures

Hyperextensive joints

Figure 14-9

digits, enlargement of the head (often greater than the 75th percentile for age), prominence of the forehead, and attenuation of the bridge of the nose. Despite the anatomic changes, the IQ of affected patients is normal with no reduction in reproductive capacity or life span. In contrast, the homozygote form results in similar but more severe morphologic changes, with rare infants surviving beyond infancy.

Fig. 14-10. Features of heterozygous achondroplasia.

Histologically, microscopic changes are noted primarily in the epiphyseal cartilaginous growth plate with disorganization of the proliferating chondrocytes and premature calcification, resulting in early closure. This premature closure of the growth plates leads to the limb shortening seen clinically.

Paget's Disease

Paget's disease is characterized by abnormal bone formation and destruction. Although the etiology remains debated, the leading suspected cause is infection with a paramyxovirus. Paget's disease arises in middle to late life, predominantly in male Caucasians.

Clinically, the presentation is quite variable, with bone pain most common. Typically, patients are mildly symptomatic and often identified through incidental findings on routine radiographs.

Two primary forms exist, depending on the extent of presenting findings. The most common form, accounting for more than three-quarters of cases, is the **polyostotic form** where multiple separate anatomic sites are involved, particularly the flat bones of the axial skeleton (e.g., the pelvis), the vertebral column, the proximal femur, and skull. In the less common **monostotic form**, a single bony site is involved.

Three stages have been identified in Paget's, depending on the degree of bone formation (osteoblastic activity) or bone destruction (osteoclastic activity). The first stage is dominated by osteoclastic activity with extensive resorption of the bone by abnormally large osteoclasts. The excessive resorption gives the bone a moth-eaten pattern.

Fig. 14-11. "Moth-eaten" appearance of Paget's disease of the bone.

As the first stage of Paget's disease comes to an end, increasing amounts of osteoblasts are noted, leading to a mixed osteoblastic and osteoclastic pattern. The osteoid (bone matrix laid down by osteocytes) in the increased bone formation is laid down in a disorganized fashion, leading to prominent cement lines displayed in a characteristic mosaic tile pattern.

Fig. 14-12. Mosaic pattern of bone in the second stage of Paget's disease.

The third stage is characterized by a "burned-out" appearance with a marked decrease in the osteoblastic and osteoclastic cellular activity. The cells and surrounding fibrovascular tissue are eventually replaced by normal and fatty marrow. The final result is transformation of the bone into a larger version of its normal self with abnormal expanded trabeculae.

The clinical expression of these histologic stages is represented by expansion and enlargement of the bones of the skull, femur, tibia, and pelvis. The changes in the bone eventually lead to weakening and can lead to fractures. Symptoms in affected patients are usually mild and consist of pain and deformity of the involved areas. Due to the increased metabolic activity in the abnormal bone, increased blood flow to the area can lead to chronic stress on the heart and eventual high-output cardiac failure.

Prognosis varies, depending on the severity and number of affected sites (polyostotic > monostotic). The most serious consequence of Paget's disease relates to the increased risk for the development of a variety of benign and malignant neoplasms in the involved sites. Benign neoplasms that are seen more frequently in pagetic patients include giant cell tumors and extramedullary

ACHONDROPLASIA

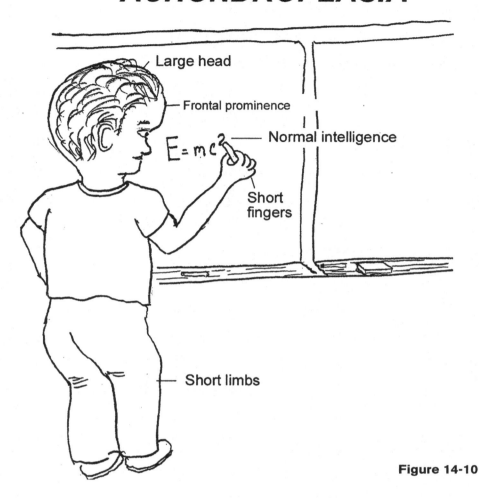

Large head

Frontal prominence

Normal intelligence

$E = mc^2$

Short fingers

Short limbs

Figure 14-10

hematopoiesis; malignant neoplasms include various sarcomas such as osteosarcoma, chondrosarcoma and malignant fibrous histiocytoma.

BONE-FORMING TUMORS
Osteoid Osteoma

Osteoid osteoma is a benign bone-forming tumor arising most commonly in patients in their second to third decades of life, with a 2:1 male:female predominance. It can arise in any bone, with a predilection for the long bones of the appendicular skeleton (femur and tibia account for half of all cases). Characteristically, osteoid osteomas are exquisitely painful, particularly at night. A useful diagnostic clue is that the pain is dramatically relieved with the use of aspirin.

Osteoid osteomas have a characteristic radiographic appearance. Plain radiographs reveal a central lucent nidus surrounded by a variably sized area of bony sclerosis.

The histologic appearance correlates with the radiographic appearance. The central nidus is composed of a mesh-like network of variably calcified bony trabeculae conspicuously lined by osteoblasts (*Slide 14.18*). The regions interspersed between the trabeculae show a highly vascular loose connective tissue stroma. Corresponding to the area of peripheral bony sclerosis, the bone surrounding the central nidus is densely sclerotic without the osteoblastic rimming or vascular connective tissue.

Simple surgical excision is curative as long as the nidus is removed completely; incomplete excision can potentially lead to recurrence.

Osteoblastoma

Osteoblastomas histologically resemble osteoid osteomas. They differ in that osteoblastoma is typically larger and lacks the surrounding rim of dense sclerotic bone. Similarly, osteoblastoma can often manifest pain, but may not have the accentuation that is seen at night

PAGET'S DISEASE OF BONE : 1ST STAGE

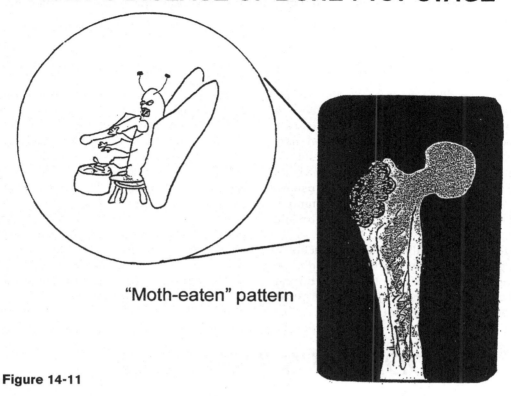

"Moth-eaten" pattern

Figure 14-11

PAGET'S DISEASE OF BONE: 2ND STAGE

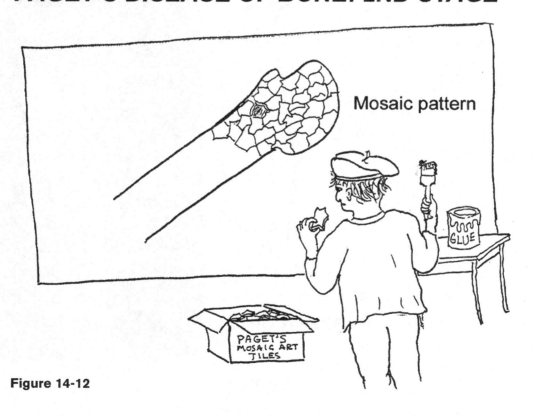

Mosaic pattern

Figure 14-12

as in osteoid osteomas. Osteoblastomas most commonly affect the vertebrae, with a similar age and gender distribution as osteoid osteomas.

Osteosarcoma

Osteosarcoma is the most common primary malignant tumor of bone. It is a tumor of adolescents and young adults, with a male predilection, but occasional examples are seen in older adults, often in association with Paget's disease or previous radiotherapy. Most cases of osteosarcoma present clinically with localized bone pain. Occasional cases may be associated with soft tissue swelling and/or a previous history of trauma in the affected area. Anatomically, osteosarcoma usually involves the metaphysis of long bones, most commonly arising in the distal femur, proximal tibia, or proximal humerus.

Radiologically, lesions usually display destruction of the surrounding bone associated with variable degrees of opacity or lucency depending on the amount of calcification present. When destruction of the cortex occurs, elevation of the periosteum may occur, associ-ated with reactive bone formation, leading to the characteristic radiologic lesion, "**Codman's triangle.**"

Fig. 14-13. Codman's triangle in osteosarcoma.

Grossly, osteosarcoma is a bulky tumor that replaces the normal medullary canal and destroys the overlying cortex. The tumor is often seen extending into the adjacent soft tissue as a soft tissue mass. Hemorrhage and areas of cystic necrosis are frequently identified.

Histologically, the neoplasm is characterized by a lace-like deposition of eosinophilic osteoid with variable degrees of calcification. Occasionally, the osteoid can be seen forming broad sheets or well-formed trabeculae, depending on the degree of differentiation. The tumor cells are variable in size, ranging from small bland spindle cells to large bizarre forms with abundant mitoses *(Slide 14.19)*. Malignant cartilage and fibrous tissue can often be identified as well.

The clinical course can be aggressive, but the prognosis has significantly improved (5-year survival rate of approximately 70%) with the development of more

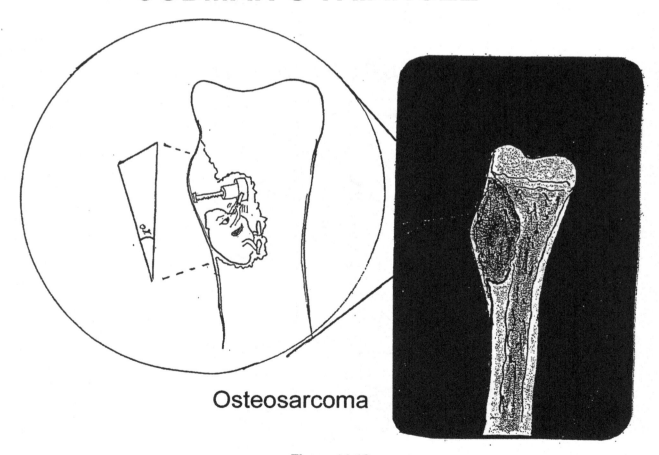

CODMAN'S TRIANGLE

Osteosarcoma

Figure 14-13

effective chemotherapeutic regimens. In addition, disability due to limb amputation has been reduced with the introduction of limb-sparing surgeries aimed at reducing the amount of tissue resected.

Cartilage-Forming Tumors

Chondroma

Chondromas are benign neoplasms composed of mature hyaline cartilage. Chondromas are typically solitary tumors arising in adults in their third through fifth decades of life. They are identified most commonly in the small bones of the hands and feet, but examples have been identified in the flat bones of the ribs and the long bones of the extremities. When chondromas are seen arising in the periosteal or adjacent tissues they are known as **juxtacortical chondromas**; when these lesions are seen to arise in the medullary cavity of the bones they are termed **enchondromas**. Regardless of the type of chondroma, the histology is similar.

Histologically, chondromas closely resemble mature hyaline cartilage, composed of bland chondrocytes arranged in closely apposed nests or diffusely distributed throughout the lesion *(Slide 14.20)*. Simple excision is curative of these benign lesions.

A small percentage of patients (approximately 30%) have multiple simultaneous enchondromas. When they arise on one side of the body, the syndrome is known as **Ollier's disease**. Cases where multiple enchondromas are present in conjunction with soft tissue hemangiomas are referred to as **Maffucci's syndrome**. The primary significance of identifying these syndromes is that there is a significant risk of malignant transformation of the enchondromas in these conditions (e.g., development of chondrosarcoma).

Osteochondroma

Osteochondroma is a benign bone and cartilage-forming tumor characterized by a mushroom-shaped outgrowth arising in the metaphyseal region of long bones of the extremities, or, less commonly, from the pelvis. Osteochondromas occur in adolescents and young adults, with a marked predilection for females. They often present with pain from pressure on the surrounding soft tissues or adjacent nerves. Although usually solitary, osteochondromas may be multiple, occurring as a hereditary syndrome known as **multiple hereditary exostosis**.

Grossly, the lesions are seen to arise from the metaphysis in the cartilaginous growth plate as a stalk of mature bone with an overlying cap of mature cartilage. Histologically, the cartilaginous cap resembles the normal growth plate, but the benign chondrocytes are often arranged in a disorganized fashion. The underlying bone consists of unremarkable appearing cortical bone with a central cavity of trabecular bone. Hematopoietic bone marrow is frequently seen occupying the central cavity.

Simple excision at the base of the bony stalk is curative, but in a small percentage of cases, malignant transformation has been identified. When this occurs, the most common neoplasm identified is a chondrosarcoma, but other sarcomas have been documented.

Chondroblastoma

Chondroblastomas are benign cartilage-forming tumors in children and young adults, with a male predilection. They most commonly occur in the epiphyseal region of the distal femur and proximal tibia, but lesions have been identified in the proximal humerus, ribs, and pelvis. Patients typically present with localized pain and/or joint stiffness. Radiographically, chondroblastomas appear as a well-circumscribed area of lucency, but variable degrees of calcification can be appreciated.

Histologically, the tumor is composed of sheets of bland chondrocytes embedded in an eosinophilic chondroid matrix distributed in a lace-like pattern. Calcification of the matrix is often present, giving the appearance of chicken-wire.

Fig. 14-14. Calcified "chicken wire" chondroid matrix in chondroblastoma. Scattered osteoclastic giant cells are frequently identified, but they are non-neoplastic. Despite the benign nature of this neoplasm, abundant mitotic figures as well as areas of hemorrhage and necrosis are often present.

Surgical excision is typically curative, but recurrences can be common.

Chondromyxoid Fibroma

Chondromyxoid fibroma is a rare cartilaginous tumor of young patients in their second and third decades of

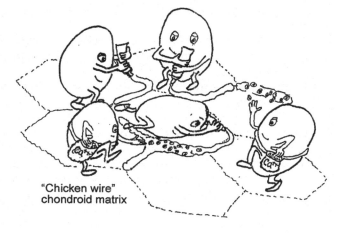

CHONDROBLASTOMA

"Chicken wire" chondroid matrix

Figure 14-14

life, with a male predilection. Clinically, patients present with localized bone pain with a radiographic presentation of a well-circumscribed lucent lesion surrounded by a rim of sclerotic bone. Anatomically, chondromyxoid fibromas arise most commonly in the metaphyseal region of the long bones of the lower extremities, but lesions have been identified in virtually every bone of the body.

Histologically, the tumors are composed of nodules of scant benign appearing spindle cells embedded in a myxoid (mucoid) cartilaginous stroma. The nodules are separated by a highly cellular connective tissue that contains numerous fibroblasts and osteoclast-like giant cells.

Surgical excision is usually curative, but recurrences may occur in approximately 20-30% of cases.

Chondrosarcoma

Chondrosarcoma is the most common malignant cartilaginous tumor. The tumor arises most often in middle-aged to older adults, with a male predilection. Clinically, the tumor presents as localized pain, often associated with a soft tissue mass. Chondrosarcomas commonly arise in the axial skeleton (e.g., the pelvis, ribs, and shoulder girdle) and demonstrate irregular areas of bony destruction, often associated with irregular areas of vague calcification radiologically. A characteristic pattern of calcification, termed "**popcorn calcification**," is frequently identified.

Four major variants of chondrosarcoma have been classified: **conventional, clear cell, myxoid,** and **mesenchymal**:

1. Conventional chondrosarcomas are the most common variant encountered. They resemble disorganized masses of gray-white cartilage grossly. Histologically, conventional chondrosarcoma closely recapitulates mature hyaline cartilage, but the malignant chondrocytes are typically more numerous and demonstrate variable degrees of cellular enlargement, nuclear hyperchromasia, and pleomorphism (variability in size and shape) *(Slide 14.21)*. Binucleation is common and mitotic activity is increased.
2. Clear cell chondrosarcomas are composed of sheets of malignant chondrocytes containing abundant clear cytoplasm.
3. Myxoid chondrosarcoma more commonly occurs in the soft tissues. When the tumor arises in the bone, the histology is similar, consisting of lobules of bland spindle or stellate chondrocytes embedded in a myxoid cartilaginous stroma.
4. Mesenchymal chondrosarcoma is seen most often in younger adults and demonstrates a hypercellular population of primitive spindle cells arranged in sheets surrounding islands or nodules of better-differentiated cartilage.

Surgical excision is the treatment of choice, but depending on the variant, chemotherapy and/or radiation therapy may be considered. Prognosis is clearly related to the variant encountered, with prognosis being significantly worse in cases of mesenchymal chondrosarcoma.

Miscellaneous Bone Neoplasms and Tumor-Like Lesions

Ewing's Sarcoma

Ewing's sarcoma is a primary malignant tumor of bone, arising almost exclusively in children and adolescents, with a slight male predominance. The neoplasm has marked predilection for Caucasians, with rare cases identified in African Americans. The tumor most commonly presents as a painful mass involving the diaphysis of long bones (e.g., the femur). Occasional cases have been identified in the flat bones of the pelvis. There may be systemic symptoms, such as fever and elevated white blood cell count, which can closely mimic osteomyelitis.

Radiographically, Ewing's sarcoma appears as an infiltrative tumor that destroys the surrounding medullary and cortical bone. A characteristic finding on plain radiographs is a prominent periosteal reaction in close proximity to the tumor's destructive margins. This reaction consists of the production of periosteal bone in a layered fashion, termed "**onion-skinning**."

Grossly, Ewing's sarcoma appears as an infiltrative tumor mass centered on the medullary cavity, with variable degrees of hemorrhage and necrosis. Microscopically, Ewing's sarcoma is included in the broad category of tumors known as "**small blue cell tumors**" in that the neoplasm consists of sheets of small malignant lymphocyte-like cells.

Fig. 14-15. Small blue cells of Ewing's sarcoma. The cells have scant amounts of cytoplasm and appear strikingly uniform from one cell to the next *(Slide 14.22)*. Despite the lack of obvious differentiation of these primitive malignant cells, evidence of neural differentiation can occasionally be identified in the form of circular arrangements of cells surrounding a central zone of fibrillar structure, known as "**Homer-Wright rosettes**."

A helpful diagnostic feature of Ewing's sarcoma is the identification of a characteristic chromosomal translocation in the malignant cells, t(11;22), involving the EWS (Ewing's sarcoma gene) on chromosome 22 and the FLI-1 gene on chromosome 11.

Surgical excision plays an important role in treating Ewing's sarcoma, but the combination of chemotherapy and radiotherapy has led to a significant improvement in survival (5-year survival of approximately 75%).

EWING'S SARCOMA

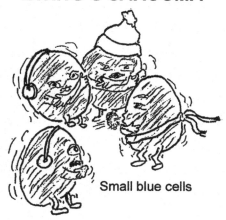

Small blue cells

Figure 14-15

Giant Cell Tumor

Giant cell tumor is a benign primary tumor of bone that arises in young to middle-aged adults, with a slight female predominance. The preponderance of lesions arise in the epiphysis and metaphysis of the long tubular bones, with the majority occurring in the region of the knee (distal femur, proximal tibia), the distal radius, and the proximal humerus. Giant cell tumors often present with symptoms of joint pain due to the close proximity of involvement to the articular surface. Radiologically, giant cell tumors appear as well-circumscribed lucent lesions, with bony destruction of the surrounding bone. Frequent destruction of the overlying cortex can be identified, leading to a bulging soft tissue mass surrounded by a reactive shell of bone.

Grossly, giant cell tumors are fleshy and frequently associated with areas of hemorrhage and cyst formation.

Microscopically, giant cell tumors consist of a relatively homogeneous population of plump spindle cells containing a prominent population of diffusely distributed multinucleated giant cells *(Slide 14.23)*. Many experts believe that the neoplastic component consists of the spindle cells, with the multinucleated giant cells representing a reactive non-neoplastic component.

Giant cell tumors are locally destructive benign lesions that often recur despite frequent attempts at surgical excision. Despite the benign behavior of most lesions, metastases are not infrequent and likely represent dislodged tumor emboli occurring from the surgical excision procedure. Metastases most commonly involve the lung; patients typically have a good prognosis if the metastatic lesions are removed.

Fibrous Dysplasia

Fibrous dysplasia is a tumor-like lesion that presents in a number of ways. Three major manifestations have been characterized:

1. The most common presentation (approximately three-quarters of cases) is a solitary lesion involving a single bony site (**monostotic fibrous dysplasia**), which affects patients in their adolescent to young adult life. The monostotic variety most commonly affects the ribs, femur, and tibia, with lesser involvement of the skull and humerus. Most cases are identified as incidental radiographic findings, but occasional cases can cause local pain and discomfort, with an area of localized bony enlargement.
2. The next most common form of fibrous dysplasia is the polyostotic form, which accounts for approximately 20-25% of cases. **Polyostotic fibrous dysplasia** typically manifests itself during childhood with involvement of the femur, tibia, humerus, skull, ribs, and distal upper extremity. Depending on the extent of involvement, polyostotic fibrous dysplasia can be a crippling disease when marked enlargement of the affected sites occurs, especially when it occurs near the major weight-bearing joints and joints of the shoulder girdle.
3. Finally, the least common pattern of fibrous dysplasia (accounting for 1-3% of cases) is the polyostotic form associated with skin pigmentation and endocrinopathies. This syndromic form of fibrous dysplasia has been termed the **McCune-Albright syndrome**. This syndrome usually manifests as the associated endocrinopathies and consists of sexual precocity, Cushing's syndrome, hyperthyroidism, and gigantism (due to growth hormone-secreting pituitary adenomas). The skin pigmentation presents as large flat macules (**café-au-lait spots**), usually distributed on one side of the body.

Fig. 14-16 (Slide 14.24). Histology of fibrous dysplasia. There is expansion of the medullary cavity by fibrous tissue and proliferating spindle-shaped fibroblasts, with embedded trabeculae and benign osteoblasts, the latter resembling "Chinese characters."

Surgical excision of symptomatic lesions cures the monostotic form of fibrous dysplasia; however, as previously mentioned, depending on the extent of involvement, the polyostotic form can be quite disabling. Progressive enlargement of the lesions is typical and with increasing bony destruction, pathologic fracture can be troubling. Rare cases of malignant transformation, most commonly as an osteosarcoma, have been described, and usually occur in the polyostotic form.

FIBROUS DYSPLASIA

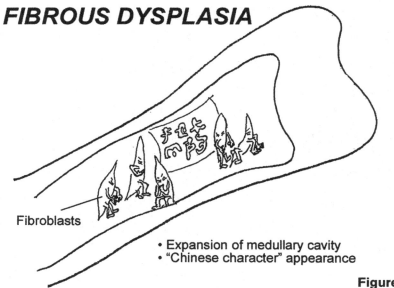

Fibroblasts

• Expansion of medullary cavity
• "Chinese character" appearance

Figure 14-16

JOINT PATHOLOGY
Arthritides

Osteoarthritis

Osteoarthritis (OA) is the most common affliction of the joints, affecting millions of people worldwide. Also known as "degenerative joint disease," OA characteristically affects older individuals, but rare cases do occur in younger individuals, often associated with a predisposing condition such as previous injury to the joint, diabetes, or obesity. OA appears to affect the sexes equally. Clinically, patients present with the insidious onset of joint pain associated with variable degrees of reduction in joint mobility. Over time, the joint pain and stiffness can become debilitating. Joints commonly affected are the knees, hips, vertebrae, wrist, and distal interphalangeal joints. A classic finding is the development of osteophytes ("new bone growth") along the distal interphalangeal joints leading to so-called "**Heberden's nodes**," These nodes are more commonly seen in women but may be present in men.

Fig. 14-17. Osteophytes protruding to form Heberden's nodes in osteoarthritis.

Radiographically, OA is characterized by a reduction in the thickness of the cartilaginous articular surface, often progressing to complete loss, with subsequent bone-on-bone apposition. Subchondral bony sclerosis and occasional subchondral cysts can be present. A typical finding in OA is the development of osteophytes. The irregular areas of bony outgrowth usually arise at the lateral edges of a joint and can be symptomatic if compression of surrounding soft tissues or nerves results.

Grossly, OA closely resembles the radiographic picture, often with marked thinning or complete loss of areas of articular cartilage. In regions where bone-on-bone friction occurs, the surface can appear shiny, smooth and polished (**eburnation** of the subchondral bone). The subchondral bone can become quite thickened and appear sclerotic, with accompanying fibrosis of the intervening medullary marrow space. Despite its name, OA typically lacks a significant inflammatory component (in contrast to rheumatoid arthritis, to be discussed), but in severe cases a degree of chronic lymphocytic inflammation can accompany the changes.

HEBERDEN'S NODES IN OSTEOARTHRITIS

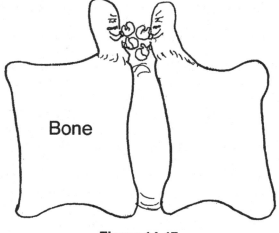

Bone

Figure 14-17

Treatment for OA is generally symptomatic through rest, non-steroidal anti-inflammatory medications and occasionally narcotics for severe pain. The disease inexorably progresses over time with continued use of the joint. When severe, it can necessitate joint replacement with plastic, metal or ceramic-based prostheses.

Rheumatoid Arthritis

Rheumatoid arthritis (RA) is a chronic deforming arthritis, most commonly arising in young adults, females most particularly. It usually presents initially with fatigue, malaise, and generalized musculoskeletal pain. Over time, specific joints are characteristically involved, becoming warm, swollen, and painful with variable degrees of stiffness. The joints most commonly involved include the metacarpophalangeal and proximal interphalangeal joints of the hands, with sparing of the distal interphalangeal joints. Other joints commonly involved are the small joints of the feet, the wrists and ankles, the knees and elbows.

Radiographically, affected joints demonstrate erosion of the joint surface and destruction of peri-articular bone with consequent joint space narrowing. With continued destruction, characteristic deformities of the joints develop. Most commonly, deviation of the fingers toward the ulna occurs with deviation of the wrist toward the radius (*Slide 14.27*). In addition, the affected joints of the fingers develop flexion deformities and hyperextension deformities such as the **swan-neck** and **boutonnière** deformities. The resultant changes lead to joints with marked range of motion loss as well as instability, occasionally leading to subluxation.

Histologically, the joint synovium shows variable degrees of edema, with hyperplasia of the synoviocytes, proliferation of synovial blood vessels and a brisk perivascular lymphocytic inflammatory infiltrate. Lymphoid follicles often form in the areas of heaviest inflammation. These changes typically transform the normally smooth synovium into an irregular surface lined by tentacle-like projections (**villi**). Over time, the hyperplastic synovium (**pannus**) grows over the articular surface, leading to further joint destruction.

Although RA is dominated by joint manifestations, RA is a systemic disease affecting many different tissues and organs. The most commonly involved organs are the skin, heart, pericardium, eyes, lungs, and pleura. Nonspecific lymphoplasmacytic inflammation of the organs can be seen, but the most characteristic histologic manifestation is the development of rheumatoid nodules. Histologically, rheumatoid nodules consist of well-circumscribed areas of fibrinoid necrosis surrounded by a rim of epithelioid histiocytes, lymphocytes, and plasma cells. Rheumatoid nodules can be identified in any organ; they lead to dysfunction due to replacement of normal tissues.

The prognosis of RA varies considerably between individuals. Certain patients manifest mild symptoms with no long-term complications while others suffer from severe, debilitating symptoms and a relentless clinical course ultimately leading to permanent disability.

Gout and Pseudogout – Crystalline Arthropathies

Crystalline arthropathies are a group of disorders characterized by the deposition of crystalline compounds in and about the joints.

Gout is the most common of these disorders. It is caused by the deposition of **uric acid crystals**, primarily in the first metatarsophalangeal joints. Gout is pathogenically related to the presence of hyperuricemia in the affected patient and is usually caused by one of two mechanisms:

1. Overproduction of uric acid (e.g., excessive consumption of purine compounds, high cell turnover, etc.)
2. Impaired excretion of uric acid

Gout occurs most commonly in adult males and postmenopausal females, primarily in the Western hemisphere. As mentioned, the first metatarsophalangeal joints are affected most commonly, but other joints may be affected, such as the smaller joints of the hands and feet, the knees, ankles, wrists, and elbows. Symptomatic patients usually present with severe pain in the affected joint accompanied by signs of significant inflammation, such as warmth, hyperemia, and swelling. Soft tissue involvement by gouty deposits of uric acid currently is rare due to effective treatment for the hyperuricemia in these patients. When present, gouty deposits usually present on extensor surfaces of the extremities as firm rock-like masses ("**tophi**") in the subcutaneous tissues.

Histologically, affected joints demonstrate neutrophils infiltrating the involved synovium in the acute stages of disease; uric acid crystals may be seen in the cytoplasm of the neutrophils after being phagocytosed. The uric acid crystals appear needle-shaped, but in many cases, the crystals may be difficult to identify due to solubilization in formalin fixative. With repeated attacks, the involved synovium appears thickened and fibrotic, with areas of villus hyperplasia similar to that seen in rheumatoid arthritis.

The prognosis of gouty arthritis is significantly influenced by the treatment of hyperuricemia in the affected patient. With treatment of hyperuricemia through medications and/or dietary manipulation, the number and severity of episodes of acute arthritis can be reduced or eliminated. Without adequate treatment, the condition can progress to a chronic phase (**chronic tophaceous gout**) (*Slide 14.25*) with or without soft tissue tophi. Despite these possible complications, most patients develop only a few episodes of acute arthritis leading to temporary disability. Long-term disability is uncommon, and patients typically have a normal life span.

Pseudogout is a crystalline arthropathy related to the deposition of **calcium pyrophosphate crystals** within affected joints. Patients with pseudogout are most commonly in their fifties to sixties, with the incidence of disease increasing with increasing age. Many patients are asymptomatic, but those with symptomatic disease present with joint pain and discomfort involving the knees, elbows, wrists, shoulders, and/or ankles.

Histologically, affected joints demonstrate deposits of large plate-like blue crystals within the articular cartilage, synovium, or menisci.

Since there is no effective treatment for the deposition of calcium pyrophosphate crystals, the disease may progress in approximately half of affected patients, leading to severe joint damage and disability.

Tumors and Tumor-like Lesions

Pigmented Villonodular Synovitis and Giant Cell Tumor of the Tendon Sheath

Pigmented villonodular synovitis (PVNS) and giant cell tumor of the tendon sheath (GCT) are closely related benign neoplasms of the joints and surrounding supporting structures (i.e., tendon sheath). The two lesions are histologically similar, but the patient demographics and sites of involvement differ. PVNS most commonly arises in young adults around the larger joints of the body (e.g., the knee, ankle, hip, shoulder, or elbow). In contrast, GCT usually arises in a younger patient population and most commonly involves the tendon sheaths of the fingers or wrists.

Pathologically, PVNS is primarily an ill-defined red-brown lesion with a shaggy (villous) surface involving the synovium and surrounding structures of the joint. GCT is primarily a well-circumscribed, localized tumor mass firmly attached to an adjacent tendon sheath. Like PVNS, GCT is often red-brown in color due to the microscopic accumulation of hemosiderin pigment within the lesion.

Histologically, both PVNS and GCT are composed of large polygonal tumor cells with abundant pink cytoplasm and uniform small nuclei arranged in sheets *(Slide 14.26)*. As previously mentioned, deposits of hemosiderin pigment can be prominent. In addition, other findings may include the presence of multinucleated giant cells, foamy macrophages, areas of hemorrhage, and fibrosis.

Despite the similarity between these lesions, the prognosis of each varies markedly. Surgical excision is the treatment of choice for each lesion, but the recurrence rate differs significantly between the two. GCT is usually easily excised due to its well-circumscribed nature and rarely recurs. PVNS, on the other hand, often recurs (approximately 15-25%) after excision due to its diffuse and often erosive character, with extension into surrounding bone and soft tissue structures.

15

Nervous System Pathology

OVERVIEW

The central nervous system (CNS) is perhaps the most complex, awe-inspiring, and fragile organ system in the body, which is quite an assertion after reviewing the beauty and vulnerability of the rest of the body. It is where we think we think. The brain is susceptible to every pathological process known, and this chapter will cover congenital disorders, infection and inflammation, metabolic disorders, vascular disease, trauma, demyelinating diseases, degenerative diseases, and neoplasia.

ANATOMY

(Slides 15.1, 15.2) Two main types of cells comprise the nervous system tissue. The main type is the **neuron**, the functional unit of the nervous system. The second type is the **glia cell**, which are the supportive cells. There are 4 main types of glia cells: **astrocytes, oligodendrocytes, ependymal cells**, and **microglia**. The glia cells have important structural and metabolic roles in the CNS.

For practical purposes, the CNS can be divided in a few ways. First, the tentorium cerebelli divides the CNS into supratentorial and subtentorial divisions. The brain also contains a right and left side. We can also divide the CNS into brain and spinal column.

Fig. 15-1. Midsagittal brain.

There are numerous important areas and divisions of the brain that can be affected by different disease processes. A disease may present with specific symptoms depending where the pathology occurs. Thus, it is important to review normal CNS anatomy.

CONGENITAL DISORDERS
Neural Tube Defects

Failure of fusion of the caudal neural tube during organogenesis results in various degrees of spinal column defects. The most benign of these is **spina bifida occulta**, a bony defect of the vertebral arch frequently accompanied by a patch of dark hair on the skin overlying it. Next in severity is the **meningocele**, a bony defect with outpouching of the meninges. It is followed by the devastating **meningomyelocele**, a defect with outpouching of the meninges, spinal cord, and spinal roots, and **myelocele**, a defect of the vertebral arch with complete exposure of spinal cord. The latter 2 often cause paraplegia. Open neural tube defects result in increased **alfa-fetoprotein** during pregnancy, which can be detected in the maternal serum and aids in the prenatal diagnosis. Folate deficiency is involved in the pathogenesis; thus daily vitamins containing folate are recommended for all women of childbearing age.

Posterior Fossa Malformations

There are 2 main categories of posterior fossa malformations: **Arnold-Chiari Types I and II** and **Dandy-Walker**. The Arnold-Chiari malformations consist of a **small fourth ventricle** and a downward displacement of specific cerebellar parts: the cerebellar tonsils in type I and the vermis in type II. The compression of the fourth ventricle results in obstructive hydrocephalus; **syringomyelia** (see below) often accompanies the malformation.

The Dandy-Walker malformation, on the other hand, consists of an enlarged fourth ventricle and a partially or completely absent vermis.

Spinal Cord Malformations

Syringomyelia is a malformation of the spinal cord consisting of a cavitation around the central canal of the spinal cord, resulting in destruction of the surrounding gray and white matter. Signs and symptoms include a bilateral loss of pain and temperature in the upper extremities with preservation of touch sensation due to damage at the crossing fibers of the spinothalamic tract. It most commonly occurs at C8-T1.

MIDSAGITTAL BRAIN

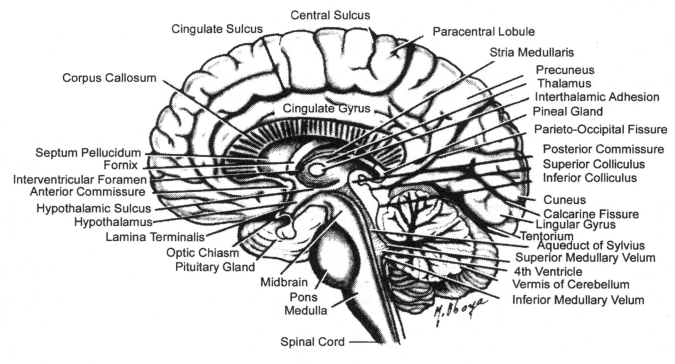

Figure 15-1

INFECTION AND INFLAMMATION
Meningitis

Meningitis is the infection and inflammation of the covering of the brain and spinal cord. It is a severe and occasionally fatal group of diseases that are difficult to treat and can occur in all age groups from neonate to the elderly. Early diagnosis and empiric treatment with broad-spectrum antibiotics are critical.

Bacterial (Septic) Meningitis (Slide 15.3)

Different organisms tend to infect the meninges of different age groups. Older adults with bacterial meningitis most commonly encounter *pneumococcus* and *Listeria monocytogenes*, while young adults are most commonly infected by meningococcus. Children primarily are affected by *H. influenzae,* and newborns by *E. coli, B-streptococcus,* and *L. monocytogenes.* Signs and symptoms include fever, headache, photophobia, nausea/vomiting, cerebrospinal fluid (CSF) changes, and a stiff neck due to irritation of the spinal roots. The presence of irritation can be confirmed with a positive **Kernig's sign**, in which the patient lying supine with hip flexed 90 degrees can't extend the knee, or a positive **Brudzinski's sign**, in which passive flexion of the neck with the patient lying supine causes flexion of the hips and knees.

Viral (Aseptic) Meningitis

Viral (aseptic) meningitis is most commonly caused by Echovirus, Coxsackie, non-paralytic poliomyelitis, and enteroviruses. The signs and symptoms resemble bacterial meningitis; however, the CSF changes differ. A definitive diagnosis is made using PCR of the CSF to detect viral DNA, but since the results of such a study are delayed by several days at most institutions and antiviral antibiotics are limited in coverage, an empiric therapy of acyclovir is begun.

Fungal Meningitis

Fungal meningitis is the third variety of meningitis, and is the least common. It occurs primarily in immunosuppressed patients and is often caused by *Cryptococcus, Coccidioides, Aspergillus* or *Histoplasma* strains. *Cryptococcus* is usually seen in AIDS; it can be identified in the CSF with an India ink preparation or with a CSF antigen agglutination test. *Coccidioides* blastocysts can be identified on CSF cytology. Signs and symptoms are similar to other varieties of meningitis but are less rapid and less severe.

Encephalitis

Encephalitis is infection and inflammation of the brain parenchyma. **Toxoplasmosis** causes congenital infections in fetuses. The causative agent is *Toxoplasma gondii*, which spreads through ingestion by the mother of foods contaminated by animal urine or feces, followed by transplacental transmission from mother to fetus. Congenital infection causes intrauterine growth retardation, **hydrocephalus**, chorioretinitis, hepatosplenomegaly, periventricular calcifications, and severe mental retardation.

Cytomegalovirus (CMV) encephalitis also causes a congenital infection through transmission from the mother to the fetus (**vertical transmission**). It causes chorioretinitis, hepatosplenomegaly, periventricular calcifications, and mental retardation similar to toxoplasmosis. CMV infection, however, causes **microcephaly** instead of hydrocephalus. Histologically, it is characterized by giant cells with eosinophilic inclusions in the nucleus and cytoplasm.

Herpes simplex encephalitis is the **most common cause** of viral encephalitis and is characterized by hemorrhagic necrosis of temporal lobes visible on MRI. The treatment of choice is acyclovir.

Progressive multifocal leukoencephalopathy (PML) occurs in **immunocompromised** patients due to infection by the JC virus, a type of polyomavirus. It attacks oligodendrocytes, resulting in a demyelinating process in the cerebrum and cerebellum. CT and MRI reveal multifocal white matter lesions.

Human Immunodeficiency Virus (HIV) can itself cause encephalitis, or more commonly, predisposes patients to infections, e.g., cryptococcosis, toxoplasmosis, cytomegalovirus (CMV), progressive multifocal leukencephalopathy (PML), tuberculosis, and syphilis. HIV dementia is seen in patients with low CD4 counts. It is characterized by progressive deterioration of cognitive function, with MRI findings of cortical and subcortical atrophy.

Creutzfeldt-Jacob disease (CJD) is caused by a prion protein. It results in a spongiform encephalopathy. 85% of cases are sporadic and 15% are familial. It clinically presents with **rapidly progressive dementia**, memory loss, and startle myoclonus.

Cerebral Abscess

Abscesses of the brain result either from penetrating injuries or from hematogenous or direct spread of infection. Sources of infection include subacute bacterial endocarditis, sinusitis, mastoiditis, and bronchopulmonary infections. Clinical presentation is classically headache, vomiting, and papilledema, all caused by increased intracranial pressure (ICP) due to the space-occupying abscess. Typical CT and MRI findings include **ring enhancing lesions** (a white center encompassed by a dark ring).

METABOLIC AND NUTRITIONAL DISORDERS
Inherited Metabolic Disorders

Wilson's disease (aka hepatolenticular degeneration) results from a defect in **copper** metabolism due to decreased levels of serum **ceruloplasmin**. It eventually causes lesions in the basal ganglia, leading to extrapyramidal tremors, psychosis, and a **Kayser- Fleischer ring** around the cornea, which is pathognomonic.

Tay-Sachs disease is a defect in **hexosaminidase A**, which causes an increase in ganglioside GM2. This leads to mental retardation, paralysis, and death by age 3. The disease primarily occurs in the Ashkenazi Jewish population. A classic finding is the cherry- red spot on the macula. There is no cure.

Acquired Metabolic Disorders

Carbon monoxide poisoning is a very dangerous condition that can cause bilateral necrosis of the globus pallidus and death. Signs and symptoms include headache, nausea and vomiting, and cherry-red lips. Lab tests show a characteristic elevation of carboxyhemoglobin levels.

Hepatic encephalopathy is seen in patients with cirrhosis. It is secondary to excess ammonia and other toxins that are no longer degraded by the damaged liver. The clinical presentation includes hyperreflexia, dementia, seizures, obtundation or coma, and asterixis (flapping of extended wrists).

Nutritional Deficiencies

Thiamine deficiency, usually secondary to alcoholism and/or malnutrition, can cause **Wernicke's encephalopathy**, a triad of **confusion** (including **confabulation**), **ophthalmoplegia**, and **ataxia**. These symptoms correspond with damage to the mamillary bodies. Untreated, severe Wernicke's can progress to Korsakoff's syndrome, which in addition to Wernicke's triad also includes frequently irreversible **antegrade amnesia** (loss of ability to retain new memories).

Chronic B12 deficiency causes subacute combined degeneration of the posterior columns and lateral corticospinal tract. Clinically this manifests itself as decreased vibration and proprioceptive (joint position) sense (with resultant ataxia), paresthesias and weakness, hyperreflexia, nighttime ataxia, personality changes, and dementia. It is easily prevented with B12 injections, but it is difficult to treat once the damage has been done.

CEREBROVASCULAR DISEASE
Epidemiology

Stroke is the **third leading cause of death** in the United States. Risk factors include older age, male sex, family history, hypertension, diabetes, smoking, hypercholesterolemia, heavy alcohol use, and cardiac or peripheral vascular disease.

Ischemic Stroke

Ischemic stroke is caused by a loss of cerebral blood supply, with or without hemorrhage, with accompanying neurological deficits corresponding to the affected area.

Ischemia causes approximately 80% of strokes. It is caused by thrombosis, embolism, or other hypoperfusion of cerebral arteries.

1. Thrombosis is an obstruction of blood flow due to a localized occlusion within a blood vessel. The most common cause of thrombus formation is **atherosclerotic disease**. Other sources include a hypercoaguable state or thrombocytosis.
2. Embolism occurs when material formed elsewhere within the vascular system travels to a distant site, in this case the cerebral arteries, where it becomes lodged, obstructing blood flow. Common sources of emboli include the heart (secondary to atrial fibrillation) or a mural thrombus originating in major arteries (e.g., the aorta, carotid, or vertebral arteries) or the systemic veins. A **paradoxical embolism** is an embolus that passes from the right side of the systemic circulation to the left side of the heart through a defect in the heart such as a patent foramen ovale or an atrial septal defect.

Emboli and thrombi cause ischemia and infarction of the area supplied by the occluded artery, although the periphery of a blocked vessel's territory may be salvaged by collaterals of an adjacent vessel. Strokes present clinically with weakness, numbness, paralysis, and/or cranial nerve abnormalities.

3. Hypoperfusion may result from hypotension due to hypovolemia or from cardiac failure caused by myocardial infarction or an arrhythmia.

Hemorrhagic Stroke

Hemorrhagic stroke is responsible for the remaining 20% of cerebovascular accidents (CVA). Hemorrhage leads to brain dysfunction by destroying tissue, causing a mass effect, or by compressing blood vessels, leading to ischemia. Two main types of hemorrhagic stroke lead to cerebrovascular dysfunction: subarachnoid and intracerebral hemorrhages:

1. **Subarachnoid hemorrhages** are caused by trauma, bleeding from aneurysms, or arteriovenous malformations. Aneurysms are commonly found in the arterial Circle of Willis. The classic presenting complaint is "This is the worst headache of my life!"

2. **Intracerebral hemorrhages** bleed directly into the parenchyma of the brain. **Trauma and hypertension are common causes**. Hemorrhages caused by hypertension are often found in the basal ganglia, thalamus, pons and cerebellum.

TRAUMA
Subdural Hematoma

Subdural hematomas result from the tearing of the bridging veins between the cerebral cortex and the venous sinuses. These frequently occur in the elderly because atrophy of the brain makes the connection of the bridging veins more tenuous, and the elderly are more likely to fall and traumatize the brain. On CT scan, subdural hematomas present with a **concave** shape that outlines the brain surface. Mental status change and death are not uncommon. Surgical evacuation of the hematoma may be necessary.

Epidural Hematoma

(*Slides 15.4, 15.5*) Epidural hematomas result from a skull fracture that lacerates the middle meningeal artery and causes blood accumulation between the dura and the skull. As arterial pressure builds, the dura dissects from the skull, causing an increasing mass effect on the brain. Patients often present with a brief loss of consciousness followed by a lucid interval. During this period the patient will seem fine, but will then experience a dramatic deterioration of mental status, requiring emergency surgery to evacuate the clot and repair the artery. On CT scan, epidural hematomas are hyperdense with a **biconvex** shape.

Contusions

Contusion are bruises of the brain parenchyma. They occur in areas where sudden deceleration of the head causes the brain to impact on bony prominences. The majority of contusions occur in the **inferior frontal or temporal lobes**. Contusions are described as either **coup** (the lesion is directly below the site of impact) or **contrecoup** (the lesion is located on the opposite side of the brain as it is thrown against the skull).

Diffuse Axonal Injury (DAI)

DAI is caused by **rotational** acceleration and deceleration of the head. It is most commonly seen in patients who have been injured in motor vehicle accidents. DAI is characterized by axonal changes in the cerebral white matter and small hemorrhagic lesions of the corpus callosum and brainstem (**Duret's hemorrhages**). Coma patients with a head injury in the absence of a space-occupying lesion on CT scan most likely have DAI. The prognosis is quite poor and treatment rather limited.

DEMYELINATING DISEASES

The demyelinating diseases are unified by the common finding of a loss of the myelin sheath that encases axons, with relative preservation of the axons themselves. The three main manifestations of this pathologic process are **multiple sclerosis**, **Guillain-Barre syndrome**, and **central pontine myelinolysis**.

Multiple Sclerosis (MS)

The cause of MS is unknown although an autoimmune reaction to a viral antigen is increasingly suspected. The disease origin is certainly multifactorial, with clear involvement of environmental and genetic factors.

MS is more common in females, usually beginning in the third and fourth decades. It is more common in patients whose first decade of life was spent in northern latitudes; the risk increases as the distance from the equator increases. Twin studies demonstrate a 25% concordance for monozygotic twins.

The signs and symptoms of MS are by definition multiple attacks separated in time and space (region of the CNS). Attacks are followed by remissions and consist of multiple lesions randomly distributed throughout the CNS. Visual disturbances are often the first symptoms and can include:

1. **optic neuritis** – This is a painful blindness due to inflammation of the optic nerve/chiasm.
2. **intranuclear ophthalmoplegia** – Diplopia results from damage to the medial longitudinal fasciculus.
3. **nystagmus** – This is due to dysfunction of the vestibular nuclei in the brainstem.

Other signs and symptoms are relapsing asymmetric limb weakness; **Lhermitte's sign** (nonspecific) characterized by electrical shocks down the spine and arms when the neck is flexed due to damage of the posterior columns; and **Charcot's triad** (diagnostic), which includes nystagmus, an intention tremor, and scanning speech. There can be many other neurologic symptoms, depending on where in the CNS the disease strikes.

Fig. 15-2. Lhermitte's sign. Electrical shock sensation on neck flexion in multiple sclerosis.

A histologic examination of an MS lesion demonstrates plaques, which are areas of demyelination *(Slide 15.6)* in both the gray and white matter of the brain and spinal cord. Periventricular plaques are most common. Lumbar puncture often reveals an increase in CSF immunoglobulins, which manifests as multiple oligoclonal bands on electrophoresis.

Treatment of MS consists of corticosteroids to ameliorate the acute phase and interferon to maintain remissions.

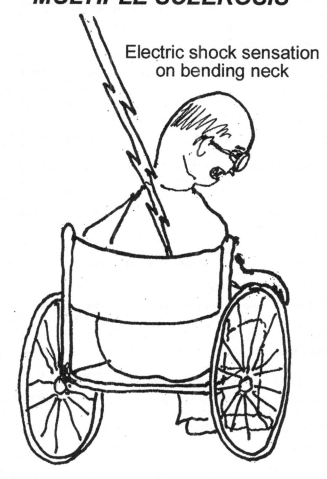

LHERMITTE'S SIGN IN MULTIPLE SCLEROSIS

Electric shock sensation on bending neck

Figure 15-2

Guillain-Barré Syndrome (GBS)

GBS is an ascending autoimmune demyelinating disease involving the **peripheral** nervous system. It is often preceded by *Campylobactor jejuni* gastroenteritis, *Mycoplasma pneumoniae* infection, viral infections, immunizations, or allergic reactions. Its incidence is highest in young adults. 80-90% of patients will spontaneously regress, but respiratory failure and death can occur in the remainder.

Signs and symptoms include paralysis ascending up from the lower limbs, muscle weakness, decreased or absent reflexes, occasional bilateral facial nerve palsy, and occasionally phrenic nerve paralysis. The CSF shows albumin-cytologic dissociation (CSF protein is elevated without an increase in cells), and histological examination shows perivenular inflammation and a loss of myelin between the nodes of Ranvier of peripheral nerves. Treatment involves corticosteroids and **intravenous immunoglobulins** (IVIG).

Central Pontine Myelinolysis (CPM)

CPM is a devastating disease that results from excessively rapid correction of hyponatremia and some liver diseases. Quadriplegia and pseudobulbar palsy develop, such that the patient experiences difficulty chewing, talking, and swallowing due to damage to several cranial nerves. In its extreme, patients suffer from the so-called "locked-in syndrome," in which sensation and comprehension are intact but only the eyes are spared from paralysis.

MRI reveals a diamond-shaped region of demyelination limited to the midpons. Histological exam demonstrates destruction of myelin and loss of oligodendrocytes, but preservation of the axons. The damage is irreparable.

DEGENERATIVE DISEASE
Alzheimer's Disease (AD)

AD is the **most common cause** of dementia (but it's not the only!). It affects 5% of people over 70; the incidence increases with age. Virtually all patients with Down's Syndrome (Trisomy 21) who live through their 30's will develop Alzheimer's.

The disease begins with short-term memory deficits and then gradually progresses to agnosia (the loss of object recognition/perception), apraxia (the inability to make purposeful movements), anxiety, hallucinations/delusions, and tremors.

Gross pathology shows diffuse cortical atrophy and a compensatory ventricular dilation. Histological exam reveals diffuse neuronal loss followed by gliosis, the increase in the number and size of astrocytes. Individual neurons contain **neurofibrillary tangles**, which are intracytoplasmic bundles of abnormal filaments made of **tau** protein. The neuropil surrounding the neurons contains numerous **senile plaques**, which are extracellular deposits present in the cerebral cortex that contain a central core of beta **amyloid** protein. Amyloid also deposits in the walls of vessels (**congophilic angiopathy**), causing them to rupture more easily. Interestingly, this same amyloid angiopathy is seen in elderly patients suffering from strokes.

Fig. 15-3. Alzheimer's disease. The man has entered a dance contest and won the neurofibrillary Tango plaque (**neurofibrillary tangle plaque**) with his partner, Amy Lloyd (**amyloid**). He is perspiring heavily, needing a towel (**tau** protein), which he'll need in order to join the next event, the Congo line (**congophilic angiopathy**).

Multi-Infarct Dementia

Multi-infarct dementia is the **second most common** cause of dementia after Alzheimer's disease. It is caused by cerebral atherosclerosis, and not surprisingly, the risk factors include coronary atherosclerosis, hypertension, diabetes, age, embolic sources, and extensive large artery atherosclerosis.

This disease differs from Alzheimer's in that the onset and progression of neurological dysfunction occur in a sudden, step-wise pattern, corresponding to new infarcts. Imaging studies show multiple strokes, lacunes, and extensive deep white matter changes.

Pick's Disease (Frontotemporal Dementia)

Pick's disease is clinically similar to Alzheimer's disease but often involves the frontal lobes first, so that personality changes are usually seen earlier than in Alzheimer's disease. Gross pathology demonstrates selective atrophy of the frontal lobe and caudal portion of the temporal lobes. The histology shows **Pick cells**, which are a swelling of cortical neurons, and **Pick bodies**, which are an accumulation of spherical intracytoplasmic inclusions consisting of neurofilaments stainable by silver.

Parkinson's Disease (PD)

Three major forms of parkinsonism exist: idiopathic, postencephalitic, and toxic. Idiopathic parkinsonism, which is referred to as Parkinson's disease, affects the elderly in a chronic and progressive fashion. It demonstrates **Lewy bodies** within the neurons of the **substantia nigra**. Postencephalitic parkinsonism was a sequela of encephalitis lethargica, which followed the "influenza epidemic" of 1914-1918, and left patients "locked-in." Toxic parkinsonism causes an acute syndrome following use of synthetic heroin (the meperidine derivative known as **MPTP**), which selectively damages the substantia nigra. All 3 forms result from a loss of dopaminergic neurons in the substantia nigra. Without those neurons, the striatum is deprived of dopamine.

Signs and symptoms of PD include the classic triad of **rigidity, bradykinesia,** and a **resting "pill-rolling" tremor of the hands,** often asymmetrically. Other signs include a shuffling gait, postural instability, and masked facies. Treatment primarily involves the use of dopamine agonists.

Huntington's Chorea

Huntington's chorea is an inherited, **autosomal dominant** disorder caused by a mutant gene localized to the short arm of **chromosome 4**. There is a high incidence of suicide due to severe depression. As the disease progresses, there is increasing destruction of the frontal

ALZHEIMER'S DISEASE

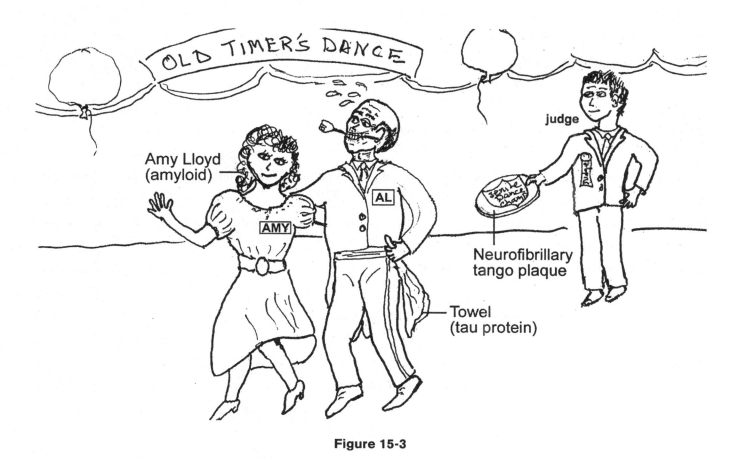

Figure 15-3

lobes and the basal ganglia, particularly the **caudate nucleus.**

Patients do not have symptoms until their 30s, after which they experience involuntary dystonic movements (chorea), progressive deterioration leading to hypertonicity and dementia, and a predilection for head trauma secondary to sudden chorea. In fact, many patients have several chronic subdural hematomas. Essentially, the disease displays a characteristic triad: **familial history, chorea,** and **dementia.**

Amyotrophic Lateral Sclerosis (ALS)

Amyotrophic lateral sclerosis (**Lou Gehrig's Disease**) involves a destruction of **both upper and lower motor neurons.** The cause is unknown, but pathological exam shows degeneration and atrophy of the lateral corticospinal tracts and anterior motor neurons. Patients develop **upper motor neuron signs,** including **hyperreflexia** and **spasticity,** and **lower motor neuron signs,** including **fasciculations** and **symmetric muscle atrophy.** There is no cure.

NEOPLASTIC DISEASE
Primary CNS Tumors

(*Slides 15.7 – 15.14*) Most brain tumors in adults are **supratentorial. Gliomas** are the most frequent tumor. They can be either benign or malignant. **Metastases** are the second most frequent and the **most common malignancy** of the adult brain. **Meningiomas** are the **most frequent benign** tumor. **Pituitary adenomas** are another common benign tumor.

On the other hand, most brain tumors in children are **infratentorial.** Cerebellar astrocytomas derived from astrocytes progress slowly and have a good prognosis. **Medulloblastoma** is a malignant tumor of the cerebellum that usually arises in the **midline** from primitive neuroectodermal cells. It is the second most common tumor of the CNS in childhood, and the **most common malignant brain tumor of children.** Medulloblastomas are sensitive to chemotherapy and radiation, but they have a poor prognosis due to quick spread through the ventricular system. Ependymomas usually arise from ependymal cells of the ventricles and present with **obstructive hydrocephalus**.

Fig. 15-4. Cerebral tumors. Most are infratentorial in children, but supratentorial in adults.

Peripheral Nerve Tumors (PNT)

PNTs are all derived from Schwann Cells and are divided into 2 types. The first is the **neurofibroma**, which occurs in **multiple foci** and lacks a capsule. It usually affects **small distal nerves**. The second is the **Schwannoma *(Slide 15.15)***, a slow-growing, **well-circumscribed** and **encapsulated** benign tumor that often localizes on the **eighth cranial nerve** and affects the **proximal aspect of larger nerves**.

Neurofibromatosis is a neurocutaneous disorder with **autosomal dominant** transmission. Like neurofibromas, it comes in two forms.

1. **Neurofibromatosis 1 (von Recklinghaus Disease)** accounts for 90% of neurofibromatoses. It presents as peripheral neurofibromatosis, multiple cutaneous neurofibromas, **café-au-lait spots** (dark macules in skin), **Lisch nodules** (freckling of the iris), and optic nerve glioma, which leads to proptosis (exophthalmos). There is a gene defect on chromosome 17.

2. **Neurofibromatosis 2** accounts for the remaining 10%. Its presents as a central neurofibromatosis, multiple meningiomas, bilateral acoustic schwannomas, spinal schwannomas, and cutaneous neurofibromatosis, with a defective gene on chromosome 22. It can be found with pheochromocytoma, medullary carcinoma of the thyroid, Wilm's tumor, skeletal lesions, and gliomas.

Metastatic Tumors

Metastatic tumors often present with multiple well-circumscribed lesions at the junction between gray and white matter. The most frequent origins are lung and breast, but skin, kidney, gastrointestinal tract, and thyroid can also metastasize. Choriocarcinoma is a malignant germ cell tumor, derived from trophoblast. It spreads hematogenously to the lungs, brain, and liver. 65% of people with melanoma will send mets to the brain; the lesion is usually dark and well demarcated from surrounding tissue.

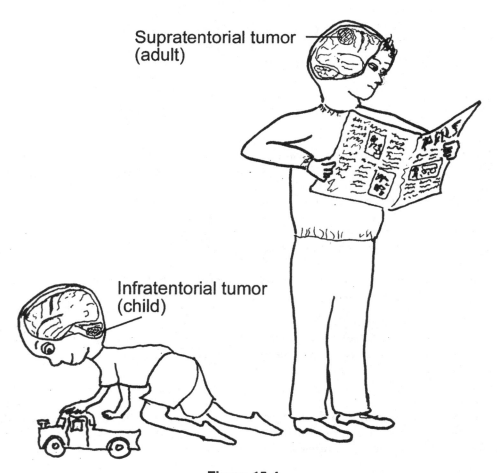

Supratentorial tumor (adult)

Infratentorial tumor (child)

Figure 15-4

INDEX